Pocket Companion to Accompany

PSYCHIATRY

Pocket Companion to Accompany

PSYCHIATRY

Allan Tasman, M.D.
Professor and Chair
Department of Psychiatry
and Behavioral Sciences
University of Louisville
School of Medicine
Louisville, Kentucky

Jerald Kay, M.D.
Professor and Chair
Department of Psychiatry
Wright State University
School of Medicine
Dayton, Ohio

Jeffrey A. Lieberman, M.D.
Vice-Chairman of Psychiatry
Professor of Psychiatry,
Pharmacology, and Radiology
University of North Carolina
School of Medicine
Chapel Hill, North Carolina

W.B. SAUNDERS COMPANY
A Division of Harcourt Brace & Company

Philadelphia   London   Toronto   Montreal   Sydney   Tokyo

W.B. SAUNDERS COMPANY
A Division of Harcourt Brace & Company

The Curtis Center
Independence Square West
Philadelphia, Pennsylvania 19106

Pocket Companion to Accompany
Psychiatry   ISBN 0–7216–5241–7

Printed in the United States of America

Last digit is the print number: 9   8   7   6   5   4   3   2   1

Preface

Pocket Companion to Accompany Psychiatry, conceived to be a useful daily guide for students, house officers, and practitioners both within psychiatry and other disciplines, reflects the tremendous advances in the knowledge base that informs clinical practice in psychiatry. This book, as the title indicates, is the companion to our textbook, *Psychiatry,* and provides core material from that work.

The emphasis in the pocket companion is on clinical practice. An introductory section on general issues related to the psychiatric interview and the doctor-patient relationship is followed by a section on psychiatric perspectives on human development and one on clinical evaluation and treatment planning. The main sections of the pocket companion follow: the first of these reviews psychiatric disorders according to the DSM-IV Criteria. Each of these clinical chapters presents practical information on diagnosis, etiology, course of illness, and treatment. The final section reviews the major treatment modalities within psychiatry.

The pocket companion is not intended to take the place of the larger textbook, *Psychiatry,* but rather is intended to fill a supplementary niche. We believe that the pocket companion will be useful on its own in the clinical setting by being a ready reference. We have especially distilled the clinical portions of the textbook so that they compose the major part of the pocket companion (i.e., the sections Disorders and Therapeutics). The table of contents helps to link the pocket companion to *Psychiatry* by indicating the corresponding chapter numbers in each work. By cross-referencing, the reader can, when time permits, review the main textbook for a more thorough, detailed, and in-depth discussion of the subject matter. The pocket companion has been sized, as the title suggests, so that it will be easy to carry on rounds and in the clinic and easy to use in the office setting. Many tables and charts highlight key information at a glance.

We thank all of the many experts in the field whose contributions to *Psychiatry* have made it an outstanding reference and have thereby provided the material in the pocket companion. We trust that the reader will find the *Pocket Companion to Accompany Psychiatry* to be a useful adjunct to *Psychiatry.*

Allan Tasman, M.D.
Jerald Kay, M.D.
Jeffrey A. Lieberman, M.D.

Contents

Section V

Therapeutics, 437

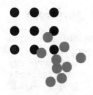

Approaches to the Patient

Listening to the Patient

The psychiatrist, more than any other physician, must constantly listen in multiple ways: symptomatically, narratively and experientially, behaviorally, interpersonally, cognitively, cross-culturally, and from a systems perspective. Symptomatic listening is what we think of as traditional medical history taking in which the focus is on the presence or absence of a particular symptom, the most overt content level of an interview. Narrative-experiential listening is based on the idea that all humans are constantly interpreting their experiences, attributing meaning to them, and weaving a story of their lives with themselves as the central character. This process goes on continuously, both consciously and unconsciously. All humans, in addition to whatever immediate external focus they have, within themselves participate in a running reaction and commentary on their lives. This commentary includes personal history, repetitive behaviors, learned assumptions about the world, and interpersonal roles. These are, in turn, the products of individual background, cultural norms and values, and family system forces.

COMMON BLOCKS TO EFFECTIVE LISTENING

Many factors influence the ability to listen. Psychiatrists come to the patient as the product of their own life experiences. Does the listener tune in to what he or she hears in a more attentive way if the listener and the patient share characteristics? What blocks to listening are posed by differences in sex, age, religion, socioeconomic class, race, or culture? What blind spots may be induced by superficial similarities in but different personal meanings attributed to the same cultural symbol? Separate and apart from the differences in the development of empathy when the dyad hold in common certain features, the act of listening is inevitably influenced by similarities and differences between the psychiatrist and the patient.

Psychiatrists discern meaning in what they hear through filters of their own—cultural backgrounds, life experience, feelings, the day's events, their own physical sense of themselves, sex roles, religious meanings systems, and intrapsychic conflicts. The filters can serve as blocks or as magnifiers if certain elements of what is being said resonate with something within the psychiatrist. When the filters block we call it counertransference or insensitivity. When they magnify, we call it empathy or sensitivity. One may observe a theme for a long time repeated with a different tone, embellishment, inflection, or context before the idea of what is happening comes to mind.

CRUCIAL ATTITUDES THAT ENABLE EFFECTIVE LISTENING

The first step in developing good listening skills involves coming to grips with the importance of inner experience in psychiatric treatment and diagnosis. The third revised edition of the *Diagnostic and Statistical Manual of Mental Disorders* (DSM-III-R) and DSM-IV have made enormous advances in reliability and accuracy of diagnosis, but their emphasis on seemingly observable phenomena has allowed the willing user to forget the importance of inner experience, even in such a basic diagnosis as major depressive disorder.

The psychiatrist must "listen to" much more than the patient's overt behavior. There are qualities in the communication, including the inner experiences induced in the listener, that are being harkened to. The experienced psychiatrist listens to the words, watches the behavior, engages in and notices the ongoing interaction, allows himself or herself to experience his or her own inner reactions to the process, and *never forgets that depression and almost all other psychiatric symptoms are exclusively private experiences*. The behavior and interactions are useful insofar as they assist the psychiatrist to infer the patient's inner experience.

Even when we make statements about brain function related to a particular patient, we use this kind of listening, generally by making at least two inferences. We first listen to and observe the patient and then *infer* some aspects of the patient's private experience. Then, if we possess sufficient scientific knowledge, we make a second inference to a disturbance in neurochemistry, neurophysiology, or neuroanatomy.

It is the constant curious awareness on the listener's part that she or he is trying to grasp the private inner experience of the patient, and the storyteller's sense of this, that impels the ever more revealing process of history taking. Empathy is this quality of listening that facilitates a growing sense of closeness between psychiatrist and patient, producing what we call rapport, without which psychiatric histories become spotty, superficial, and even suspect. There are no bad historians, only patients who have not yet found the right listener.

We now know that just as there is a neurobiological basis for empathy and countertransference, there is a similar biological basis for the power of listening to heal, to lift psychological burdens, to remoralize, and to provide emotional regulation to patients who feel out of control of their rage, despair, terror, or other feelings. Attachment and social support are psychobiological processes that provide necessary physiological regulation to human beings.

LISTENING IN SPECIAL CLINICAL SITUATIONS

Children

Listening to children involves inviting them to play, then engaging them in describing what is happening in the play action. The psychiatrist pays careful attention to the child's feelings. These feelings are usually attributed to a doll, puppet, or other humanized toy. If a child describes Raggedy Andy as being scared, the psychiatrist may say, "I wonder if you, too, are scared when . . ." or "That sounds like you when. . . ."

For a child to be heard and the child's inner experience understood, the language of play and fantasy is used. Healing occurs in being listened to and understood. To hear the voice of a child telling her story, one listens in on the child's play. At the same time, one must be with the child in play to observe, guide, and provide labels for the emotional experience of the child. With the help of imagination, one is free to explore what this child's world is like, and that imagination is aided by also having been a child once.

Geriatric Patients

It is difficult to pull the elements of a story together, especially when they span years that compose a generation or more. The elderly are often stoic and noncomplaining. In the face of losses that mark the closing years of life, denial often becomes a healthy tool allowing one to proceed in the time of decline for oneself and loss through death and debilitation of one's circle of friends and loved ones. The psychiatrist must keep in mind the processes of grief and how these processes both resemble and differ from depression. Careful listening requires tracking the story, keeping in mind the person represented while one is also differentiating among and between diagnoses that sometimes overlap in characteristics.

CHRONICALLY MENTALLY ILL

Listening to the chronically mentally ill can be especially challenging, too. The unique choice of words characteristic of many who have a thought disorder requires that the psychiatrist search for the meanings of certain words and phrases that may be peculiar to that particular person.

The chronically psychiatrically disabled patient has a unique way of presenting the inner world experience. Sometimes the link to outer world experience is not so apparent. However, increases in psychotic symptoms are often linked in a reality-based way to patients' experience of themselves, persons close to them, and their world. The psychiatrist is regularly challenged with making sense of the meanings of the content and changes in intensity or frequency of the hallucinations, and the patient has the opportunity to be heard and understood as a person with schizophrenia, not as a schizophrenic.

PHYSICALLY ILL PATIENTS

In the work of psychiatry, one is often listening to a patient who has a physical illness, either chronic or acute. The invitation to listen to these persons often comes in the form of a request for consultation from a colleague in a medical or surgical specialty. If the patient is hospitalized, the communication from the primary physician may alter how the psychiatrist will experience the patient and what the psychiatrist will hear from the patient. It falls to the psychiatrist, then, not only to listen to the story of the patient but also to keep in mind the story as reflected in the hospital records, the nursing staff's notes, and the medical or surgical team's findings. Thus the psychiatrist truly serves as the liaison not only between psychiatry and the rest of the medical profession but also between the patient (who may not have been adequately heard) and the medical or surgical team providing primary care.

DEVELOPING AS A LISTENER

There is increasing recognition that to be a healing listener, one must be able to bear the burden of hearing what is told. There is often a fear of what might be heard. The story may be one of rage in response to early childhood attachment ruptures, sadness as personal losses are remembered, or terror in response to disorganization during the experience of perceptual abnormalities accompanying psychotic breaks. The hearing may invoke anger, shame, guilt, abject helplessness, or sexual feelings within the listener. These feelings, unless attended to, appreciated, and understood, will block the listening that is essential for healing to take place.

The physician-patient relationship is essential to the healing process and is the foundation on which an effective treatment plan may be negotiated, integrating the best of what medical technology and human caring can provide. The centrality of this relationship is particularly true for psychiatric physicians and their patients. In the psychiatrist-patient relationship, empathy, compassion, and hope frequently serve as major means of alleviating pain and enhancing active participation in all treatment interventions: biological, psychological, and social.

The development of the physician-patient relationship depends on skilled assessment, the development of rapport through empathy, a strong reality-based therapeutic alliance, and the effective understanding of transference, countertransference, and defense mechanisms.

The development of the physician-patient relationship is influenced by numerous factors, including the phase of treatment, the treatment setting, transitions between inpatient and outpatient care, managed care, and changes in the physician's health. The astute physician is attuned to the needs and characteristics of specific populations of patients, adopting the therapeutic approach that most effectively bridges the gap between physician and patient and that leads to a healing relationship.

Psychiatric Interview: Settings and Techniques

The interview is the principal means of assessment in clinical psychiatry. Despite major advances in neuroimaging and neurochemistry, no laboratory procedures are as informative as observing, listening to, and interacting with the patient, and none as yet is more than supplementary to the information gathered by the psychiatric interview.

The psychiatric interview systematically surveys subjective and objective aspects of illness and generates a differential diagnosis and plan for further evaluation and treatment. It differs from other medical interviews in the wide range of biological and psychosocial data that it must take into account and in its attention to the emotional reactions of the patient and the process of interaction between the patient and the interviewer. The nature of the interaction is informative diagnostically as well as being a means of building rapport and eliciting the patient's cooperation.

GOALS OF THE PSYCHIATRIC INTERVIEW

Table 2–1 lists the questions that the interview addresses and the implications of each for understanding and treating the patient.

THE PSYCHIATRIC DATABASE

The body of information to be gathered from the interview may be termed the psychiatric database (Table 2–2). Whose questions are to be answered—the patient's concern about himself or herself, a family's or friend's concern about the patient, another physician's diagnostic dilemma, a civil authority's need to safeguard the public safety, or a research protocol's requirement? Who will have access to the data gathered and under what circumstances? Is the interview to be the first session of a psychotherapy regimen, or is it a one-time-only evaluation? What is the nature of the disorder? For example, negative responses regarding the presence of major psychotic symptoms, coupled with a history of good occupational function, generally preclude detailed inventory of psychotic features. A missed orientation or memory question requires careful cognitive testing. Patients with personality disorder symptoms warrant careful attention to their history of significant relationships, to their work history, and to the feelings evoked in the interviewer during the evaluation process. The database should be expanded in areas of diagnostic concern, to support or rule out particular syndromes.

TABLE 2–1	Issues to Be Addressed in a Psychiatric Assessment

Question	Implications
Does the patient have a psychiatric disorder?	Need for treatment
How severe is the disorder?	Need for hospitalization Need for structure or assistance in daily life Ability to function in major life roles
What is the diagnosis?	Description of the illness Prognosis and treatment response
Are there abnormalities of brain function?	Degree of dysfunction of major mental processes, such as perception, cognition, communication, regulation of mood and affect Responsivity of symptoms to environmental and motivational factors Responsivity of symptoms to biological treatment
What is the patient's baseline level of functioning?	Determination of onset of illness State versus trait pathology Goals for treatment Capacity for treatment
What environmental factors contribute to the disorder?	Prediction of conditions that may trigger future episodes of illness Need for focus on precipitating stressors Prevention of future episodes through amelioration of environmental stressors or increased environmental and social support
What biological factors contribute to the disorder?	Need for biological therapy Place of biological factors in explanation of illness presented to the patient Focus on biological factors as part of ongoing therapy
What psychological factors contribute to the disorder?	Responsivity of symptoms to motivational, interpersonal, and reinforcement factors Need to deal with psychological or interpersonal issues in therapy
What is the patient's motivation and capacity for treatment?	Decision to treat Choice of treatment

TABLE 2–2	Core Database

Identifying Data	**Chief Complaint**	**History of Present Illness**
Name Age/date of birth Next of kin	Reason for consultation	Major symptoms Time course Stressors Change in functioning Current medical problems and treatment

Psychiatric History	**Medical History**	**Family History**
Any previous psychiatric treatment History of suicide attempts Functioning problems secondary to psychiatric symptoms Alcohol or drug abuse	Ever hospitalized Surgery Medications	Psychiatric illness

Personal History	**Mental Status**
Educational level Ever married or in a committed relationship Work history Means of support Living situation	Appearance Attitude Affect Behavior Speech Thought process Thought content Perception Cognition Insight Judgment

Database Components

IDENTIFYING DATA

This information establishes the patient's identity, especially for the purpose of obtaining history from other contacts and, when necessary, to fix the patient's position in society.

CHIEF COMPLAINT

The chief complaint is the patient's response to the question, What brings you to see me/to the hospital today? or some variant. It is usually quoted verbatim, placed within quotation marks, and should be no more than one or two sentences.

HISTORY OF THE PRESENT ILLNESS

MINIMAL ESSENTIAL DATABASE. The present illness history should begin with a brief description of the major symptoms that brought the patient to psychiatric attention. The most troubling symptoms should be detailed initially; later, a more thorough review will be stated. At a minimum, the approximate time since the patient was last at her or his baseline level of functioning, and in what way she or he is different from that now, should be described, along with any known stressors, the sequence of symptom development, and the beneficial or deleterious effects of interventions.

EXPANDED DATABASE. A more expanded description of the history of the present illness would include events in a patient's life at the onset of symptoms as well as exactly how the symptoms have affected the patient's occupational functioning and important relationships. Any concurrent medical illness symptoms, medication use (and particularly changes), alterations in sleep-wake cycle, appetite disturbances, and eating patterns should be noted; remarks about significant negative findings should be recorded.

PSYCHIATRIC HISTORY

MINIMAL ESSENTIAL DATABASE. Most of the major psychiatric illnesses are chronic in nature. For this reason, patients have often had previous episodes of illness with or without treatment. New onset of symptoms without any previous psychiatric history becomes increasingly important with advancing age in terms of diagnostic categories to be considered. At a minimum, the presence or absence of past psychiatric symptoms and diagnoses should be recorded, along with psychiatric interventions taken as the result of such interventions. An explicit statement about past suicide attempts should be included.

EXPANDED DATABASE. A more detailed history would include names and places of psychiatric treatment, dosages of medications used, and time course of response. The type of psychotherapy, the patient's feelings about former therapists, the patient's compliance with treatment, and the circumstances of termination are also important. Note what the patient has learned about his or her biological and psychological predisposing factors to illness and whether there were precipitating events.

MEDICAL HISTORY

MINIMAL ESSENTIAL DATABASE. In any clinical assessment, it is important to know what a patient's general health status has been. In particular, any current medical illness and treatment should be noted, along with any major past illness requiring hospitalization. Previous endocrine or neurological illness is of particular pertinence.

EXPANDED DATABASE. An expanded database could include significant childhood illnesses, how these were handled by the patient and the family, and therefore the degree to which the patient was able to develop a sense of comfort and security about his or her physical well-being. Illnesses later in life should be assessed for the degree of regression produced. A careful medical history can also at times bring to light a suicide attempt, substance abuse, or dangerously careless behavior that might not be obtained any other way.

FAMILY HISTORY

MINIMAL ESSENTIAL DATABASE. Given the evidence for familial, genetic factors in so many psychiatric conditions, noting the presence and type of mental illness in biological relatives of the patient is a necessary part of any database. It is important to specify during questioning the degree of family to be considered, usually to the second degree: aunts, uncles, cousins, and grandparents as well as parents, siblings, and children.

EXPANDED DATABASE. A history of familial medical illness is a useful part of an expanded database. A genogram (pedigree), including known family members with dates and causes of death, as well as other known chronic illnesses, is helpful. Questioning about causes of death also occasionally brings out hidden psychiatric illness—sudden, unexpected deaths that were likely suicides, or illness secondary to substance abuse, for example.

PERSONAL HISTORY

MINIMAL ESSENTIAL DATABASE. Recording the story of a person's life can be a daunting undertaking, and this is often where a database can expand dramatically. At a minimum, this part of the history should include where a patient was born and raised, and in what circumstances (whether there was an intact family, number of siblings, degree of material comfort). Note how far the patient went in school, how well she or he did there, and what her or his occupational functioning has been. If the patient is not working, why not? Has the patient ever been involved in criminal activity, and with what consequences? Has the patient ever married or been involved in a committed relationship? Are there any children? What is the patient's current source of support? Does he or she live alone or with someone? Has he or she ever used alcohol or other drugs to excess, and is there current use? Has the patient ever been physically or sexually abused or the victim of some other trauma?

EXPANDED DATABASE. An expanded database can include a great deal of material beginning even before the patient's conception. The kinds of data that may be gathered about a patient, along with an organizational framework, include the following: family of origin, prenatal and perinatal history, early childhood, later childhood, adolescence, identity (sexual, gender, ethnic), sexual history, adulthood (especially level of educational attainments, employment history), history of significant relationships (including duration, typical roles in relationships, patterns of conflict, marital history), legal entanglements and criminal history, major medical illness as an adult, and substance abuse history.

MENTAL STATUS EXAMINATION

Table 2–3 gives a summary of areas to be commented on, along with common terms.

TABLE 2–3	Mental Status Examination

Appearance

Level of consciousness (alert, hypervigilant, somnolent, stuporous)

Dress (casual, appropriate for weather, eccentric, careless, disheveled)

Grooming (style of hair, degree of makeup, shaven or unshaven, clean, malodorous)

Idiosyncrasies (tattoos, professional or amateur; prominent scars; religious emblems)

Attitude

Cooperative, hostile, evasive, threatening, obsequious

Affect

Range (restricted, expansive, blunted, flat)
Appropriateness to items discussed
Stability (labile, shallow)
Quality (silly, anxious)

Mood

Response to question, How are you feeling/How's your mood been?

Behavior

Psychomotor agitation or retardation

Speech

Rate (rapid, slowed, pressured, hard to interrupt)
Volume (loud, soft, monotone, highly inflected or dramatic)
Quality (neologisms, fluent, idiosyncratic)

Thought Process

Goal directed, disorganized, loose associations, tangential, circumstantial, flight of ideas

Thought Content

Major preoccupations, ideas of reference, delusions (grandiose, paranoid, bizarre; state exactly what it is the patient appears to believe)

Thought broadcasting, insertion, or withdrawal

Suicidal or homicidal ideation; plan and intent to carry out ideas

CONDUCT OF THE INTERVIEW

Factors that affect the interview include the: patient's physical or emotional distress, cognitive capacities of the patient, emotionally based biases of the patient (transference), emotionally based biases of the interviewer (countertransference), and situational factors (patient reluctance, civil commitment, disability evaluation, press of time).

General Features of Psychiatric Interviews

SETTING

The ideal interview setting is one that provides a pleasant atmosphere and is reasonably comfortable, private, and free from outside distractions. Such a setting not only provides the physical necessities for an interview but conveys that the patient will be well cared for and safe.

VERBAL COMMUNICATION

Speech may be straightforward imparting of information, or may convey information indirectly through metaphor or use of words for noninformational purposes, such as to express or contain emotions or create an impact on the interviewer.

Language may be used by influencing the process of the interview. Patients may shift topics, make offhand remarks or jokes, ask questions, and compliment or belittle the interviewer as a way of expressing feelings. The process of the interview frequently expresses the patient's feelings about her or his immediate situation or interaction with the interviewer.

Language also may be used in the service of psychological defense mechanisms to contain rather than express emotions.

Another form of process communication is the use of language to make an impact on the interviewer. A statement such as "If you can't help me I'm going to kill myself" might convey suicidal intent, but it may also serve to stir up feelings of concern and involvement in the interviewer.

NONVERBAL COMMUNICATION

Emotions and attitudes are communicated nonverbally through facial expressions; gestures; body position; movements of the hands, arms, legs, and feet; interpersonal distance; dress and grooming; and speech prosody. Some nonverbal communications, such as gestures, are almost always conscious and deliberate; others often occur automatically outside one's awareness. The latter type are particularly important to observe during an interview because they may convey messages entirely separate from or even contradictory to what is being said.

Facial expression, body position, tone of voice, and speech emphasis are universal in the way they convey meaning. The interviewer will automatically decode these signals but may ignore the message because of countertransference or social pressure from the patient.

Nonverbal communication proceeds in both directions, and the nonverbal messages of the interviewer are likely to have a considerable effect on the patient. Thus, the interviewer who sits back in the chair and looks down at notes communicates less interest and involvement than one who sits upright and makes eye contact. Similarly, an interviewer who gives a weak handshake and sits behind a desk or far across the room from the patient communicates a sense of distance that may interfere with establishing rapport.

LISTENING AND OBSERVATION

The complexity of communication in the psychiatric interview is mirrored by the complexity of listening. The interviewer must remain open to literal and metaphorical messages from the patient, to the impact the patient is trying to make, and to the degree to which nonverbal communication complements or contradicts what is being said. Doing this optimally requires that the interviewer also be able to listen to her or his own mental processes throughout the interview, including both thoughts and emotional reactions.

Another important issue in listening is maintaining a proper balance between forming judgments and remaining open to new information and new hypotheses.

ATTITUDE AND BEHAVIOR OF THE INTERVIEWER

The optimal attitude of the interviewer is one encompassing interest, concern, and intention to help the patient. Although the interviewer must be tactful and thoughtful about what he or she says, this should not preclude behaving with natural warmth and spontaneity. Indeed, these qualities may be needed to support patients through a stressful interview process. Similarly, the interviewer must try to use natural, commonly understood language and avoid jargon or technical terms. The interviewer must communicate an intention to keep the patient as safe as possible, whatever the circumstances. Thus, although one must at times set limits on the behavior of an agitated, threatening, or abusive patient, one should never be attacking or rejecting.

Empathy is an important quality in psychiatric interviewing. Whereas sympathy is an expression of agreement or support for another, empathy entails putting oneself in another's place and experiencing her or his state of mind. Empathy comprises both one's experiencing of another person's mental state and the expression of that understanding to the other person.

As a mode of listening, empathy is an important way of understanding the patient; as a mode of response, it is important in building rapport and alliance. Patients who feel great emotional distance from the interviewer may make empathic understanding difficult or impossible. Thus, the interviewer's inability to empathize may itself be a clue to the patient's state of mind.

Structure of the Interview

The overall structure of the psychiatric interview is generally one of reconnaissance and detailed inquiry. In reconnaissance phases, the interviewer inquires about broad areas of symptoms, functioning, or life course: Have you ever had long periods when you felt low in mood? How have you been getting along at work? What did you do between high school and when you got married? In responding to such questions, patients give the interviewer leads that must then be pursued with more detailed questioning. Leads may include references to symptoms, difficulty functioning, interpersonal problems, ideas, states of feeling, or stressful life events. Each such lead raises questions about the nature of the underlying problem, and the interviewer must attempt to gather enough detailed information to answer these questions.

The patient's emotional state and attitude may impede a smooth flow of information. If the patient shows evidence, for example, of anxiety, hostility, suspiciousness, or indifference, the interviewer must first build a working alliance before trying to collect information. This usually requires acknowledging the emotions that the patient presents, helping the patient to express his or her feelings and related thoughts, and discussing these concerns in an accepting and empathic manner.

In the usual clinical situation, although the interviewer may have a standardized general plan of approach, she or he must adapt the degree of structure to the individual patient. Open-ended, nondirective questions derive from the psychoanalytic tradition. They are most useful for opening up and following emotionally salient themes in the patient's life story and interpersonal history. Focused, highly structured questioning derives from the medical-descriptive tradition and is most useful for delineating the scope and evolution of pathological signs and symptoms. In general, one uses the least amount of structure needed to maintain a good flow of communication and cover the necessary topic areas.

Phases of the Interview

The typical interview comprises opening, middle, and closing phases. In the opening phase, the interviewer and patient are introduced, and the purposes and procedures of the interview are set. It is generally useful for the interviewer to begin by summarizing what he or she already knows about the patient and proceeding to the patient's own account of the situation.

The opening phase may also include clarification of what the patient hopes to get from the consultation. Patients may sometimes state this explicitly but often do not, and the interviewer should not assume that her or his goals are the same as the patient's. A question such as "How were you hoping I could help you with the problem you have told me about?" invites the patient to formulate and express his or her request and avoids situations in which the patient and interviewer work at cross-purposes.

The middle phase of the interview consists of assessing the major issues in the case and filling in enough detail to answer the salient questions and construct a working formulation. Most of the work of determining the relative importance of biological, psychological, environmental, and sociocultural contributions to the problem is done during this phase. The patient's attitudes and transferential perceptions are also monitored during this phase so that the interviewer can recognize and address barriers to communication and collaboration.

When appropriate, formal aspects of the mental status examination are performed during the middle phase of the interview. Whereas most of the mental status evaluation is accomplished simply by observing the patient, certain components, such as cognitive testing and review of psychotic symptoms, may not fit smoothly into the rest of the interview. These are generally best covered toward the end of the interview, after the issues of greatest importance to the patient have been discussed and the rapport has been established. A brief explanation that the interviewer has a few standard questions that need to be answered before the end of the interview serves as a bridge and minimizes the awkwardness of asking questions that may seem incongruous or pejorative.

In the third or closing phase of the interview, the interviewer shares his or her conclusions with the patient, makes treatment recommendations, and elicits reactions. Summing up allows the patient to correct or add to the salient facts as understood by the interviewer and contributes to the patient's feeling of having gotten something from the interview. All treatment plans must be negotiated with the patient, including discussion of mutual goals, expected benefits, liabilities, limitations, and alternatives, if any.

Dimensions of Interviewing Technique

Although many systems have been suggested for classifying interviewing techniques, it is convenient to think about four major dimensions of interviewing style: degree of directiveness, degree of emotional support, degree of fact versus feeling orientation, and degree of feedback to the patient (Tables 2–4 to 2–8). The interviewer must seek a balance among these dimensions to best cover the needed topics, build rapport, and arrive at a plan of treatment.

Text continued on page 21

TABLE 2–4	Supportive Interventions
Intervention	**Examples**
Encouragement	*Patient:* I'm not sure I'm making any sense today, doctor. *Interviewer:* You're doing very well at describing the troubles you've been having.
Approval	You did the right thing by coming in for an appointment. You've been doing your best to keep going under very difficult circumstances.
Reassurance	What you are telling me about may seem very strange to you, but many people have had similar experiences.

Table continued on following page

TABLE 2–4	Supportive Interventions *(Continued)*
Intervention	**Examples**
Reassurance *(Continued)*	You feel like you will be sick forever, but with treatment you have a very good chance of feeling better soon.
Acknowledgment of affect	You look very sad when you talk about your brother.
	I have the impression that my question made you angry.
	I can see that you don't feel very safe here.
Empathic statements	When your boyfriend doesn't call you, you feel completely helpless and unloved.
	It seems unfair for you to get sick so many times while others remain well.
Nonverbal communication	Smiling, firm handshake, attentive body posture.
Avoidance of affect-laden material	Interviewer elects to defer discussion or probing of topics that arouse intense feelings of anxiety, shame, or anger.

TABLE 2–5	Obstructive Interventions
Intervention	**Examples**
Suggestive or biased questions	You haven't been feeling suicidal, have you?
	You've had six jobs in the last 2 years. I guess none of them held your interest?
Judgmental questions or statements	How long have you been behaving so selfishly?
	What you've told me is typical of delusional thinking.
Why questions	Why can't you sit still?
	Why do you keep choosing men who can't make a commitment to you?

TABLE 2–5	Obstructive Interventions *(Continued)*
Intervention	**Examples**
Ignoring the patient's leads	*Patient:* I'm afraid I'm going to fall apart. *Interviewer:* Have you had any odd experiences, such as hearing voices? *P:* No, but I just feel as though I can't cope and I wanted to talk to someone about it. *I:* Has your sleep pattern or appetite changed? *P:* Well, I don't sleep as well as I used to, but it's getting through the days that's the hardest. *I:* Have you had any suicidal thoughts?
Crowding the patient with questions	*P:* I just can't get it out of my mind that this cancer of mine is a punishment of some kind because I . . . *I:* Have you been in a low mood or been tearful?
Compound questions	Have you ever heard voices or thought that other people were out to harm you?
Vague questions	Do you feel socially self-conscious a lot? How much trouble do you have with your memory?
Minimization or dismissal	*P:* I don't seem to be able to enjoy my life as much as I think I should. *I:* You're doing well at your job and have a family—you're probably just feeling some minor stress.
Premature advice or reassurance	*P:* I've been having terrible headaches and I forget a lot of things. There's nothing wrong with my brain, is there? *I:* Headaches and forgetfulness are common and are probably due to some minor cause in your case. *P:* I've started to have thoughts that I married the wrong man and I should leave my husband. *I:* Maybe the two of you ought to take some time away together.
Nonverbal communication	Sitting at a distance, yawning, looking at watch, fidgeting, frowning, rolling of eyes.

TABLE 2–6	Fact-Oriented Interventions in the Psychiatric Interview

Intervention	Examples
Questions about symptoms	Do the voices seem to come from within your own head or from outside?
	When did you first begin to check your door lock many times before going out?
Questions about behavior	What do you do when you fly into a rage—do you yell, hit the furniture, or hit people?
	Since you've had your pain, how is your daily routine different from what it used to be?
Questions about events	What was the next thing you did after you took the overdose of medication?
	What led up to your decision to move out of your parents' home?
Requests for biographical data	Who lived with you when you were growing up?
	How many times have you been in a psychiatric hospital?
	Tell me about your close relationships with women.
Requests for medical data	What medicines do you take?
	What conditions do you see a doctor for?

TABLE 2–7	Feeling-Oriented Interventions in the Psychiatric Interview

Intervention	Examples
Questions about feelings in specific situations	Some people might have been angry in the situation you told me about. Did you feel that way?
	How did you feel when your doctor told you that you had had a heart attack?
	I noticed your voice got much quieter when you answered my last question. What were you feeling just then?
Questions or comments about emotional themes or patterns	Growing up, you never felt like you measured up to your mother's expectations. Do you feel that same way in your marriage?
	You've had a very competitive relationship with your brother. When you were asking about my qualifications just now, I wonder if you were feeling competitive with me also.
Questions or comments about the personal meaning of events	You are concerned about becoming enraged at your daughter. When she disregards your wishes, what do you feel it means about you as a parent?
	From what you have said, I think your becoming ill means to you that you will no longer have the respect of the people who depend on you.

TABLE 2–8	Feedback in the Psychiatric Interview
Intervention	**Examples**
Sharing of ongoing thoughts	As you were talking I began to wonder whether you had ever lost anyone very close to you. As I hear your story, it occurs to me that you've been an outsider every place you've lived.
Sharing of subjective reactions	What you are saying makes me feel quite sad. You've told me how you left treatment with your last psychiatrist, but I still feel a bit confused about what happened. I notice I'm feeling somewhat tense right now and I wonder if you might be feeling it too.
Imparting of information	About 75% of people with your condition respond well to medication. The tendency to have the kind of symptoms you described runs in families and is probably inherited.
Proposing a formulation	I think the immediate cause of your depression and insomnia is your heavy drinking. When you are under stress, you tend not to think clearly and to have unrealistic fears. It seems as though your present stress comes from the way you and your family are getting along at home.
Making treatment recommendations	For you to keep safe and begin treatment, I think it would be best to go into the hospital for a while. Medication should help you get out of your depression much faster. When you are feeling better, it would be a good idea for us to try to understand how you got so isolated from your friends and family.
Advice	It might be better not to decide about changing jobs until you're feeling back to your regular self.

TABLE 2–8	Feedback in the Psychiatric Interview *(Continued)*
Intervention	**Examples**
Response to questions	*Patient:* What type of psychiatrist are you, doctor? *Interviewer:* I'm a general psychiatrist who uses medication and psychotherapy. I also have a special interest in anxiety disorders. *P:* Have you ever seen another patient like me? *I:* I can answer your question better if you tell me what there is about you that I might never have seen before. *P:* Do you think I'm a terrible person? *I:* I don't think you're terrible, but I wonder what you think about yourself that you would ask me that.

SPECIAL PROBLEMS IN INTERVIEWING

The Delusional Patient

Psychotic patients often present with a variety of delusions—fixed, false beliefs that are not consistent with their cultural milieu. Delusions may be persecutory, grandiose, or a variety of other types.

The interviewer must walk a fine line between giving reassurance and at the same time not validating the delusions.

It is important to keep in mind that delusions are by definition unresponsive to logical argument. Whatever psychological or neurobiological purpose they serve will not be easily abandoned. The interviewer risks losing any chance of alliance, with almost no chance of benefit, by trying to persuade a patient that he or she is mistaken.

The Violent, Agitated Patient

In conducting an interview with an unpredictable or potentially violent person, it is appropriate to make the patient aware of one's concern that he or she might be unable to control himself or herself and find out whether the patient agrees. If so, then the patient and interviewer together must ensure a safe environment. Most potentially violent people fear the violence as much as anyone and are relieved by efforts to help them maintain control—even the use of four-point leather restraints.

If a patient is unable to agree with needed measures, and the potential for violence mandates their use, the intervention should proceed in an orderly manner. Explanation should be given to the patient concurrently, including exactly what will be done, the reason for it, assurance of the patient's safety, and what behavioral requirements there are for the cessation of the intervention.

Sometimes patients refuse to conduct an interview after safety measures have been instituted. They will insist that the interview room door not be left open, that security personnel leave, that they be permitted out of a seclusion room, or that restraints be removed. Assuming that the initial decision for such intervention was appropriate, it is useful to remind the patient that a valid assessment is the quickest way to achieve what he or she and you wish. No one should accept an unsafe situation as part of a bargain to get questions answered.

The Hostile Patient

A therapeutic alliance is the sine qua non of most interviews. Without an agreed basis on which to work, anything an interviewer says can be interpreted as intrusive and provoke an angry response. Overt hostility must be acknowledged right at the onset, or the patient may perceive further things to feel hostile about. Pointing out the incongruity of the anger, once it is acknowledged, can be the next step; after all, the psychiatrist is presumably conducting an evaluation in the service of the patient.

Clearly, responding to hostile provocation with hostility has no place in an interview. Ignoring it or being too accommodating to provocative acts can have deleterious effects as well, by breaking the usual interview frame of two people working together to solve the problems of one of them.

Talking to a profoundly depressed patient can sap the energy of the interviewer. The patient often has the classic symptom of prolonged latency of response; it can be difficult to avoid repeating the question, suggesting responses, or simply changing the line of inquiry. An occasional rephrasing or seeking to find out whether the patient understands the question is all the interviewer can do. A great deal of patience is required in conducting an evaluation of someone who is extremely depressed.

Crying is a frequently encountered behavior in the interview of a depressed patient, which is sometimes a problem. Especially when the patient's first priority is expressing the depth of his or her emotion, it may be difficult to get needed information. At times, the patient must be told of this difficulty and the importance of completing the assessment in a timely manner to reduce the pain.

The Confused Patient

Assessing a patient with cognitive loss requires a lowering of expectations for historical data and the realization that the going will be slow. Most confused patients will not be able to respond to open-ended questions reliably; the unstructured stimulus requires too much secondary processing on the patient's part. Instead, simple yes or no questions, of no more than about 10 words, are likely to yield the most reliable responses.

Patients with memory problems also need to be frequently reoriented to their surroundings as well as to the task at hand. It is helpful to query these patients about their current situation at times and provide the reassurance of their being in a treatment situation dedicated to their welfare.

The mental status examination of the confused patient deserves special attention. It is important that the patient's performance be characterized precisely; both the requested task as well as the patient's response should be included. The format of most standard tests (serial sevens, remembering three objects, naming of presidents from the present backward, digit span, spelling *world* backward) does not require explication; it is important, however, to describe exactly how the patient responded to which test, rather than just to note poor memory or concentration.

With confused patients, more than any other, the setting of the interview can markedly affect the results. Patients with impaired cognitive processing are susceptible to extraneous distractions—the capacity to focus attention is often lost. As much as possible, stimuli other than the interviewer should be at a minimum.

The Seductive Patient

Psychiatric assessment requires that the interviewer display a degree of emotional openness and support that can stimulate a powerful longing in some patients. Few aphrodisiacs can compare in potency with the sincere, nonjudgmental interest from another person, especially one in a position of relative power. In particular, patients who have been sexually abused as children, or those who have been unable to achieve close relationships, sometimes find the interview an invitation to greater intimacy. A good psychiatrist will try to foster an atmosphere wherein the patient can feel comfortable sharing anything, including such deeply personal things as sexual attraction. Therefore, the interviewer must maintain the boundary between expression of sexual feelings and acting on them.

The interviewer's emotional reaction to the patient, including at times sexual attraction (or repulsion), can play a part in how she or he responds to seductiveness. An awareness that the patient is usually responding more to what he or she needs to see or hear (that is, to transferential perceptions) rather than to the actual person of the interviewer can help keep the interaction in perspective.

Seductiveness in an initial interview is rare. It may signify a frontal lobe dysfunction or hypomania, or a misunderstanding of the clinical situation. Pointing out this misunderstanding is an effective way of management. "My understanding is that you're here for help with some things that are troubling you. Helping as a doctor is something I can do, but that is a specifically limited relationship."

Cultural Disparity

Significant cultural, religious, ethnic, racial, language, and other differences between the patient and the interviewer create at least three major problems, which are closely related: the basic problem of obtaining information, the interpretation of information in the appropriate cultural context, and finally the establishment of necessary rapport.

The use of an interpreter deserves special mention. Whenever possible, an unbiased third party should be used, rather than a family member. The interpreter must be explicitly instructed to interpret verbatim, as much as possible, except perhaps in the fortuitous circumstance when the interpreter is also a psychiatrist. The purpose of the interview, how long it will last, and of course the need to respect confidentiality should all be explained. Confidentiality is especially important in dealing with members of small minority groups because the likelihood of common business or social ties is high.

Membership in subcultures creates problems for understanding "peculiarities" of word choice and concept. Assessment for delusional beliefs in particular must take the patient's background into account; a delusion cannot be diagnosed if the belief is shared by a significant percentage of the patient's peers.

The final issue is the degree of comfort a patient can have with an "outsider." The wish to be understood, to be accepted, and to be valued is part of the human condition and is at work in nearly every interview. When there are cultural discrepancies between the patient and the psychiatrist, the fears of being misunderstood can be overwhelming. It is the interviewer's responsibility to give reassurance of a commitment to understanding the patient as best as possible and to take steps to minimize the chance of distortion.

The Deceitful Patient

One basic expectation of the physician-patient relationship is honesty. There are many different reasons for deception. Most commonly, the patient has a different agenda, which he or she feels must be kept hidden from the interviewer and which is often directed toward achieving the secondary gains of illness. At times, the patient hides symptoms, because of fear of them or because of fear of what treatment might be required. Patients who mistrust the medical establishment may be unwilling to share important information, believing themselves to be the best judge of what care they need and couching their replies in the way they think will best achieve their own ends.

Malingering and factitious disorder must be distinguished from that of the patient who is unaware that she or he is giving misinformation. Patients with conversion disorder experience neurological symptoms purely on a psychological basis and may be unable to speak, walk, or see but have no organic defect. These patients are not being deceitful; they truly cannot function and will not until their illness is treated.

A Developmental Perspective on Normal Domains of Mental and Behavioral Function

CHAPTER
3

A Psychiatric Perspective on Human Development

In this chapter, an overview of five prominent lines of human development is presented so that the reader can quickly obtain a sense of the timetable of normal development. These five lines of development are 1) biological development, 2) cognitive development, 3) emotional development, 4) social development, and 5) moral development. In addition, a longitudinal review of developmental periods associated with an increased risk for specific psychiatric disturbances is provided.

Psychoanalysis focused on the influence of early experience on development and may well have been a forewarning of the probable importance of intense early experience in gene expression that is only now becoming well appreciated.

BIOLOGICAL DEVELOPMENT

A time line of biological development over the course of the life span is presented in Figure 3–1.

Neurological Considerations

Brain growth is a basic indicator of neurological development. The brain is already at approximately one third of its adult size at birth, and it grows rapidly, reaching 60% by approximately 1 year and 90% by 5 years of age. The final 10% of growth occurs during the next 10 years with attainment of full weight by 16 years of age. The processes of myelinization, synapse proliferation, and synaptic pruning occur in the course of the life span, but they are particularly active in the first years of life, when the functional structure of the brain is becoming defined. The visual cortex reaches peak synaptic density by 6 months of age; the frontal cortex does not peak until

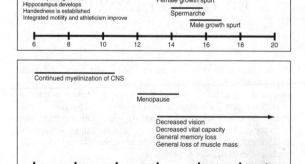

Figure 3–1 *Time line (in years) of biological development across the life span.*

TABLE 3–1	New York Longitudinal Study Dimensions of Temperament
Temperament Dimensions	**Description**
Activity level	Overall level of motor activity
Rhythmicity*	Regularity of the infant's biological functioning
Approach-withdrawal*	Tendency for the infant to approach or withdraw around unfamiliar people
Adaptability*	Flexibility to adjust to changes in routine and to new environments
Intensity*	Intensity of the infant's emotional reactions, whatever their content
Mood*	Infant's tendency to display predominantly positive or negative moods
Distractibility	Tendency to react to sensory stimulation
Sensory threshold	Ease with which the infant can be distracted into more socially desirable responses
Persistence	Tendency to sustain attention

*Negative poles describe dimensions of difficult temperament.

Modified from Chess S, Thomas A: Temperament in Clinical Practice, New York: Guilford Press, 1986.

1 year. The density of dendritic spines decreases to adult levels by the end of the second year of life, at which time glucose metabolism is also fully developed. The establishment of biological rhythms occurs in early infancy, and sleep becomes more organized and of shorter nocturnal duration.

A stable pattern of temperament cannot be documented in the first months of life, but it gradually becomes established during the second year. During the preschool period, individual neurons and neural networks are preferentially preserved if they receive stimulation. Motor skills develop and activity levels increase, rapidly reflecting underlying neural development (Table 3–1).

By the age of 7 years, considerable sensory integration has occurred. Handedness has been clearly established, and brain plasticity has decreased. By 10 years of age, limitations in the ability to learn to speak an unaccented second language reflect further changes in the development of the motor linguistic pathways. In the years of adolescence, full brain weight is achieved, but myelinization continues well into the fourth decade. By the end of the fifth decade, there is often evidence of the beginning of decline in specific neuronal functions, with vision and memory being particularly vulnerable. However, integrative capacities may reach a peak during the later decades.

Endocrinological Considerations

Although interesting changes in hormonal development occur in the first years of life, dramatic changes in both physical and emotional functions are triggered by the striking hormonal shifts associated with puberty that usher in the adolescent years. In girls, estradiol and progesterone production results in the onset of breast development, followed by the onset of pubic hair development and vaginal elongation. Axillary hair subsequently develops during stage 3 of pubic hair development. Menarche is usually attained 2 years after the onset of breast development and has been reported to occur at an average of 12.8 years of age in population studies, with wide variability in different cultural environments. In boys, puberty begins when rising levels of pituitary hormones result in enlargement of the testes and subsequent increases in circulating testosterone. Spermatogenesis occurs after testicular enlargement at approximately 14 years of age. Pubic hair development is triggered by adrenal androgens and occurs in five stages during the course of about 2.5 years. Facial hair tends to develop between 14 and 15 years of age.

Sexual function peaks early in the adult years in men, but there is only a gradual decline in sexual function as measured by frequency of orgasm from 20 to 70 years. Women have consistent sexual functioning throughout the childbearing years and frequently become more orgasmic in their 30s. However, decreases in estrogen levels associated with menopause usually occur between 45 and 54 years of age. Men have no comparable menopausal change in hormonal levels.

COGNITIVE DEVELOPMENT

A time line of cognitive development during the course of the life span is presented in Figure 3–2.

The study of cognitive development provides a perspective on the evolution of the capacity to think. Increased cognitive abilities are an integral component required for the onset of language, and changes in thinking shape the course and ultimate level of emotional, social, and moral development. However, the acquisition of mental abilities has been charted as an independent sequence of mental accomplishments. Piaget (1969) established the field of cognitive development, and his stage theory of the evolution of cognitive processes has dominated this field. Although specific aspects of his four primary stages have been modified by subsequent empirical experiments as well as by the development of a greater appreciation of the role of emotions and context in the utilization of cognitive abilities, his careful observations and brilliant deductions have provided the framework on which much of our knowledge of cognitive development has been built.

Piaget both introduced the concept of schemas, which represent units of cognition, and defined processes that result in schema modification, such as the classical interaction of assimilation and

Cognitive Development

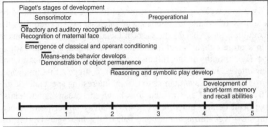

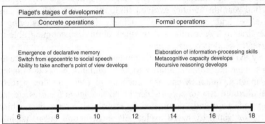

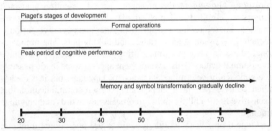

Figure 3–2 *Time line (in years) of cognitive development across the life span.*

accommodation of new stimuli. A particularly important piagetian concept has been that of a decalage within cognitive development. In cognitive terms, this refers to an unevenness in development. For example, a child demonstrating cognitive abilities at the concrete operational stage of development with regard to conservation of volume while retaining preoperational forms of thinking as manifested by a persistent egocentrism demonstrates an unevenness in performance. Such distortion can also be seen across lines of development, and is termed an interlineal decalage.

Even newborns have the ability to learn through making associations between different states or experiences. There is evidence that cognitive "prewiring" exists that allows for the perceptual capacities of infants that are necessary to seek stimulation and interaction with adult caregivers. A key capacity required for these early cognitions is recognition of the invariant features of perceptual stimuli coupled with the ability to translate these invariant features across sensory modalities, an ability known as cross-modal fluency. Interestingly, infants can innately differentiate the human voice from other sounds and do not have to "learn" the complex characteristics of the structure and pitch of speech.

By 2 to 3 weeks of age, cross-modal fluency is demonstrated by the ability of infants to imitate facial expression. This requires the recognition of a visual schema of a facial expression to be linked with a proprioceptive tactile schema of producing a facial expression. By 3 months of age, infants can be classically conditioned, and their interest in stimuli led Piaget (1969) to suggest that this was a period dominated by attempts to make "interesting spectacles last."

By 6 months of age, associations between "means" and "ends" have been demonstrated. This is followed by object permanence, which evolves during the second half of the first year. During the second year, the abilities evolve both to infer cause after observing an effect and, conversely, to anticipate effects after producing a causal action. A corollary of this new ability is becoming able to correctly sequence past events.

By the third year of life, children enter the preoperational stage. This stage has some similarity to adult thinking but is dominated by magical qualities and the tendency to focus on one perceptual attribute at a time. Idiosyncratic cosmological theories are the rule and are usually dominated by transductive reasoning, which attributes causality based exclusively on temporal or spatial juxtaposition. Throughout the preschool period, attention span and memory are limited and pretend play and fanciful thinking are common. Therefore, it is not surprising that this cognitive period is characterized by imaginary friends and talking pets. The preoperational stage is also the time during which explosive language development occurs. This development appears to be made possible by a genetically determined capacity for language, but it is clearly enhanced by experiential support and parental communication that is sensitive to the child's ability to process new words and language structure.

By age 6 or 7 years, children begin to use operational thinking. The concrete operational child has the ability to conserve both volume and quantity and can appreciate the reversibility of events and ideas. A shift from an egocentric perspective results in a new capacity to appreciate the perspectives of others. These new cognitive skills are the result of new cognitive structures that are required to engage in logical dialogue and to develop an appreciation for more complex causal sequences. These are precisely the abilities that are required to benefit from the grade school curriculum.

Adolescence results in the development of a new processing capacity that involves the manipulation of ideas and concepts. Furthermore, the informational fund of knowledge is dramatically expanded and serves as a referent for verification of new data that are assimilated. A final major transition is to the new ability to reflect on cognition as a process. This is referred to as the development of a metacognitive capacity. This capacity allows adolescents to understand and empathize with the divergent perspectives of others to a greater degree. Furthermore, recursive thinking is now possible whereby the awareness that others can think about the domain of the adolescent's own thought is achieved. These cognitive skills represent the transition into the final stage of cognitive ability, referred to as the use of formal operations. This form of thinking is complex and is not achieved by many adults who remain at the stage of concrete operations. A specific product of this process is the ability to understand complex combinatorial systems that require a well-developed sense of reversibilities including inversion, reciprocity, and symmetry. New levels of problem solving are achieved that include the ability to recognize a core problem isomorph that previously has been solved within a new problem. Through the use of previously successful solutions, efficient parallel solutions can be developed and applied.

EMOTIONAL DEVELOPMENT

A time line of emotional development during the course of the life span is presented in Figure 3–3.

The emotional state of the newborn is largely assessed by facial expression and accompanying vocalizations. However, the communicative capacity of young infants has become increasingly well appreciated. In the first weeks of life, contentment and distress have been reliably monitored, and they further differentiate during the first months of life. By 7 to 9 months, a transition occurs that is based on the earliest attainment of intersubjectivity. At this point infants

Emotional Development

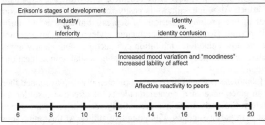

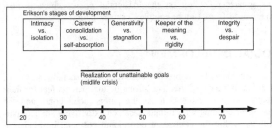

Figure 3–3 *Time line (in years) of emotional development across the life span.*

begin to understand that their own inner experiences and feelings can be appreciated by other individuals. This leads to the possibility of developing affect attunement as parents match their own behavior with the behavior of their infant, which is accompanied by some sharing of internal feeling states. Furthermore, the instrumental use of emotions is evidenced by an infant pouting to elicit a parental response. Social referencing occurs by 12 months of age, as illustrated by infants' turning to examine their mothers' facial expressions when they are confronted with potentially fearful situations or objects.

In the second year of life, a period of mixed emotions evolves and the rapprochement crisis occurs as infants become aware of their separateness from their primary attachment object and the limitations of their control on the primary object's behavior. After the infant has attained self-cognition, new more complex emotions of embarrassment and envy emerge that further evolve to create shame, pride, and then guilt by the end of the second year. Furthermore, object constancy, or the ability to reduce anxiety in response to the separation from the primary caretaker, reflects the association of an emotional state with the memory of the affect modulation provided by the attachment figure.

During the preschool years, children begin to learn more effectively the nature of the relationship between emotions and behaviors. They begin to understand the culturally defined rules associated with affect expression and consequently begin to mask their emotions. This is also the period when the Oedipus complex is most evident, and the child must deal with conscious desire for the parent of the opposite sex and the potential retaliation from the same-sex parent. Clearly, this links positive effects with fearful and angry emotions.

As children move into the school years, they experience the full range of adult emotions, although there is at least a qualitative sense that during the prepubertal period there is less intense expression of affect. Although sadness is easily recognized from the second year of life, prolonged periods of depressed affect are rare during this period. However, temperamental styles tend to emerge and, specifically, behavioral inhibition can become more clearly appreciated within the context of increasing social and educational demands.

In adolescence, emotions are more intensely displayed, and there is an emergence of a greater incidence of affective disorder and anxiety. Similarly, there is a dramatic increase in suicidal behavior that is in part associated with cognitive ability. At this point, there is a greater reflection on the existential crisis, which is now experienced from a more complex vantage point.

SOCIAL DEVELOPMENT

It has become widely appreciated that infants are socially interactive from the first days of life. The strong tie that parents feel for their infants has been referred to as the parent-infant bond, and the process of bonding with infants has been extensively studied, particularly within the context of developing postnatal hospital procedures. Between 7 and 9 months of age, infants develop separation protest and a negative reaction to the approach of a stranger.

TABLE 3–2	Patterns of Attachment			
Characteristics	Secure Pattern	Avoidant Pattern	Resistant Pattern	Disorganized Pattern
Distress	Open display of distress and need for comfort	Inhibited display of distress	Exaggerated display of distress	Odd or contradictory display of distress
Soothing	Effective soothing; positive greeting	No soothing; avoidance instead of greeting	Ineffective soothing; no positive greeting because of distress	Ineffective soothing; usually no positive greeting; often odd or ambivalent greeting
Anger	Little angry behavior	Displaced anger	Angry, resistant behaviors	No predictable pattern
Stress	Low cortisol secretion	High cortisol secretion	No cortisol data	No cortisol data
Strategy for obtaining comfort	Coherent strategy of seeking comfort directly when needed	Coherent strategy of minimizing distress by displaced attention	Coherent strategy of exaggerating distress to mobilize caregiver	Incoherent strategy or significant lapse in organization of strategy
Parental characteristics	Sensitive, emotionally available caregiving, balanced perspective on childhood relationship experiences	Emotionally restricted caregiving; dismissing of painful relationship experiences and their effects	Inconsistent caregiving; unintegrated emotional response to relationship experiences	No data on caregiving; unresolved losses or traumatic childhood experiences

Social Development

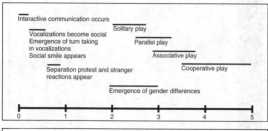

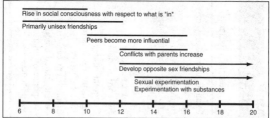

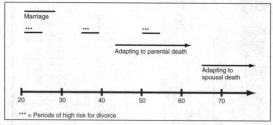

*** = Periods of high risk for divorce

Figure 3–4 *Time line (in years) of social development across the life span.*

During the second half of the first year, the attachment of the infant to his or her parents evolves. The primary role of the attachment figure is the provision of a secure base from which the infant can begin to explore a wider social environment. It is within the context of the attachment relationship that the first eriksonian state of "basic trust" is achieved (Table 3–2).

A summary of social development is presented in Figure 3–4.

MORAL DEVELOPMENT

The newborn infant lives in an interactive world but one that is free of moral directives or structure. However, by the second year of life the emergence of "moral emotions," such as embarrassment, shame, and guilt, demonstrates that the beginning of a code of moral behavior in the most primitive sense is being established. By 36 months, children demonstrate the internalization of parental standards even when their parents are not available to provide cues or reinforcement. The importance of emotions in the early evolution of moral behavior represents a distinct departure from the more traditional perspective that moral development does not occur until the establishment of concrete operations.

A time line of moral development during the course of the life span is presented in Figure 3–5.

DEVELOPMENTAL PSYCHOPATHOLOGY

Risk and Protective Factors

The risk and protective factor model is a paradigm that facilitates the understanding of developmental deviations. It can be applied at any stage of development. Risk factors have been divided into three large categories: those at the level of the individual, the family, and the community.

The first category of risk factors is defined at the level of the individual. Both physical and emotional considerations are relevant. Examples include vulnerable genes, deficits in perception, and intense anxiety.

Moral Development

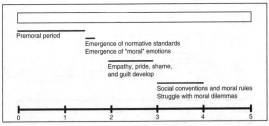

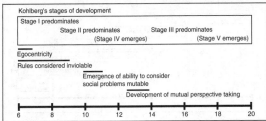

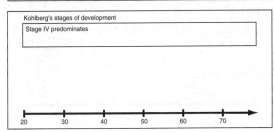

Figure 3–5 *Time line (in years) of moral development across the life span.*

The second category of risk factors is conceptualized at the level of the family. One classical example of a familial risk factor is a child being raised by a parent with a serious mental illness.

The third category of risk factors is defined at the level of the community. Discrimination based on any ethnic or racial condition falls into this group of risk factors, as does social disadvantage.

Resilient children represent a most fascinating opportunity to understand the mechanism by which risk and protective factors interact. Of particular interest for psychiatrists is the study of the children of schizophrenic mothers. It is striking that some children turn out to be productive and happy adults despite what appear to be overwhelming odds.

High-Risk Periods for Psychopathology

Psychiatrists who treat children and adolescents are particularly aware of the precursors and onset of psychiatric illnesses. Figure 3–6

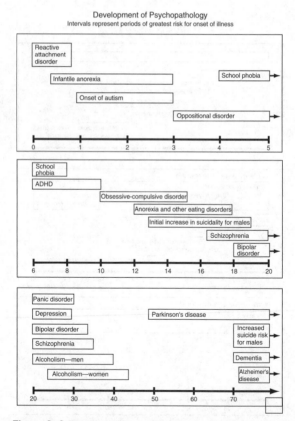

Figure 3–6 *Time line (in years) showing the development of psychopathology across the life span.*

gives an overview of the periods of most probable onset for many of the major psychiatric disorders.

THE PSYCHIATRIST AS A DEVELOPMENTALIST

All psychiatrists inevitably become students of development. The life histories of their patients demand developmental formulations to achieve a sense of understanding of the origins of the presenting symptoms and disturbing behaviors that bring the patients to psychiatric treatment. Anticipating the challenges of later life and understanding the origins of the strengths and weaknesses of each patient are at the core of the therapeutic process, whether it involves influencing the balance of the patient's central neurotransmitters or identifying and supporting available community resources.

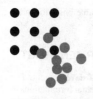

Manifestations of Psychiatric Illness

CHAPTER 4

Clinical Evaluation and Treatment Planning: A Multimodal Approach

The complete psychiatric evaluation for a hospitalized patient consists of the psychiatric interview; physical examination, including neurological assessment; laboratory testing; and, as appropriate, neuropsychological testing, structured interviews, and brain imaging. The results of the evaluation are then used to assess risk, reach tentative and definitive diagnoses if possible, and complete initial and comprehensive treatment plans. Clearly, the length, detail, and order of the evaluation need to be modified when it is conducted in different settings. The clinician needs to assess the goals of the interview, the patient's tolerance for questioning, and the time available. Table 4–1 shows the variation of the psychiatric evaluation with the type of setting.

TABLE 4–1	Psychiatric Evaluation and Treatment Planning		
Setting	**Psychiatric Interview and Mental Status Examination**	**Physical or Neurological Examination, Laboratory Assessments, Brain Imaging**	**Treatment Planning**
Emergency room	Most often lengthy and extensive, except as limited by patient's ability or willingness to communicate.	Physical examination is often performed; other tests and examinations are ordered as indicated.	Primary focus is on disposition.
Psychiatric inpatient unit	Extensive, but complete information may be obtained in a series of interviews over time.	Physical and neurological examinations and laboratory tests are always performed. Other tests and examinations are ordered as indicated.	Comprehensive and formal plans are developed.
Consultation liaison service	Depth of interview is highly variable depending on reasons for referral and patient's medical condition. An attempt is made to obtain a complete MSE.	Most medical information is obtained from the chart. Psychiatric consultant may request further assessment.	Recommendations focus on reasons for referral and are made to the primary treatment team.

TABLE 4–1	Psychiatric Evaluation and Treatment Planning *(Continued)*		
Setting	Psychiatric Interview and Mental Status Examination	Physical or Neurological Examination, Laboratory Assessments, Brain Imaging	Treatment Planning
Outpatient office or clinic	Urgency of situation is assessed. In nonurgent situations, the initial interview usually focuses on the chief complaint and MSE.	Medical information is obtained as needed, usually by referral to a general practitioner or specialist.	Planning may be formal or informal, depending on applicable regulatory and reimbursement requirements.
Third-party interviews (e.g., for court, disability determinations)	Interview addresses the reason for referral and may be narrowly focused but contains a complete MSE.	Assessments are ordered according to the purpose of the interview.	Not usually relevant except for recommendations pertaining to the purpose of the interview.

PSYCHIATRIC INTERVIEW

Despite the advent of brain imaging tests, standardized diagnostic criteria, and structured rating scales, the psychiatric interview (Table 4–2) remains the cornerstone of clinical evaluation in psychiatry.

Identifying Information

Most interviewers find it helpful to begin with a few questions designed to identify the patient in a general way. Asking the patient's name, age, address, marital status, and occupation provides a quick general picture and begins the interview with emotionally neutral material.

Chief Complaint

At the start, the interviewer wants to ascertain exactly why the patient is seeking psychiatric help at this time.

History of Present Illness

Having obtained the chief complaint, the interviewer should clarify the nature of the present illness. By definition, the present illness begins with the onset of signs and symptoms that characterize the current episode of illness.

Past Psychiatric History

The interviewer should ask for information regarding any previous episodes of psychiatric illness or treatment, including hospitalization, medications, outpatient therapy, substance use treatment, self-help groups, and consultation with culture-specific healers such as shamans. The duration and effectiveness of treatment should be ascertained, as well as the patient's general experience of psychiatric treatment to date.

Personal History

No interview is complete without some understanding of the patient's background and life circumstances (Table 4–3).

Family History

The interviewer should ask the patient specifically about any relatives with a history of psychiatric illness or treatment, suicide, or substance use.

Medical History

A careful review of a patient's medical history is an important part of the psychiatric interview because medical conditions can dra-

TABLE 4–2	Psychiatric Interview
Greeting	
Identifying information	
Chief complaint	
History of present illness	
Past psychiatric history	
Personal history	
Family history	
Medical history	
Substance use history	
Mental status examination	

TABLE 4–3	Personal History

Prenatal History

Wanted versus unwanted pregnancy

History of maternal malnutrition or maternal drug use (including prescription drugs)

Circumstances of birth (vaginal delivery versus cesarean section)

History of birth trauma

Birth order

Early Childhood (0–3 y)

Temperament

Major milestones, including speech and motor development

History of toilet training

Early feeding history, including breast-feeding

Early behavioral problems, (e.g., nightmares and night terrors, enuresis and encopresis, aggressive behavior)

Early relationships with parents and siblings

History of significant early illnesses or hospitalizations

History of early separations from caregivers

Middle Childhood—Latency (3–11 y)

Early school history, including any evidence of cognitive impairment

Relationships with siblings and peers

Early personality development

History of behavioral problems (e.g., separation anxiety, school phobia, aggressive behavior)

Adolescence (12–18 y)

Psychosexual development, including experience of puberty and menarche, masturbatory history, and early sexual behavior

Later school history

Later personality development

History of behavioral or emotional problems (e.g. substance abuse, eating disorders)

Adulthood

Marital history or history of relationships with significant others

History of child-rearing

Sexual history

Occupational and educational history

Religious history

Current living situation

matically affect psychiatric status. Many medical disorders, such as endocrinological conditions (thyroid disease, pheochromocytomas, pituitary adenomas), neurological disorders (Parkinson's disease, neoplasms, Wilson's disease, stroke syndromes, head trauma), and infectious diseases (HIV infection, meningitis, sepsis) can have manifestations that include psychiatric symptoms. When a medical disorder is suspected, rigorous inquiry is essential. A review of all of the patient's medications, including over-the-counter preparations, is important, because many of these substances can produce or exacerbate psychiatric symptoms.

Substance Use History

The interviewer should inquire about which substances are used, under what circumstances, and the quantity, variety, and duration of use. The interviewer must be sure to ask about past and current drug injection, including the sharing of injection equipment, to assess for HIV risk factors (Table 4–4).

Mental Status Examination

The MSE is a structured way to assess a patient's mental state at a given time. Unlike the parts of the interview that focus on the history, the MSE provides a descriptive snapshot of the patient at the interview. Much of the information needed for the evaluation of appearance, behavior, and speech is gathered without specific questioning during the course of the interview. However, the interviewer generally wants to ask specific questions to assess the patient's mood, thought process and content, and cognitive functioning. Keeping the outline of the MSE (Table 4–5) in mind ensures that the interview is comprehensive. The components of the MSE are described in the following paragraphs.

APPEARANCE. The interviewer should note the patient's general appearance, including grooming, level of hygiene, and attire.

BEHAVIOR. This includes patient's level of cooperativeness with the interview, motor excitement or retardation, abnormal movements (e.g., tardive dyskinesia, tremors), and maintenance of eye contact with the interviewer.

SPEECH. The psychiatrist should carefully assess the patient's speech for rate, fluency, clarity, and softness or loudness (Table 4–6).

MOOD AND AFFECT. The interviewer should be aware of the patient's mood and affect. *Affect* is the observable behavior seen in the expression of emotion, which responds to changes in emotional states. *Mood* is a sustained and pervasive emotion (Tables 4–7 through 4–10).

THOUGHT. The clinician should assess the patient's thought process and content. Thought process is the form of the patient's thoughts—are they organized and goal directed or are they tangential, circumstantial, or loosely associated (Table 4–11).

COGNITION. Every psychiatric interview should include some assessment of the patient's cognitive functioning (Table 4–12). This includes the patient's level of awareness, alertness, and orientation (to person, place, and time). If there is a question about the patient's memory, formal memory testing may be done to assess short-term, intermediate, and long-term memory.

Text continued on page 49

TABLE 4–4	Human Immunodeficiency Virus Risk Factors

Parenteral Factors

Use of shared needles or drug works in the course of drug injection or amateur tattooing

Receipt of blood, blood products, or organ transplant in the United States between 1978 and 1985

Maternal-fetal transmission (pediatric cases)

Occupational exposure among health care workers and laboratory technicians through needle-stick injuries and other significant exposures (uncommon)

Unsafe Sexual Activity

Most common for men: unprotected anal intercourse with other men; unprotected vaginal or anal intercourse with women who are known to be HIV-positive, engage in prostitution, or are injection drug users or sexual partners of injection drug users; multiple heterosexual partners

Most common for women: unprotected anal or vaginal intercourse with men who are known to be HIV-positive, are injection drug users, are the sexual partners of injection drug users, are bisexual, or have hemophilia or coagulation disorder; multiple heterosexual partners

Cofactors

Compromise of the skin or mucous membranes, especially through the presence of sexually transmitted diseases, which increases the likelihood of transmission on exposure to HIV-infected body fluids

Use of noninjection drugs, especially alcohol and crack cocaine, through association and high-risk sexual activity

Environmental Context

Risk behavior while living or traveling in geographic areas with high rates of HIV infection, through increased likelihood of exposure to HIV-infected body fluids

TABLE 4–5	Mental Status Examination

   I. Appearance
  II. Behavior (includes attitude toward the interviewer)
 III. Speech
  IV. Mood and affect
   V. Thought
       A. Thought process
       B. Thought content
  VI. Perception
       A. Hallucinations
           1. Auditory
           2. Visual
           3. Other (somatic, gustatory, tactile)
       B. Illusions
 VII. Cognition
       A. Level of awareness
       B. Level of alertness
       C. Orientation
           1. Person
           2. Place
           3. Time
       D. Memory
           1. Immediate
           2. Short term
           3. Long term
       E. Attention (digit span)
       F. Calculations
       G. Fund of knowledge
       H. Abstractions
           1. Similarities
           2. Proverbs
       I. Insight
       J. Judgment

TABLE 4–6	Disorders of Speech

Disorder	Definition
Looseness of association	Idiosyncratic shifts in frame of reference, failure in elaborating topic
Flight of ideas	Shifts in frame of reference but greater coherence and meaning within the frame
Clang association	Shift in frame of reference driven by phonetic similarity of words rather than topical relationships

Table continued on following page

TABLE 4–6	Disorders of Speech *(Continued)*
Disorder	**Definition**
Pressured speech	Speech produced at an abnormally high rate
Tangentiality	Less abrupt shifts in frame of reference; at any given time, message is coherent, with deviation from initial topic
Circumstantiality	Similar to tangentiality but with return to the original topic
Illogical thinking	Breakdowns in reasoning
Perseveration	Inappropriate repetition of words or phrases
Poverty of speech	Reduced conversational output
Neologism	Nonword phonetic combinations used as words
Paragrammatism	Ungrammatical word sequences
Word salad or incoherence	Combination of words or phrases that renders utterance devoid of decodable meaning
Mutism	Persistent total absence of speech
Thought blocking	Episodic interruption of speech

TABLE 4–7	Disturbances in Affect
Blunted	Severe reduction in the intensity of emotional expression
Fixed	Display of only one particular emotion, and absence of range and mobility of affect
Flat	Near-absence of affective expression
Inappropriate	Emotional expression and thought content that do not coincide
Labile	Repeated, rapid, and abrupt variability in affective expression
Restricted or constricted	Mild to moderate reduction in emotional expression

TABLE 4–8	Description of Affect	
Parameter of Affect	Normal	Abnormal
Appropriateness	Appropriate Congruent	Inappropriate Incongruent
Intensity	Normal	Blunted Exaggerated Flat Heightened Overly dramatic
Mobility	Mobile	Constricted Fixed Immobile Labile
Range	Full range	Restricted range
Reactivity	Reactive Responsive	Nonreactive Nonresponsive

Adapted from Trzepacz PT, Baker RW: The Psychiatric Mental Status Examination. New York: Oxford University Press, 1993:46.

TABLE 4–9	Mood States
Dysphoric	Includes sustained emotional states, such as sadness, anxiety, or irritability
Elevated	Exaggerated feeling of well-being, euphoria, or elation
Expansive	Lack of restraint in expressing feelings
Irritable	Easily annoyed or angered
Euthymic	Mood in the normal range

TABLE 4–10	Clinical Assessment of Mood
Evaluate its quality	How do you feel? What is your mood like?
Evaluate its stability	Do you always feel like this?
Evaluate its reactivity	Does your mood ever change? When does your mood change?
Evaluate its intensity	What is it like to feel this way? On a scale of 1 to 10, how would you rate your mood?
Evaluate its duration	How long have you felt this way?
Evaluate whether the mood is congruent with the thought content	

TABLE 4–11	Disorders of Thought Content
Disorder	**Definition**
Delusion	False belief not endorsed by social group, relatively impervious to invalidation
Obsession	Preoccupation acknowledged by patient to be irrational and associated with anxiety
Compulsion	Repetitive actions based on obsession
Rumination	Preoccupation generally associated with the irreversibility of past events
Overvalued idea	Frequently endorsed idea, often imposed on others
Grandiosity	Belief that one's ideas, capacities, or actions are generally superior to those of others
Suspiciousness	A cautious attitude based on possible malevolent intentions of others
Phobia	Persistent and irrational fear of delineated aspects of nonhuman environment (e.g., "germs," heights)
Paranoia	Level of suspiciousness altering thinking and behavior in nonadaptive ways

TABLE 4–12	Alterations of Consciousness
State*	**Definition**
Hypervigilance	Increased scanning of environment, arousal
	Difficulty in focusing or shifting attention
Alert wakefulness	Subject responds immediately in all sensory modalities
Lethargy	State of drowsiness, inaction, indifference
	Responses delayed or incomplete
	May need increased stimulation to respond
Obtundation	More indifferent
	May maintain wakefulness but little more
Stupor	Subject can be aroused by vigorous and continuous external stimulation

TABLE 4–12	Alterations of Consciousness (Continued)
State*	**Definition**
Coma	Psychological and motor responses to stimulation either completely lost or reduced to rudimentary responsiveness, e.g., withdrawal, sucking, chewing, swallowing
Catatonia	Dramatic reduction of psychomotor activity presenting as rigidity, waxy flexibility, mutism, and negativism
Partial Alterations of Consciousness	
Dissociation	Unintegrated perceptions
Depersonalization	Feels detached from world
Derealization	Environment seems unreal
Déjà vu	Feeling of familiarity
Jamais vu	Feeling of unfamiliarity
Unilateral neglect	Unawareness of a body part

*The causes are the same for all states: anxiety, stress, paranoia, drugs, and central nervous system damage.

The interviewer should gain a full understanding of the patient's insight into the illness by asking why, in the patient's opinion, he or she is currently in need of psychiatric care and what has caused the problems. Finally, the interviewer should learn about the patient's judgment. This is best assessed in terms of the patient's life circumstances—for example, asking a mother how she would deal with a situation in which she had to leave her children to go to the store or asking a chronically ill person what he does when he sees that he is running out of medicine.

PHYSICAL EXAMINATION

The physical examination is an important part of the comprehensive psychiatric evaluation for several reasons. First, many patients who present with psychiatric symptoms may have underlying medical problems that are causing or exacerbating the presenting symptoms. Second, the patient's physical capacity to tolerate certain psychiatric medications, such as tricyclic antidepressants or lithium, must be assessed. Finally, many patients who present to a psychiatrist have had inadequate medical care and should be routinely examined to assess their general level of physical health.

Certain aspects of the information obtained in the psychiatric interview should alert the psychiatrist to the need for a physical examination. Any indication from the history that the psychiatric symptoms followed physical trauma, infection, medical illness, or drug ingestion should prompt a full physical examination. Similarly, the acute onset of psychiatric symptoms in a previously psychiatrically healthy individual, as well as symptoms arising at an unusual age, should raise questions about potential medical causes (Table 4–13).

TABLE 4–13	Physical Illnesses That May Present with Psychiatric Symptoms

Neurological	**Metabolic**
Amyotrophic lateral sclerosis	Acute intermittent porphyria
Epilepsy—particularly partial complex seizures (e.g., temporal lobe epilepsy)	Electrolyte imbalance
	Hepatic encephalopathy
	Hepatolenticular degeneration (Wilson's disease)
Huntington's disease	Hypoxemia
Multiinfarct dementia	Uremic encephalopathy
Normal-pressure hydrocephalus	**Nutritional**
Parkinson's disease	
Pick's disease	Vitamin B_{12} deficiency
Stroke syndromes (cerebrovascular disease)	Central pontine myelinolysis
	Folate deficiency (megaloblastic anemia)
Rheumatological (Autoimmune)	General malnutrition
	Nicotinic acid deficiency (pellagra)
Systemic lupus erythematosus	Thiamine deficiency (Wernicke-Korsakoff syndrome)
Temporal arteritis	
Infectious	**Traumatic, Particularly Head Trauma**
Acquired immunodeficiency syndrome	**Toxic**
Brain abscess	
Encephalitis	Environmental toxins
Meningitis	Intoxication with alcohol or other drugs
Syphilis, particularly neurosyphilis	
Tuberculosis	**Neoplastic**
Viral hepatitis	
	Carcinoma (general)
Endocrine	Central nervous system tumors (primary or metastatic)
	Endocrine tumors
Adrenal hypoplasia (Cushing's syndrome)	Pancreatic carcinoma
Diabetes mellitus	
Hypo- or hyperparathyroidism	
Hypo- or hyperthyroidism	
Hypothalamic dysfunction	
Panhypopituitarism	
Pheochromocytoma	

NEUROLOGICAL EXAMINATION

In the hospital setting, every patient should have a thorough neurological examination. Patients who have a history of neurological disturbances, such as strokes, seizure disorders, central nervous system neoplasms, dementias, and movement disorders, should be carefully evaluated.

Patients with acquired immunodeficiency syndrome should also be carefully evaluated neurologically, because many neurological manifestations of advanced HIV-related illness (including HIV encephalopathy, toxoplasmosis, and cryptococcal meningitis) and the medicines administered to treat these illnesses may produce psychiatric symptoms, including depression, delirium, dementia, mania, and psychosis.

Psychological and Neuropsychological Testing

Psychological and neuropsychological tests are standard instruments used to measure specific aspects of mental functioning. They are usually administered by psychologists or other professionals who have been trained in their use and interpretation. In most cases, several tests, often referred to as a battery, are performed together. These test results must then be interpreted in the context of the broad clinical picture of the patient.

Table 4–14 lists some of the most commonly used tests.

TABLE 4–14	Common Psychological and Neuropsychological Tests
Name of Test	**General Purpose**
Bender Gestalt Test	Subject's reproduction of geometric designs used to screen for neuropsychiatric impairment
Halstead-Reitan Battery	Complex battery of tests that give a detailed picture of neuropsychiatric functioning
Minnesota Multiphasic Personality Inventory*	Multiple true-false questions designed to assess psychopathology and personality
Rorschach Test	Ten inkblot designs; subject's associations used to assess thinking disturbances and psychological conflicts and defenses

*Can be self-administered.

Table continued on following page

TABLE 4–14	Common Psychological and Neuropsychological Tests *(Continued)*
Name of Test	**General Purpose**
Thematic Apperception Test	Emotionally suggestive pictures portraying one or more people; used to elicit stories that reveal psychological development and motivation
Wechsler Adult Intelligence Scale Revised	Eleven subscales; used to assess verbal and performance IQ in adults
Wechsler Intelligence Scale for Children Revised	Twelve subscales; used to assess verbal and performance IQ in children 6 to 16 y old

Structured Clinical Instruments and Rating Scales

Although most practicing clinicians do not commonly use structured instruments to assess or follow up patients, a small number of rating scales have come to be used routinely in clinical practice.

Table 4–15 shows some of the most commonly cited structured instruments and rating scales.

TABLE 4–15	Common Structured Instruments and Psychiatric Rating Scales
Name of Scale	**General Purpose**
Abnormal Involuntary Movement Scale	Brief structured assessment of abnormal movements; used to rate presence and severity of tardive dyskinesia
Beck Depression Inventory*	Twenty-item rating scale for depression; focuses on mood and cognition
Brief Psychiatric Rating Scale	Eighteen-item scale that rates current severity of psychopathology
Diagnostic Interview Schedule	Diagnostic instrument developed for use by nonclinicians to conduct community surveys

*These instruments are self-administered.

TABLE 4–15	Common Structured Instruments and Psychiatric Rating Scales *(Continued)*

Name of Scale	General Purpose
Global Assessment of Functioning Scale	Overall psychosocial functioning rated on a scale from 0 to 100; used as Axis V of DSM-IV
Hamilton Depression Rating Scale	A 17- to 21-item scale that rates the severity of depressive symptoms; strong focus on somatic problems
Nurses' Observation Scale for Inpatient Evaluation	Eighty items used to rate the behavior of hospitalized patients by staff
Overt Aggression Scale	Rates aggression in four categories: verbal, physical against self, physical against objects, physical against other people
Personality Disorder Examination	Items that rate six areas of personality functioning, which are analyzed by computer with a series of algorithms to generate personality disorder diagnoses
Present State Examination	Continually updated semistructured diagnostic interview used in international research and tied to the manual on the International Classification of Diseases (most recently ICD-10)
Schedule for Affective Disorders and Schizophrenia	Semistructured questions, similar to the Structured Clinical Interview for DSM-IV but more detailed, for establishing diagnoses of affective disorders and schizophrenia
Structured Clinical Interview for DSM-IV	Semistructured questions used to establish DSM-IV Axis I and Axis II diagnoses
Symptom Checklist*	Ninety-item self-report instrument used to assess psychopathology

*These instruments are self-administered.

TABLE 4–16	Common Laboratory Tests for Evaluation of Psychiatric Patients

Serologic

Toxicology screen (blood)
Complete blood count
Blood glucose
Kidney function tests
Liver function tests
Thyroid function tests
Syphilis serology
HIV antibody test
Pregnancy test
Blood cultures
Vitamim B_{12} and folate levels

Urine

Toxicology screen (urine)
Dipstick for protein and glucose
Pregnancy test

Lumbar Puncture

Electrocardiogram

Chest Radiograph

TABLE 4–17	Toxicology Screens	

Drug	Amount per mL	Approximate Duration of Detectability (d)*
Alcohol	300 µg	1
Amphetamines	500 ng	2
Barbiturates	1000 ng	1–3
Benzodiazepines	300 ng	3
Cocaine	150 ng	2–3
Opiates	300 ng	2
Phencyclidine	25 ng	8
Tetrahydrocannabinol carboxylic acid	<15 ng	3–20

*May vary widely depending on amount ingested, compound, physical state of subject, and other factors.
Modified from Council on Scientific Affairs, The American Medical Assocation: Scientific issues in drug testing. JAMA 1987;257:3110–3114. Copyright 1987, American Medical Association. See also Gold MS, Dackis CA: Role of the laboratory in the evaluation of suspected drug abuse. J Clin Psychiatry 1986;47 (suppl):17–23.

TABLE 4–18	Indications for Lumbar Puncture (Cerebrospinal Fluid Evaluation) in Psychiatric Patients

Rapid onset of new psychiatric symptoms, including dementia, delirium, psychosis

New-onset psychiatric symptoms with fever

New-onset neurological symptoms (e.g., seizures, paralysis)

Suspected neuroleptic malignant syndrome (e.g., while taking antipsychotics, patient develops fever, tremor, anemia, obtundation)

New-onset psychiatric symptoms with a known history of HIV infection or neoplasm (if space-occupying lesion is suspected, brain imaging should precede lumbar puncture)

LABORATORY ASSESSMENTS

A variety of laboratory tests can aid in the clinical evaluation of the psychiatric patient (Tables 4–16 through 4–19).

BRAIN IMAGING

Several methods of brain imaging are available when routine laboratory examination proves insufficient for diagnostic purposes. Table 4–20 lists the indications for brain imaging.

Abrupt onset of psychiatric symptoms such as psychosis, mania, or personality change suggests a medical etiology and may be an indication for electroencephalography.

SPECIAL ASSESSMENT TECHNIQUES

In certain situations, special assessment techniques may be indicated in the psychiatric evaluation of patients who are unable or unwilling to cooperate. These situations include the assessment of patients who are mute, have amnesia, or intentionally provide false information. In general, special techniques are employed only

TABLE 4–19	Indications for Electrocardiography

Assessment of cardiac functioning before beginning
    Tricyclic antidepressants
    Lithium
    Thioridazine
    β-Blockers
    Electroconvulsive therapy

Drug overdoses (need varies with substance or substances ingested)

TABLE 4–20	Indications for Brain Imaging

History of head trauma

Focal neurological findings on physical examination

New-onset psychiatric systems after age 40 y (including psychosis, affective disorder, personality change)

Rapid onset of psychiatric symptoms

History of neurological symptoms (including seizures)

Evidence of cognitive impairment

Abnormal electroencephalogram

Abnormal lumbar puncture

after all conventional ways to obtain the necessary information have been exhausted. Techniques include hypnosis and use of sedatives (i.e., IV sodium amobarbital).

TREATMENT PLANNING

The psychiatric evaluation is the basis for developing the case formulation, initial treatment plan, initial disposition, and comprehensive treatment plan.

Case Formulation

The case formulation is the summary statement of the immediate problem, the context in which the problem has arisen, the tentative diagnosis, and the assessment of risk.

ASSESSMENT OF RISK

The assessment of risk is the most crucial component of the formulation because the safety of the patient, the clinician, and others is the foremost concern in any psychiatric evaluation. Four areas are important: suicide risk, assault risk, life-threatening medical conditions, and external threat.

SUICIDE RISK. The risk of suicide is the most common life-threatening situation mental health professionals encounter. Its assessment is based on both an understanding of its epidemiology, which alerts the clinician to potential danger, and the individualized

TABLE 4–21	Estimated Lifetime Rates of Completed Suicide by Diagnosis

Major affective disorders: 10%–15%

Alcoholism: 10%–15% (comorbid depression usually present)

Schizophrenia: 10% (often during a postpsychotic depressive state)

Borderline and antisocial personality disorders: 5%–10%

assessment of the patient. Suicide is the eighth leading cause of death in the United States.

In certain psychiatric disorders, there is a significant lifetime risk for suicide, as listed in Table 4–21.

The most consistent predictor of future suicidal behavior is a prior history of such behavior, which is especially worrisome when previous suicide attempts have involved serious intent or lethal means. Table 4–22 lists risk factors for suicide.

TABLE 4–22	Risk Factors for Suicide
Category	**Risk Factors for Suicide**
Demographic	White Male Older age Divorced, never married, or widowed Unemployed
Historical	Previous suicide attempts, especially with serious intent, lethal means, or disappointment about survival Family history of suicide Victim of physical or sexual abuse
Psychiatric	Diagnosis: affective disorder, alcoholism, panic disorder, psychotic disorders, conduct disorder, severe personality disorder (especially antisocial and borderline) Symptoms: suicidal or homicidal ideation; depression, especially with hopelessness, helplessness, anhedonia, delusions, agitation; mixed mania and depression; psychotic symptoms, including command hallucinations persecutory delusions Current use of alcohol or illicit drugs Recent psychiatric hospitalization
Environmental	Recent loss such as that of a spouse or job Social isolation Access to guns or other lethal weapons Social acceptance of suicide
Medical	Severe medical illness, especially with loss of functioning or intractable pain Delirium or confusion caused by central nervous system dysfunction
Behavioral	Antisocial acts Poor impulse control, risk taking, and aggressiveness Preparing for death (e.g., making a will, giving away possessions, stockpiling lethal medication) Well-developed, detailed suicide plan Statements of intent to inflict harm on self or others

TABLE 4–23	Risk Factors for Violence
Category	**Risk Factors**
Demographic	Young
	Male
	Limited education
	Unemployed
Historical	Previous history of violence to self or others, especially with high degree of lethality
	History of animal torture
	Past antisocial or criminal behavior
	Violence within family of origin
	Victim of physical or sexual abuse
Psychiatric	Diagnosis: substance-related disorders, antisocial personality disorder; conduct disorder; intermittent explosive disorder; pathological alcohol intoxication; psychoses (e.g., paranoid, toxic)
	Symptoms: physical agitation; intent to kill or take revenge; identification of specific victim(s); psychotic symptoms, especially command hallucinations to commit violence and persecutory delusions
Environmental	Access to guns or other lethal weapons
	Living under circumstances of violence
	Membership in violent group
Medical	Delirium or confusion caused by central nervous system dysfunction
	Disinhibition caused by traumatic brain injuries and other central nervous system dysfunctions
	Toxic states related to metabolic disorders (e.g., hyperthyroidism)
Behavioral	Antisocial acts
	Agitation, anger
	Poor impulse control; risk taking or reckless behavior
	Statements of intent to inflict harm

It is essential to be clear about whether the patient has passive thoughts about suicide or actual intent. Is there a plan? If so, how detailed is it, how lethal, and what are the chances of rescue? The possession of firearms is particularly worrisome, because nearly two thirds of documented suicides among men and more than a third among women have involved this method.

In addition to the assessment of risk factors, it is important to decide whether the possibility of suicide is of immediate concern or represents a long-term ongoing risk.

RISK OF ASSAULT. Unlike those who commit suicide, most people who commit violent acts have not been diagnosed with a mental illness, and data clarifying the relationship between mental illness and violence are limited. The most common psychiatric diagnoses associated with violence are substance-related disorders. Conduct disorder and antisocial personality disorder, by definition, involve aggressive, violent, and/or unlawful behavior.

Table 4–23 lists risk factors for violence. As with suicide, the best predictor of future assault is a history of past assault.

LIFE-THREATENING MEDICAL CONDITIONS. It is essential to consider life-threatening medical illness as a potential cause of psychiatric disturbance. Clues to this etiology can be found in the present illness (e.g., physical complaints), family history (e.g., causes of death in close family members), medical history (e.g., previous medical conditions and treatments), physical examination (e.g., abnormalities identified), and MSE (e.g., confusion, fluctuation in levels of consciousness).

Probably the most common life-threatening situations that the psychiatrist evaluates are acute central nervous system changes caused by medical conditions and accompanied by mental status alterations. These include increased intracranial pressure or other cerebral abnormalities, severe metabolic alterations, toxic states, and alcohol withdrawal. Patients may be at risk of death if these states are not quickly identified.

EXTERNAL THREAT. Some patients who present for psychiatric evaluation are at risk as a result of life-threatening external situations. Such patients can include battered women, abused children, and victims of catastrophes who lack proper food or shelter. Information about these conditions is usually obtained from the present illness, the personal history, the medical history, and the physical examination.

DIFFERENTIAL DIAGNOSIS

A complete diagnostic evaluation includes assessments on each of the five axes of DSM-IV (Table 4–24).

Disturbances of speech, thinking, perception, and self-experience are common in psychotic states that can be seen in patients with such diagnoses as schizophrenia and mania, as well as in central nervous system dysfunction caused by substance use or a medical condition.

TABLE 4–24	DSM-IV Multiaxial System
Axis I:	Clinical disorders Other conditions that may be a focus of clinical attention
Axis II:	Personality disorders Mental retardation
Axis III:	General medical conditions
Axis IV:	Psychosocial and environmental problems
Axis V:	Global assessment of functioning

From American Psychiatric Association: Diagnostic and Statistical Manual of Mental Disorders, 4th ed. Washington, DC: American Psychiatric Association, 1994.

Disturbances in self-experience are also common in dissociative disorders and certain anxiety, somatoform, and eating disorders. Cluster A personality disorders may be associated with milder forms of disturbances in this domain (Table 4–25).

Disturbances of emotion are most typical of affective and anxiety disorders.

Physical signs and symptoms and any associated abnormalities revealed by diagnostic medical tests and medical history are used to establish the presence of general medical conditions, which are coded on Axis III.

TABLE 4–25	Descriptive Features of Personality Disorders in Three Clusters	
Cluster	**Specific Disorder**	**Descriptive Features**
Odd-eccentric	Paranoid	Distrust and suspiciousness; others' motives interpreted as malevolent
	Schizoid	Detachment from social relationships; restricted range of emotional expression
	Schizotypal	Discomfort in close relationships; cognitive or perceptual distortions; eccentricities of behavior
Dramatic-emotional	Antisocial	Disregard for and violation of the rights of others
	Borderline	Instability in interpersonal relationships, self-image, and affects; marked impulsivity
	Histrionic	Excessive emotionality and attention seeking
	Narcissistic	Grandiosity, need for admiration, lack of empathy
Anxious-fearful	Avoidant	Social inhibition, feelings of inadequacy, hypersensitivity to negative evaluation
	Dependent	Submissive and clinging behavior; need to be taken care of
	Obsessive-compulsive	Preoccupation with orderliness, perfectionism, and control

Adapted from American Psychiatric Association: Diagnostic and Statistical Manual of Mental Disorders, 4th ed. Washington, DC: American Psychiatric Association, 1994:629–673.

TABLE 4–26	Areas Covered by Comprehensive Treatment Plan

Mental health
   Diagnoses on five axes
   Psychiatric management, including medications
Physical health
   Medical diagnoses
   Medical management, including medications
Personal strengths and assets
Rehabilitation needs
   Educational
   Occupational
   Social
   Activities of daily living skills
   Use of leisure time
Living arrangements
Social supports and family involvement
Finances
   Personal finances
   Insurance coverage
   Eligibility for social service benefits
Legal or forensic issues
Central goals and objectives
Listing of treatment team members
Evidence of participation by patient and, as appropriate,
   family members and others
Criteria for discharge from treatment

Information about behavior and adaptive functioning is useful for diagnosing personality disorders, documenting psychosocial and environmental problems on Axis IV, and assessing global functioning on Axis V.

Initial Treatment Plan

The initial treatment plan follows the case formulation, which has already established the nature of the current problem and a tentative diagnosis. The plan distinguishes between what must be accomplished now and what is postponed for the future. Treatment planning works best when it follows the biopsychosocial model (Table 4–26).

Initial Disposition

The primary task of the initial disposition is to select the most appropriate level of care after completion of the psychiatric evaluation. Disposition is primarily focused on immediate goals. After referral, the patient and the treatment team develop longer term goals.

Disorders

Childhood and Adolescent Manifestations of Adult Disorders

MOOD DISORDERS

Major Depressive Disorder

Although major depressive disorder (MDD) is relatively less common in children, its point prevalence approaches adult rates of 6% to 9% by late adolescence. Diagnostic criteria for MDD in children and adolescents are identical to those in adults apart from two caveats. First, in children and adolescents, depressed mood may manifest primarily as irritability. Second, calculations regarding weight loss may be made from failure to establish normal developmental weight gain, rather than actual loss. Especially for adolescents, care must be taken to distinguish fluctuating developmental problems accompanied by strong and variable feeling states from actual psychopathological processes.

In prepubertal children prevalence rates for boys and girls are roughly equal, and by late adolescence, the sex ratio approximates that of adults, with rates for girls about twice those for boys.

Onset of MDD in childhood or adolescence is often the first episode of a chronic mood disorder characterized by relapse and functional impairments. Furthermore, investigations suggest a cohort effect; younger cohorts show both an earlier age at onset and an increased prevalence of the disorder.

The relatively specific risk factors for onset of MDD can be understood to be parental history of MDD, female sex, persistent subsyndromal depressive symptoms, and dysthymia.

Depressive disorders in children and adolescents are associated with cognitive difficulties, poor academic achievement, social-personal-family difficulties, and increased use of psychoactive substances. Some of these may persist after the acute symptoms have improved or remitted and are hypothesized to increase the risk for further depressive episodes. Suicide in adolescents is strongly associated with unrecognized and untreated depressive disorders.

Evidence for familial aggregation is strong, with high rates of affective disorders in first-degree relatives of youngsters with MDD. One study suggested that by the age of 20 years, more than 50% of the offspring of depressed patients report having at least one major depressive episode themselves, and there is some evidence for the temporal association of major depressive episodes of mothers and children.

Neuroendocrine investigations have essentially identified that abnormalities of the hypothalamic-pituitary-adrenal axis and the hypothalamic-pituitary-thyroid axis are found relatively infrequently in children and adolescents.

As with adults, the presence of disorders comorbid with major depression is striking (Table 5–1).

Depressive disorders in children and adolescents are persistent in spite of treatment, and their long-term course is characterized by relapse. Although a variety of psychosocial and biological interventions may be applied, the optimal method of treatment has not been identified. No long-term studies of either psychosocial or biological treatments are available.

Pharmacological treatments have not demonstrated efficacy of tricyclic antidepressants in childhood and adolescent depression. Specific serotonin reuptake inhibitors seem to be more promising and are usually better tolerated. Of particular importance in this group, the toxicity of specific serotonin reuptake inhibitors is significantly less than that of tricyclic antidepressant, particularly in overdose. Desipramine use has been associated with sudden death in children, although the causal relationship of its use in this rare event has not been clearly established. Electroconvulsive therapy or combined neuroleptic and selective serotonin reuptake inhibitor pharmacotherapy may be of value in psychiatrically depressed children and adolescents.

Dysthymic Disorder

The defining characteristic of dysthymic disorder is chronically depressed mood, which in children may be manifested as irritability "most of the day, more days than not" for a period of at least a year, with symptom-free periods lasting no longer than 2 months. The

TABLE 5–1	Common Patterns of Comorbidity in Adolescence

Disorder Type or Specific Disorder	Comorbid Disorders
Mood disorders	Anxiety disorders Substance use disorders Eating disorders
Anxiety disorders	Other anxiety disorders Mood disorders
Substance use disorders	Substance-induced disorders Other substance use disorders Conduct disorder
Conduct disorder	Substance use disorders Mood disorders
Pathological gambling	Mood disorders Substance use disorders Anxiety disorders
Trichotillomania	Substance use disorders Mood disorders Anxiety disorders
Eating disorders	
Anorexia nervosa	Major depressive disorder Obsessive-compulsive disorder Substance use disorders Avoidant personality disorder General medical conditions
Bulimia nervosa	Major depressive disorder Dysthymic disorder Anxiety disorders Substance use disorders Borderline personality disorder
Narcolepsy	Mood disorders Substance-related disorders Generalized anxiety disorder Sleepwalking disorder Enuresis
Body dysmorphic disorder	Mood disorders Anxiety disorders Personality disorders

Adapted from American Psychiatric Association: Diagnostic and Statistical Manual of Mental Disorders, 4th ed. Washington, DC: American Psychiatric Association, 1994.

initial 1-year period must be free of a major depressive episode. If such episodes occur later, it is justified to diagnose both dysthymic disorder and MDD, the so-called double depression.

Prevalence rates for dysthymic disorder ranging from 4% to 8% are roughly comparable to those associated with MDD in childhood and adolescence and are associated with significant morbidity, often signaling the onset of a chronic mood disorder. Compared to MDD, dysthymic disorder in school-aged children is associated with an earlier age at onset, more frequent symptoms of affective dysregulation, and greater overall risk of subsequent affective disorder, and represents an early marker for recurrent affective illness.

There are no placebo-controlled studies of psychopharmacological interventions for dysthymic disorder in children and adolescents.

No psychosocial interventions are known to affect either the syndrome or the outcome of dysthymia in children and adolescents.

Bipolar Disorder

To meet criteria for bipolar I disorder, children and adolescents must have experienced a clinical course characterized by the occurrence of one or more manic episodes or mixed affective episodes (both manic and depressed). Bipolar II disorder criteria require that young people have experienced one or more depressive episodes accompanied by at least one hypomanic episode. In young people bipolar disorder is often confused with schizophrenia, which has somewhat different precursors and outcome, or with personality disorders, especially borderline personality disorder. Mixed episodes with both depression and mania are also more likely to occur in adolescents, and psychiatric symptoms are common.

Especially in younger adolescents, differential diagnosis also may be complicated by nonaffective psychoses, unipolar depression, organic syndromes, attention-deficit disorder, and disruptive behavior disorders.

The existence of major depressive episodes in prepubertal children may be an early marker of bipolar disorder; more than 30% of such youngsters were found to have bipolarity on 2- to 5-year follow-up, especially those children with family histories loaded for bipolar disorder. Similarly, 20% of adolescents hospitalized for depression had a subsequent manic episode at 3- to 5-year follow-up. There is also evidence that children with dysthymic disorder are at increased risk for the later emergence of bipolar disorder. Rapid onset of depression, psychiatric symptoms while depressed, and a history of bipolarity in first-degree relatives are features that might predict a bipolar course.

As with adults, lithium treatment is the therapy of choice for children and adolescents with bipolar disorder, even though its efficacy has not been subject to rigorous double-blind investigation. Ordinarily, dosage is similar to that in adults (i.e., 600 to 2700 mg/d, in divided doses). The therapeutic level is between 0.8 and 1.2 mEq; common adverse side effects in children are weight gain, stomachache, vomiting, nausea, tremor, enuresis, acne, and weight loss. Weight gain and acne are often of particular concern to adolescents, especially because gains of up to 30 lb have been reported. These gains may reverse within a year of maintenance medication, however. The presence of comorbid personality disorder in adolescents may also have treatment implications because adolescents with bipolar illness and personality disorder have differed significantly from a purely bipolar group in terms of increased lithium unresponsiveness. As with adults, premature discontinuation of lithium maintenance therapy can have adverse effects for adolescent patients with bipolar disorder. It has been found that bilateral brief-pulse electroconvulsive therapy is a useful treatment of pharmacologically unresponsive acute adolescent manias, which suggests, as in adults, that this treatment modality should be considered for a subgroup of seriously ill patients. Much further study of this and other biological interventions is necessary.

ANXIETY DISORDERS

Anxiety disorders in children and adolescents include panic disorder, generalized anxiety disorder (GAD), obsessive-compulsive disorder (OCD), specific phobia, social phobia, and SAD. These are relatively common, affecting some 10% to 15% of the population. They often occur comorbidly with other anxiety disorders or other psychiatric illness, particularly MDD, dysthymia, attention-deficit/ hyperactivity disorder, and Tourette's disorder. High rates of familial prevalence have been reported, and all the anxiety disorders are associated with significant disturbances in social, academic, and interpersonal functioning. Behaviorally inhibited children may be more likely to have an anxiety disorder, and anxiety disorders may predate the appearance of a mood disorder in some cases. The common problem of school refusal in children is often a symptom of an underlying anxiety disorder. Among behaviorally inhibited children, rates of anxiety disorders and psychiatric disorders in general are higher than those for control children.

Specific Phobia

DSM-IV defines specific phobia as a "marked and persistent fear of clearly discernible, circumscribed objects or situations." Responses to these stimuli "almost invariably" provoke an anxiety response, a situationally specific panic attack, and avoidance behavior, leading to marked distress or some functional impairment. To meet criteria, individuals older than 18 years also need to recognize that the fear is excessive or unreasonable. Subtypes are now specified: animal, natural environment (e.g., heights, water), blood-injection-injury, situational (e.g., airplanes, elevators), and other (e.g., loud sounds, vomiting). For individuals younger than 18 years, the duration of such symptoms must be at least 6 months.

Childhood fears and anxieties are among the most common psychological characteristics of youth and may be expressed in ways typical of children: crying, tantrums, freezing, or clinging. Objects of fear may also be developmentally idiosyncratic (e.g., anxiety about masks, balloons, or costumed figures). More commonly, fears of the dark, blood, strangers, dogs, thunderstorms, and the like may reflect typical developmental phenomena and warrant nothing more than parental reassurance, talk, patience, and, perhaps, setting of limits.

When are such symptoms significant enough to meet diagnostic criteria or warrant specialized treatment approaches? DSM-IV warns that fears do not warrant a diagnosis of specific phobia unless "there is significant interference with social, educational, or occupational functioning." Does the fear of a dog en route prevent the child from attending school? Does concern about insects stand in the way of the child's going outside to play? Does fear of the physician prevent the child from having routine physical examinations or being examined when ill? When such functional impairments are clearly present, the psychiatrist should entertain the possibility of diagnosis and specialized intervention.

Behavioral interventions are the treatment of choice for specific phobias. Techniques of systematic desensitization and progressive relaxation offer benefit, especially when done in the presence of the threatening stimulus. Modeling and flooding have also been employed with success, as have operant procedures employing contingency management programs. Pharmacotherapy is not indicated, although short-term use of low-dose benzodiazepines may be of value in assisting the care with exposure therapy.

Social Phobia

Social phobia is defined in DSM-IV as a "marked and persistent fear" of social or performance situations in which one is exposed to unfamiliar people or when one's actions are witnessed by others. For children, this presumes the capacity for age-appropriate relationships with familiar people and the existence of the fear in peer-related situations, not simply with adults. As with specific phobia, social phobia in children may take the form of crying, tantrums, freezing, or shrinking from social contact. Socially phobic children may refuse to participate in group play, prefer the periphery of peer activities, or attempt to remain close to adults with whom they are familiar and feel safe. School functioning is often affected. Socially phobic children exhibit an avoidance of speaking in front of others in class, writing on a blackboard where others may see, or even eating in a cafeteria with other children. Aversion to the use of a shared bathroom may also be seen, not for fear of contamination, as might be present in OCD, but for fear of being seen, heard, or smelled by other children when using the facility.

Current clinical wisdom states that the course of this disorder appears to be chronic and unremitting, with a continuing fear of social scrutiny and evaluation.

Fluoxetine and buspirone appear to be effective in children and adolescents with overanxious disorders, social phobia, and SAD (excluding OCD, panic, and depression). MAOIs are not recommended for use in children and adolescents. Psychotherapeutic approaches have traditionally included insight-oriented psychodynamic therapy, but there are no known studies demonstrating its effectiveness. Cognitive-behavioral approaches, including social skills training, show promise of enhancing social competence but await proper evaluation.

Panic Disorder

The diagnosis of panic disorder, in children and adolescents as well as in adults, requires the presence of recurrent, unexpected panic attacks followed by at least 1 month of persistent concern or worry about the possible recurrence of an attack, the consequences of the attack, or behavioral change related to the attacks. Agoraphobia may or may not be present, and the attacks must not be a function of a medical condition, substance use, or other mental disorder.

Age at onset of panic disorder varies fairly widely (ages 3 to 18 years). The frequency of panic disorders increases with ascending pubertal stage and peaks in adolescence and young adulthood.

SAD and depression have been widely reported to co-occur with panic, as has comorbidity of behavioral disorders (i.e., attention-deficit/hyperactivity disorder, oppositional defiant disorder) and eating symptoms with panic disorder. In keeping with research on adult panic disorder, mitral valve prolapse has also been found to occur in some children with panic disorder.

Psychopharmacological studies of panic disorder treatment in adults have suggested the efficacy of tricyclic antidepressants, monoamine oxidase inhibitors, and benzodiazepines, but few studies have addressed their efficacy in children and adolescents in placebo-controlled, double-blind trials. Open trials and case studies have pointed to the potential usefulness of clonazepam for panic symptoms in prepubertal children and panic disorder in adolescents. Evidence of the usefulness of combined pharmacological and cognitive-behavioral interventions has been reported for adults with panic disorder, but no scientifically valid studies of psychological treatments have been reported for children and adolescents.

Obsessive-Compulsive Disorder

OCD often has onset during childhood and adolescence. As in adults, OCD in children and adolescents is characterized by ego-dystonic intrusive, recurrent, and persistent thoughts, images, or impulses and repetitive, purposeful, intentional behaviors performed in response. These are accompanied by various degrees of distress and functional impairments.

The most common obsessions are fears of contamination, fears of harm to self, and fears of harm to a familiar person (often a parent). Common compulsions are washing, cleaning, checking, and counting. In most cases, OCD is found comorbidly with another Axis I disorder, most frequently an anxiety disorder, a tic disorder, major depression, or a specific developmental disability.

The natural history of OCD is that of a chronic psychiatric disorder characterized by periodic waxing and waning of symptom severity. Changes in symptom hierarchy may occur as well. With treatment, symptoms and functioning may in most cases be improved, although most patients will continue to be somewhat symptomatic.

Familial-genetic studies suggest heritability for OCD, particularly in association with Tourette's disorder.

A number of neurobiological studies suggest that central nervous system serotonin dysfunction is a pathoetiological feature of OCD. Sydenham's chorea (autoimmune inflammation of the basal ganglia) may be associated with OCD in children, which suggests that antibody-mediated disturbance could underlie some cases of this disorder.

Cognitive-behavioral therapy is the psychological treatment of choice when exposure, response prevention, and anxiety management constitute the essential therapeutic components. Pharmacotherapy with medications that inhibit serotonin reuptake (clomipramine, fluoxetine, fluvoxamine, and sertraline) is well established as an effective treatment for childhood and adolescent OCD. Doses smaller than those used for adults may be beneficial in children. Combination therapy with clonazepam may be useful in optimizing response. The use of concomitant cognitive-behavioral therapy and medication treatments has been demonstrated to increase the magnitude of the initial treatment response and improve long-term outcome.

Separation Anxiety Disorder

SAD is a childhood-onset psychiatric disturbance characterized by "developmentally inappropriate and excessive anxiety concerning separation from home or from those to whom the individual is attached—usually parents." It is accompanied by functional impairment and must be distinguished from developmentally appropriate fears, such as "stranger anxiety." This core cognitive feature is associated with various behaviors designed to avoid separation (tantrums, bed avoidance, school refusal) and symptoms of autonomic arousal when separation has occurred or is anticipated.

The reported prevalence of SAD is 3% to 5%; the peak age at onset occurs at 7 to 9 years. About 40% to 60% of children with SAD will demonstrate a comorbid psychiatric diagnosis, with other anxiety disorders and MDD being the most common. The presence of comorbidity, later age at onset, and serious family psychiatric illness may be associated with a greater risk of chronicity. Furthermore, childhood-onset SAD may be associated with an increased risk for development of panic disorder, depression, social phobia, or agoraphobia in adolescence and adulthood. SAD has shown a familial pattern. Treatment of SAD is primarily that of behavioral therapy, although controlled clinical trials are lacking. A variety of pharmacological interventions have been reported, usually as an adjunct to behavioral interventions. In the main, these also were uncontrolled. Currently, buspirone, fluoxetine, or low-dose clonazepam may be considered as part of a comprehensive medication plan. Family counseling may be of benefit in those cases in which family dysfunction complicates the clinical picture. Often, identification and effective treatment of an anxious parent also will help to decrease functional impairment in a child with SAD.

Generalized Anxiety Disorder

GAD often has onset in childhood. The core feature of GAD is excessive and functionally impairing worries across a variety of domains, including such things as personal safety, social interactions, and past and future events. Somatic disturbances are extremely common, with headaches and stomachaches predominating. In some cases, these children may be needlessly subjected to repeated and unnecessary medical investigations in an attempt to determine whether a specific medical diagnosis underlies their somatic complaints.

Prevalence rates of stringently diagnosed GAD are found to range between 2% and 4% with a female predominance.

Those few controlled studies that are available support the short-term efficacy of combined self-control and relaxation training.

Pharmacological treatments of GAD have included buspirone

("first line"), low-dose benzodiazepines such as lorazepam, and selective serotonin reuptake inhibitors. The results are difficult to interpret given the uncontrolled nature of these investigations.

SCHIZOPHRENIA

Age at onset of schizophrenia is commonly noted to be in adolescence, but cases in younger children have been described. Presentation of the disorder in these children is similar to that in adults, including negative and positive signs; the most commonly reported symptoms are auditory hallucinations, affective disturbance, thought disorder, and delusions. Early-onset schizophrenia is more common in boys and is more frequently preceded by a premorbid schizotypal personality and by a high frequency of neurodevelopmental abnormalities. In children, hallucinations and delusions may be less elaborated than those in adults, and some care must be taken to differentiate some hallucinatory phenomena that occur in some normal children from true schizophrenic hallucinations. Similarly, disordered speech can be found in other childhood disorders (e.g., communication disorders, pervasive developmental disorder) and is not pathognomonic of schizophrenia. When schizophrenia does occur in childhood and adolescence, diagnostic, prognostic, and treatment ramifications are similar to those noted with adult-onset schizophrenia.

Studies suggest that children with schizophrenia are deficient at several stages of information processing regarding cognitive control and strategic allocation of various control processing resources.

Children with schizophrenia have been shown to improve with neuroleptic medication, and successful double-blind, placebo-controlled studies of haloperidol have been conducted with the use of sound psychometric measures. Clozapine also has been found effective in single-case studies and open trials; clozapine concentrations were demonstrated to bear a consistent linear relationship to clinical benefit in children with schizophrenia.

Psychoeducational programs have produced some positive results, but parents' cooperation is a critical component to a good outcome.

CHAPTER 6

Mental Retardation

MENTAL RETARDATION

CONCEPT OF MENTAL RETARDATION

The five basic concepts this chapter uses concerning mental retardation and the psychiatric approaches to it are as follows:

1. Mental retardation is not a specific disease. The term refers to a behavioral syndrome, describing the level of a person's functioning in defined domains. It does not have a single cause, mechanism, course, or prognosis and does not necessarily last a lifetime.

2. Mental retardation is not a unitary concept. Persons diagnosed as having mental retardation are not a homogeneous group but represent a wide spectrum of abilities, clinical presentations, and behavioral patterns.

3. Persons with mental retardation do not have unique personalities or behavioral patterns.

4. Maladaptive behaviors should not automatically be seen as part of the retardation or as an expression of "organic personality disorder." As in all individuals, these behaviors may be related to life experiences; they can also be a symptom of comorbid mental illness existing with the retardation.

5. Mental disorders seen in persons with mental retardation are the same as those in the general population.

Some common misconceptions about mental retardation are that it is a specific and lifelong disorder with a characteristic behavioral phenotype associated with specific personality patterns and that comorbid mental disorders existing with mental retardation are different from those encountered in other individuals. Although mental retardation is listed as a mental disorder in the *Diagnostic and Statistical Manual of Mental Disorders,* Fourth Edition (DSM-IV), it is not a unique nosological entity with specific pathognomonic features. Instead, mental retardation describes the level of a person's intellectual and adaptive functioning below a cutoff point that is not even natural but arbitrarily chosen in relation to the average level of functioning of the population at large. The condition is not necessarily lifelong. Strictly speaking, mental retardation is not a medical term. Its chief function is administrative, defining a group of persons in need of support and educational services. Thus, mental retardation does not have a single cause, mechanism, course, or prognosis. It has to be differentiated from the diagnosis (if known) of the underlying medical condition.

DSM-IV Definition

DSM-IV Criteria

Mental Retardation

A. Significantly subaverage intellectual functioning: an IQ of approximately 70 or below on an individually administered IQ test (for infants, a clinical judgment of significantly subaverage intellectual functioning).

B. Concurrent deficits or impairments in present adaptive functioning (i.e., the person's effectiveness in meeting the standards expected for his or her age by his or her cultural group) in at least two of the following areas: communication, self-care, home living, social/interpersonal skills, use of community resources, self-direction, functional academic skills, work, leisure, health, and safety.

C. The onset is before age 18 years.

Severity	Approximate IQ Range	Code
Mild	50–55 to approx. 70	317
Moderate	35–40 to approx. 50–55	318
Severe	20–25 to approx. 35–40	318.1
Profound	Below 20–25	318.2
Undiagnosed		319

Mental retardation is coded on Axis II.

In terms of age, the highest prevalence of mental retardation is in the school-age group, when the child cannot meet the expectations of academic learning. Conversely, some persons diagnosed at school with mild mental retardation lose that diagnosis in adulthood, when their good adaptive skills are more relevant than their academic achievement.

THE CAUSES OF MENTAL RETARDATION

The prevalence of diagnosable biomedical causes of mental retardation varies with the degree of the disability. When the retardation is severe, a prenatal cause can be identified in 59% to 73% of patients, but in mild mental retardation, such a cause can be identified in only 23% to 43% of patients. Tables 6–1 and 6–2 illustrate some syndromes associated with mental retardation.

DIAGNOSIS AND DIFFERENTIAL DIAGNOSIS OF MENTAL RETARDATION

Phenomenology and Variations in Presentation

The clinical presentation of persons with mental retardation is influenced by multiple factors, which can be grossly divided into biological (such as syndromes underlying the retardation), psycho-

TABLE 6-1	Examples of Various Malformation Syndromes Connected with Mental Retardation
Syndrome	Features
Chromosomal Aberrations	
Trisomy 21: Down syndrome	Mean IQ = 50; CHD, GI abnormality
Trisomy 13 syndrome	IQ <50; growth retardation; polydactyly; holoprosencephaly; ear, eye, and scalp defects; CHD
Deletion 5p: cri du chat syndrome	IQ 20–50, growth retardation, microcephaly, cat-like cry, hypertelorism, epicanthus
Malformation Syndromes Due to Microdeletions	
Prader-Willi syndrome	IQ 20–80, almond-shaped eyes, small hands and feet, cryptorchidism, hypotonia, obesity
Angelman's (happy puppet) syndrome	IQ <50, ataxia, seizures, microbrachycephaly, large mouth, prognathism, jerky gait
Williams' syndrome	IQ 40–80, long philtrum, prominent lips, supravalvular aortic stenosis, loquatious, "cocktail party manners," hypercalcemia in infancy
Rubinstein-Taybi syndrome	IQ 20–85; growth retardation; beaked, long nose; broad thumbs, narrow palate

CHD, Congenital heart disease.

Table continued on following page

TABLE 6-1	Examples of Various Malformation Syndromes Connected with Mental Retardation *(Continued)*
Syndrome	**Features**
Malformation Syndromes of Unknown Cause	
de Lange's syndrome	IQ <50, growth retardation, microcephaly, hirsutism, synophrys, anteverted nostrils
Sotos' syndrome	Sometimes mental retardation, large size, macrocephaly, prognathism, downward-slanting palpebral fissures
Prenatal Infections	
Congenital rubella	± Mental retardation, microcephaly, hearing loss, cataracts, CHD, microphthalmia, retinal pigmentation
Toxoplasmosis	± Mental retardation, hydrocephalus microcephaly, chorioretinitis, cataracts, intracranial calcifications, hepatosplenomegaly
Toxic Agents	
Fetal hydantoin syndrome	± Mental retardation, growth retardation, short nose, hypertelorism, cleft lip, CHD

Data from Jones KL: Smith's Recognizable Patterns of Human Malformation, 4th ed, Philadelphia: WB Saunders, 1988.

TABLE 6–2 Examples of Inborn Errors of Metabolism Causing Mental Retardation*

Disorder	Enzyme Defect	Onset/Life Expectancy	Clinical Features	Laboratory Diagnosis/Treatment
Aminoacidurias				
PKU	Phenylalanine hydroxylase	I/A	If not on diet: vomiting, musty odor, eczema, seizures, tremors, psychosis	U: ferric chloride test; gene locus 12q22–24; diet: low in phenylalanine
Homocystinuria	Cystathionine β-synthetase	I/A	Seizures, venous thromboses → cerebrovascular accidents, Marfan's habitus, malar flush, lens subluxation, often MR	U: cyanide-nitroprusside test
Lysosomal Disorders/Glycoproteinoses				
Mannosidosis	Mannosidase	6–36 mo/A	Coarse facial features, short stature, skeletal changes, hepatosplenomegaly, loose joints, hearing loss, ataxia	U: oligosaccharides
I-cell disease	Multiple lysosomal hydrolases	I/2–8 y	Early facial feature coarsening, short stature, stiffness of joints, gum hyperplasia	U: sialyl oligosaccharides

Table continued on following page

*All disorders cause mental retardation except that in homocystinuria it does not occur in every case. Dietary treatment benefits patients with PKU and galactosemia. Prenatal diagnosis is available for all disorders. Inheritance is autosomal recessive, except for MPS II and Lesch-Nyhan, which are X linked. I, Infancy; A, adulthood; U, urinary; MR, mental retardation.

TABLE 6-2 Examples of Inborn Errors of Metabolism Causing Mental Retardation *(Continued)*

Disorder	Enzyme Defect	Onset/Life Expectancy	Clinical Features	Laboratory Diagnosis/Treatment
Mucopolysaccharidoses				
MPS I (Hurler's)	L-Iduronidase	I/10 y	Early facial feature coarsening, hepatosplenomegaly, growth failure, corneal clouding, skeletal changes	U: heparan sulfate, dermatan sulfate
MPS II (Hunter's)	Iduronidate sulfatase	I/15 y	Symptoms milder and progression slower than in MPS I	U: heparin sulfate, dermatan sulfate
Sphingolipidoses				
Tay-Sachs (GM$_2$)	GM$_2$ ganglioside-*N*-acetylhexosaminidase	3–6 mo/2–3 y	Hypotonia → rigidity, macular cherry red spot → blindness, seizures, hyperacusis	Serum hexosaminidase assay
Metachromatic leukodystrophy	Arylsulfatase A deficiency	1–4 y/10–15 y	Gait disturbance, ataxia, motor incoordination	U: metachromatic cells, sulfatase A assay; sural nerve biopsy

Adapted from Nellhaus G, Stumpf DA, Moe PG: Neurologic and muscular disorders, and Robinson A, Goodman SI, O'Brien D: Genetic and chromosomal disorder. In Kempe CH, Silver HK, O'Brien D (eds): Current Pediatric Diagnosis and Treatment, 8th ed. Los Altos, CA: Lange Medical Publications, 1984:628–711 and 992–1030. Copyright by Appleton & Lange.

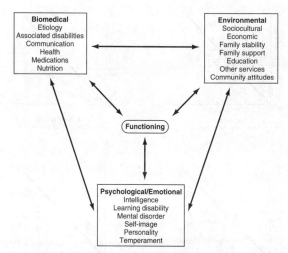

Figure 6–1 *Schematic representation of transactional relationship of various factors influencing the development of adaptive and maladaptive behaviors in persons with mental retardation.*

logical (the level of the person's intellectual and adaptive functioning), and environmental (such as cultural expectations and services received). Their mutual relationship is illustrated in Figure 6–1.

Assessment of Mental Retardation

The American Association on Mental Retardation has published a new manual for the classification of mental retardation, which includes the following outline:

A. Step one: diagnosis of mental retardation
   Dimension I: intellectual and adaptive skills
B. Step two: classification and description
   Dimension II: psychological and emotional considerations
   Dimension III: physical-health-etiology considerations
   Dimension IV: environmental considerations

COURSE AND NATURAL HISTORY OF MENTAL RETARDATION

The development of an individual with mental retardation depends on the type and extent of the underlying disorder, the associated disabilities and disorders, environmental factors (such as general health, education, treatment, and other services), and psychological factors (cognitive abilities, comorbid psychopathological condition). Some general principles concerning the developmental trajectories of various mental retardation–associated disorders and syndromes are seen in Figure 6–2.

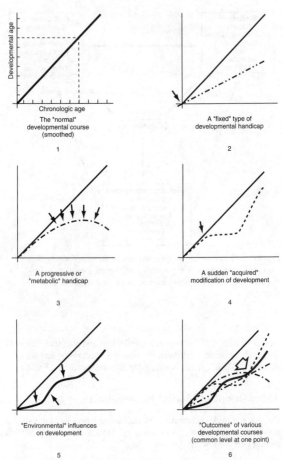

Figure 6–2 *Schematic representation of patterns of developmental disorders (arrows refer to point of insult): 1) normal developmental course; 2) fixed, nonprogressive, type of developmental disorder; 3) metabolic type of disorder of development in which the manifestations of the underlying process (e.g., Tay-Sachs disease) occur after birth and evolve into a progressively deteriorating course; 4) acquired developmental disorder: the curve represents normal development up to a point of insult (arrow) to the CNS; 5) environmental disorder of development: a fluctuating course, with periods of stress (downward arrows) and periods of nurturance or positive intervention or both (upward arrows); 6) outcomes: the convergence (arrow) of the various developmental courses represents the point at which the physician becomes aware of the developmental disorder. (Adapted from Szymanski LS, Rubin LL, Tarjan G: Mental Retardation. In Tasman A, Hales RE, Frances AJ [eds]: Review of Psychiatry, Volume 8, Washington, DC: American Psychiatric Press 1989:227.)*

OVERALL GOALS OF TREATMENT OF MENTAL RETARDATION

Strictly speaking, there is no specific treatment of mental retardation itself, although there might be treatments of underlying mental retardation–associated syndromes (e.g., PKU) and of comorbid disorders (e.g., seizure disorder), if such are present. The interventions targeted at the mental retardation itself include a variety of educational, habilitative, and supportive approaches, depending on the person's individualized needs.

The current approach to the services for persons with mental retardation is based on the following principles:

- The *normalization principle,* which refers to "making available to the mentally retarded patterns and conditions of everyday life that are as close as possible to the norms and patterns of the mainstream of society."
- The *right to community living,* which includes
  - Right to live with a family, preferably one's own or a substitute one if necessary (foster or adoptive).
  - No institutionalization of children, regardless of the level of retardation, and generally not of adults either. At present, some children are placed in special residential schools (usually private) for specific reasons, typically medical or behavioral needs that require specialized treatment.
  - Deinstitutionalization of adults and placement in as normal a setting as possible, for example, community residences, supervised apartments, and foster homes.
  - Education and training for all children, regardless of their disability and its degree, to a maximally possible extent in community-based programs. Mainstreaming, which refers to placement in special classes in regular schools but with participation in some activities of regular classes, rather than segregation in separate schools, has been the rule so far. The current trend is toward inclusion, which refers to full-time placement in an age-appropriate regular classroom, with the educational program being individualized according to the child's needs. Services of special educators and therapists, as necessary, are also provided in these programs.
  - Employment of adults in the community according to their abilities, ranging from sheltered workshops to the competitive job market, or occupational-recreational day programs for those with the most significant retardation.
  - Training to the maximal possible degree in the use of normal community services and facilities (shopping, banking, transportation).
  - Advocacy and appropriate protective measures, for example, against inappropriate use of pharmacological and behavioral measures as substitutes for active education and treatment.
  - Movement toward full inclusion, meaning the end of segregated services and education and the provision of the specialized services in regular educational, living, and work settings.

MENTAL DISORDERS IN PERSONS WITH MENTAL RETARDATION

Persons with mental retardation have the same mental disorders as persons in the general population.

DIAGNOSIS OF MENTAL DISORDERS IN PERSONS WITH MENTAL RETARDATION

Although there is no evidence that mental disorders seen in persons who have mental retardation are basically different from mental disorders seen in the general population, the clinical manifestations may be modified by the cognitive impairment; communication skills; associated sensory, motor, and other disabilities; and life experiences and circumstances. The most important factor is the presence or absence of verbal language. Many diagnostic criteria are based on a person's verbal communications.

In most cases, if not all, careful consideration and assessment can find an appropriate DSM-IV category that best categorizes the patient's clinical presentation.

A common concern and the reason for referral for psychiatric consultation is whether a person with mental retardation also has a behavioral or mental disorder (dual diagnosis). Although there is no clear definition of behavioral disorder, it is usually meant to refer to a deliberate misbehavior, learned response, and attention-getting behavior. However, in the clinical presentation of every defined mental disorder, there might be elements of learned behavior—for example, caused by the responses of persons in the patient's environment.

Assessment

SPECIAL ISSUES IN THE PSYCHIATRIC HISTORY AND EXAMINATION

The basic principles of the psychiatric diagnostic assessment of persons who have mental retardation are the same as those of persons who do not have mental retardation. What is needed is the modification of usual clinical techniques, according to the patient's discrete developmental levels in various domains, and in particular communication skills.

THE "MULTI" PRINCIPLE

This principle refers to the fact that persons with mental retardation usually depend on multiple providers for multiple services because of multiple needs and problems (Table 6–3). Not all needs and problems listed in Table 6–3 apply at all times to all individuals, but their relevance to the particular situation has to be carefully considered. In accordance with the principle of biopsychosocial integration, all these factors as well as their mutual interaction and contribution to the patient's problems and general functioning must be considered. Thus, the presenting problems must be assessed in the comprehensive context of a patient's abilities and disabilities and not as an isolated issue.

TABLE 6–3	The Multi Principle (Persons with Mental Retardation Have Multiple Needs)
Caregivers and providers	Parents, family, teachers, attendants, counselors, supervisors, physicians
Disabilities	Cognitive, specific learning, sensory, motor, language, associated medical
Need to learn	Self-care, communication, use of community services, recreation, self-direction, social skills
Need therapies	Various medical, language, physical, occupational, vocational
Need opportunities	Work or education, or both, recreation, social, coordinated health care

APPROACHES TO OBTAINING A HISTORY

All involved caregivers should be interviewed if possible (parents, teachers, direct care workers, supervisors in workshops). Direct care staff members (e.g., from the group home and workshop supervisors) are particularly important because they can provide a firsthand description of a person's behavior. Exploring the following areas is important:

1. Reasons for current referral
2. Behavioral symptoms
3. Psychotropic medication history
4. Nature of the disability
5. Past and current services
6. Milieu events
7. The family

Evaluation of Clinical Data

The clinical observations should be interpreted in light of a patient's life experiences, learning, understanding, and communication level. The global IQ or overall mental age alone is not a good guide here. In particular, the psychiatrist should

1. Differentiate between behaviors appropriate for an earlier age and those that are pathological in any age (e.g., true hallucinations).
2. Avoid over- or underdiagnosing mental disorders.
3. Try to make a formal Axis I and/or Axis II DSM-IV diagnosis (besides mental retardation) whenever clinically justified. The diagnostic criteria can usually be adapted to the patient's developmental level (just as one does with child patients).
4. Assess the strengths, impairments, and need for supports and services in each discrete domain of the patient's functioning, as well as in the environment (community and family).
5. Obtain, if needed, evaluations and consultations with those in other disciplines—for example, language pathologists, psychologists, and neurologists.

6. Assess and understand, most importantly, the dynamic, ongoing transactional relationships among the various factors contributing to the person's development.

Aggression

"Aggression" is one of the most frequent reasons (if not the most frequent) for referring persons with mental retardation to a psychiatrist. On closer investigation, the actual behavior ranges from occasional swearing (verbal aggression) to serious violence. However, there is no single entity called aggression in this population that would have just one explanation. It would be a gross mistake for a psychiatrist to talk about a single treatment for aggression (except for emergency measures). Different factors must be considered in assessing the cause of aggressive behavior. Such behavior might be associated with a defined mental disorder, for example, aggression following a command hallucination, paranoid delusion, anxiety, borderline or antisocial personality, or depression. The factor of learning will reinforce aggressive behavior if it brings a desired response by the caregivers. A pathological brain condition, such as rage attacks after brain trauma or associated with temporolimbic seizure disorder, may also lead to aggression. Often, the causation follows the multi principle, and several factors are involved, all of which require evaluation and intervention.

The DSM-IV has a category of intermittent explosive disorder that can be used provided other mental disorders have been ruled out.

OVERALL GOALS OF PSYCHIATRIC TREATMENT OF PERSONS WITH MENTAL RETARDATION

The most common mistake made by psychiatrists treating persons with mental retardation is to treat (usually with medications) single problems (usually disruptive behaviors leading to referral) and to ignore other possible problems and interventions or, at best, to assume that they are taken care of by someone else. This can be avoided by performing an adequate diagnostic assessment that follows the multi principle and considering the interaction of the various factors (see Fig. 6–1). The goal of treatment, like that of any other medical intervention, should not be simply to remove the offending symptom but to help the patient achieve a realistically optimal quality of life.

Prerequisites for a Successful Treatment Program

1. Comprehensive diagnostic understanding
2. Developing goals of treatment
3. Developing treatment priorities
4. Monitoring treatment results
5. Avoidance of indefinite treatment
6. Team collaboration

PHARMACOTHERAPY

The use of psychotropic drugs for persons with mental retardation does not differ from that for persons without mental retardation. There is no evidence that there is a different response to psychotropic drugs in persons with and those without mental retardation, all other factors being equal. Yet, most of the existing studies refer to the effectiveness of a drug in "the retarded" with a particular problem, as if the effectiveness were different in the presence of retardation. What is different is the difficulty of making an accurate diagnosis and the need for several concurrent interventions.

Persons not identified as having mental retardation are treated for major depression, schizophrenia, and so on. Unfortunately it is still a common practice to prescribe psychotropic agents for persons with mental retardation nonspecifically "for behaviors."

Another unfortunate practice is that of adding another drug, often of the same class, when the first drug fails to reduce the undesirable behavior, without evidence that it will have a synergistic effect. Some individuals, especially those in institutions, may end up taking many drugs, without evidence that any one of them is effective. The proper approach is to institute a follow-up system. However, it should not focus on a single behavior but on a person's global functioning. Periodic tapering of the drug (unless clinically contraindicated) should be performed to ascertain its effectiveness.

PSYCHOSOCIAL INTERVENTIONS

Programmatic and Educational Approaches

The goal of these interventions is to provide a proper living and programmatic environment. For instance, certain persons easily become overstimulated, anxious, and disruptive in noisy and confused large workshops; thus arranging for a smaller and quieter workroom is preferable to a prescription for thioridazine. The vocational and educational program should focus on developing a person's strengths and providing an opportunity for success rather than continuous failure. In turn, this will lead to such results as an improvement in self-image.

Psychotherapies

Psychotherapy in this population is not different in nature from psychotherapy in persons with average intelligence and is similar to that in treating children, inasmuch as in both cases the techniques and the therapist must adapt to the developmental needs of the patient. The treatment should be driven by the patient's needs and responses and not by the therapist's theoretical orientation.

Behavioral Treatment

The focus should not be on eliminating objectionable behaviors only but on teaching appropriate replacement behaviors. Aversive techniques involving active punishment (electric shocks, spraying of noxious substances into a person's face) are not used except in a few controversial settings. There is a professional consensus that these techniques should not be used at all, or only when all other techniques have failed and the patient's behavior poses severe danger to herself or himself or to others.

Learning and Motor Skills Disorders

For children and adolescents, school is their "workplace." Successful school performance is essential for psychological growth and development. Social competency and social skills are developed and then shaped in the family and school but are practiced and mastered in the school. The development of self-image and self-esteem is based on successes in school. Feedback from the school concerning academic performance and social interactions influences the parents' image of their child or adolescent. Thus, if something interferes with success in school, the impact will affect the emotional, social, and family functioning of a child or adolescent.

Academic performance requires the integrated interactions of the cognitive, motor, and language functions of the brain. As detailed in the *Diagnostic and Statistical Manual of Mental Disorders,* Fourth Edition (DSM-IV), if brain dysfunction results in cognitive difficulties, it is called a learning disorder; in motor difficulties, a motor skills disorder; and in language difficulties, a language disorder.

EDUCATIONAL CRITERIA

The most recent federal guidelines for determining whether a student in a public school is eligible for special programs for learning disabilities list four criteria:

1. Documented evidence indicating that general education has been attempted and found to be ineffective in meeting the student's educational needs.
2. Evidence of a disorder in one or more of the basic psychological processes required for learning. A psychological process is a set of mental operations that transform, access, or manipulate information. The disorder is relatively enduring and limits ability to perform specific academic or developmental learning tasks. It may be manifested differently at different developmental levels.
3. Evidence of academic achievement significantly below the student's level of intellectual function (a difference of 1.5 to 1.75 standard deviations between achievement and intellectual functioning is considered significant) on basic reading skills, reading comprehension, mathematical calculation, mathematical reasoning, or written expression.
4. Evidence that the learning problems are not due primarily to other handicapping conditions (i.e., impairment of visual acuity or auditory acuity, physical impairment, emotional handicap, mental retardation, cultural differences, or environmental deprivation).

The presence of a central nervous system processing deficit is essential for the diagnosis of a learning disability. A child might meet the discrepancy criteria, but without central processing deficits in functions required for learning, he or she is not considered to have a learning disability.

The question of the significant discrepancy between potential and actual achievement determines eligibility for services. Different school systems use different models for determining the extent of discrepancy.

DIAGNOSIS OF A LEARNING DISORDER OR MOTOR SKILLS DISORDER

The child or adolescent experiencing academic difficulty would normally be referred to the special education professionals within the school system. However, the student with academic difficulties often presents with emotional or behavioral problems and is more likely to be referred to a mental health professional. It is critical to understand this potential referral bias. This mental health professional must clarify whether the observed emotional, social, or family problems are causing the academic difficulties or whether they are a consequence of the academic difficulties and the resulting frustrations and failures experienced by the individual, the teacher, and the parents.

The evaluation of a child or adolescent with academic difficulties and emotional or behavioral problems includes a comprehensive assessment of the presenting emotional, behavioral, social, or family problems as well as a mental status examination. The psychiatrist should obtain information from the child or adolescent, parents, teachers, and other education professionals to help clarify whether there might be a learning disorder or a motor skills disorder and whether further psychological or educational studies are needed. Descriptions by teachers, parents, and the child or adolescent being evaluated will give the psychiatrist clues that there might be one of the learning disorders or a motor skills disorder.

DSM-IV Criteria 315.00

Reading Disorder

A. Reading achievement, as measured by individually administered standardized tests of reading accuracy or comprehension, is substantially below that expected given the person's chronological age, measured intelligence, and age-appropriate education.

B. The disturbance in criterion A significantly interferes with academic achievement or activities of daily living that require reading skills.

C. If a sensory deficit is present, the reading difficulties are in excess of those usually associated with it.

Children who experience problems in reading typically have difficulty in decoding the letter-sound associations involved in phonic analysis. As a result, they may read in a disjointed manner, knowing a few words on sight and stumbling across other unfamiliar words. They might guess. If they have difficulty with visual tracking, they might skip words or lines. If comprehension is a problem, they commonly report that they have to read material over and over before they understand.

Children with mathematical difficulties often display problems in attention, which is reflected in the types of errors they make in computations. They may leave a problem partially completed and move on to the next. They might make impulsive mistakes, yet be able to complete the problem correctly when this is brought to their attention. They may have difficulty shifting from one operation to the next and, as a result, add when they should subtract. They might have visual-spatial difficulties and thus misalign columns or rows and make "careless mistakes."

DSM-IV Criteria 315.1

Mathematics Disorder

A. Mathematical ability, as measured by individually administered standardized tests, is substantially below that expected given the person's chronological age, measured intelligence, and age-appropriate education.

B. The disturbance in criterion A significantly interferes with academic achievement or activities of daily living that require mathematical ability.

C. If a sensory deficit is present, the difficulties in mathematical ability are in excess of those usually associated with it.

Children who have difficulties with writing may have a problem with handwriting. They grasp the pencil or pen differently and tightly. They write slowly, and their hand gets tired. Often, they prefer printing rather than cursive writing. Most also have problems with the language of writing. They have difficulty with spelling, often spelling phonetically. They may have problems with grammar, punctuation, and capitalization.

Many, if not most, students with a learning disorder also have difficulties with memory or organization. The child or adolescent with a memory problem has difficulty following multistep directions or reads a chapter in a book but forgets what was read. Others might have sequencing problems, performing instructions out of order. In speaking or writing, the facts might come out but in the wrong sequence. Students with organizational difficulties may not be able to organize their lives (notebook, locker, desk, bedroom); they forget or lose things; they have problems with time planning; or they have difficulty using parts of information from a whole concept or putting parts of information into a whole concept.

DSM-IV Criteria 315.2

Disorder of Written Expression

A. Writing skills, as measured by individually administered standardized tests (or functional assessments of writing skills), are substantially below those expected given the person's chronological age, measured intelligence, and age-appropriate education.

B. The disturbance in criterion A significantly interferes with academic achievement or activities of daily living that require the composition of written texts (e.g., writing grammatically correct sentences and organized paragraphs).

C. If a sensory deficit is present, the difficulties in writing skills are in excess of those usually associated with it.

DSM-IV Criteria 315.4

Developmental Coordination Disorder

A. Performance in daily activities that require motor coordination is substantially below that expected given the person's chronological age and measured intelligence. This may be manifested by marked delays in achieving motor milestones (e.g., walking, crawling, sitting), dropping things, "clumsiness," poor performance in sports, or poor handwriting.

B. The disturbance in criterion A significantly interferes with academic achievement or activities of daily living.

C. The disturbance is not due to a general medical condition (e.g., cerebral palsy, hemiplegia, or muscular dystrophy) and does not meet criteria for a pervasive developmental disorder.

D. If mental retardation is present, the motor difficulties are in excess of those usually associated with it.

Children and adolescents with a developmental coordination disorder may show evidence of gross or fine motor difficulties. The gross motor problems might result in difficulty with walking, running, jumping, or climbing. The fine motor problems might result in difficulty with buttoning, zipping, tying, holding a pencil or pen or crayon, arts and crafts activities, or handwriting. Both gross and fine motor difficulties might result in the individual performing poorly in certain sports activities.

DIFFERENTIAL DIAGNOSIS

The presenting problem is academic difficulty. The differential diagnostic process must clarify the reason for the academic difficulty. A "decision tree" for academic difficulties developed by Silver and Ostrander (1993) is useful for exploring all of the possible reasons for such difficulties (Fig. 7–1).

Three principal areas of inquiry concerning the factors contributing to the student's learning difficulties are explored. The first involves considerations related to the child or adolescent's psychiatric, medical, or psychoeducational status. The second area of inquiry is family functioning. The third area to explore involves the environmental and cultural context in which the student functions. The true prevalence of these disorders is not known.

COMORBIDITY

Individuals with a learning disorder or a motor skills disorder might have other mental disorders or a related neurological disorder. They might also have social problems.

For many, psychological problems are secondary to the frustrations and failures experienced because learning disabilities were not identified or were inadequately treated. For others, these conditions may be another reflection of a dysfunctional nervous system. The presenting behavioral or emotional issues might be the individual's characterological style for coping with a dysfunctional nervous system.

Studies of youth diagnosed as having a conduct disorder or young adults diagnosed as having a personality disorder, especially the borderline type, show that about one third have unrecognized or recognized and poorly treated learning disabilities (learning disorders). Similar findings have been observed with adolescent boys in detention centers.

Social Problems

The learning disabilities that result in learning disorders or motor skill disorders may directly contribute to peer problems by interfering with success in activities required for interaction with certain age groups (e.g., visual perception and visual-motor problems interfering with ability to perform quickly such eye-hand activities as catching, hitting, or throwing a ball).

Many children and adolescents with learning disorders have difficulty learning social skills and being socially competent. These individuals do not pick up such social cues as facial expressions, tone of voice, or body language and thus do not adapt their behaviors appropriately.

Other Psychiatric or Medical Disorders

The first neurologically based disorder to be recognized as frequently associated with a learning disability (learning disorder) was attention-deficit/hyperactivity disorder (ADHD). Studies suggest that there is a continuum of disorders associated with neuro-

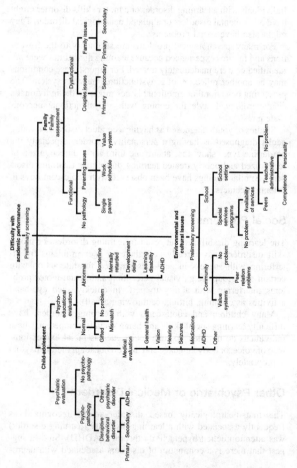

Figure 7-1 *Academic underachievement and the clinical decision-making process. ADHD, Attention-deficit/hyperactivity disorder.* (From Ostrander R: Clinical observations suggesting a learning disability. Child Adolesc Psychiatr Clin North Am 1993; 2:249–263.)

logical dysfunction that are often found together. Thus, when one is diagnosed, the others also must be considered in the diagnostic process.

There may be a spectrum of disorders caused by prenatal, perinatal, and postnatal brain damage. Depending on location, extent of damage, time of life, and developmental stage at the time of damage, the stress from this damage might cause fetal or neonatal death, cerebral palsy, epilepsy, or mental retardation. The less severe forms might produce a variety of learning disorders.

Microscopic studies of brains of individuals known to have learning disabilities have demonstrated a consistent pattern of cortical cells that maintained an earlier developmental stage of migration and development, suggesting that something had an impact on the brain during development, halting or slowing down the normal developmental stages. Some factors studied as possibly contributing to the stress that results in neurological dysfunction are maternal cigarette smoking during pregnancy, convulsions during pregnancy, low fetal heart rate during the second stage of labor, lower placental weight, breech presentations, and chorionitis. Also noted is a history of maternal alcohol consumption (two to three drinks daily) during pregnancy.

Research has also focused on the genetic basis for these disorders. Several studies have shown a familial pattern in approximately 40% to 50% of children with learning disabilities. In longitudinal studies of twins, identical pairs are more likely than fraternal pairs to be concordant for academic difficulties. These studies support the possibility that this is a heterogeneous disorder.

TREATMENT

Treatment is directed at the underlying disabilities by use of educational interventions. Psychological interventions are also directed at any existing emotional, social, or family difficulties. In addition, social skills training may be helpful.

Educational Interventions

The goal of special educational interventions is to help children and adolescents overcome or compensate for their learning disorders or motor skills disorder so that they can succeed in school. These efforts involve remedial and compensatory approaches and use a multisensory approach that facilitates building on all areas of strength while compensating for any areas of weakness. These efforts are to be provided in a setting as nearly like a regular classroom as possible. It is essential that the classroom teacher know how to adapt the classroom, curriculum, and teaching style to best accommodate each student's areas of difficulty.

Psychotherapeutic Interventions

Learning disorders affect all aspects of the child or adolescent's life. The same processing problems that interfere with reading, writing, mathematics, and language may also hinder communicating with peers and family, success in sports and activities, and such daily life skills as dressing oneself or cutting food.

Lack of success in school can lead to a poor self-image and low self-esteem. Individuals with learning disorders might feel that they have minimal control over their lives and may compensate by trying to be more in control. Some individuals might become anxious or depressed, or a disruptive behavior disorder may develop.

The initial psychological interventions focus on educating the child or adolescent and the family about his or her difficulties. The psychiatrist must help parents learn to advocate for the necessary services in school. The next level of interventions focuses on helping the family understand and work with the child or adolescent with a learning disorder.

Some children or adolescents may need specific individual, behavioral, group, or family therapy. If so, it is critical that the therapist understand the impact that the learning disorder has had on the individual and how this disability might affect the process of therapy. As noted earlier, many students with a learning disorder have social skills problems and difficulties with peers. Therefore, social skills training might be helpful.

USE OF MEDICATIONS

No medication has been found to be effective for treating the learning disorders or motor skills disorder. If the individual with these disorders also has ADHD, it is important that medication be used to minimize the hyperactivity, distractibility, or impulsivity so that the student can be available for learning.

Autistic Disorder and Other Pervasive Developmental Disorders

The pervasive developmental disorders (PDDs) are a group of clinical syndromes that have two fundamental elements: developmental delays and developmental deviations. It is the presence of the deviation in combination with delays that differentiates PDDs from mental retardation and other specific developmental disorders. Thus, PDDs are not merely an arrest or delay in development but a unique set of deviant behaviors and aberrant functioning on several levels. Most often, these conditions are congenital, but all certainly begin before the third year of life. The common developmental disturbances include disruption in social interactions and communication along with the presence of stereotyped behaviors, activities, and interests as well as cognitive impairment. The prototypical PDD is autistic disorder. The other PDDs, including Rett's disorder, childhood disintegrative disorder, Asperger's disorder, and PDD not otherwise specified (NOS), share certain core features with autistic disorder.

The current criteria for autistic disorder and other PDDs are summarized in Table 8–1.

EPIDEMIOLOGY

Autistic disorder is relatively rare, with prevalence rates in the range of 2 to 5 per 10,000 children. When broader definitions of autistic disorder are used, however, the prevalence rate increases to 10 to 20 per 10,000.

Like most forms of childhood and adolescent psychiatric illness, autistic disorder is four times more prevalent in boys than in girls. The other PDDs seem to be similar to autistic disorder, with a greater ratio of affected boys, except in the case of Rett's disorder, which has been diagnosed only in girls.

The majority of children with autistic disorder are mentally retarded. This appears to be the case in other PDDs as well. Approximately 25% to 30% of autistic children have an IQ of less than 50; 20% to 30% have an IQ of 70 or greater. Overall, intelligence levels range from profoundly retarded to above average in autistic disorder and the other PDDs. A notable exception is childhood disintegrative disorder, in which all affected children are mentally retarded. In addition, follow-up studies of autistic disorder have demonstrated that mental retardation, when present, persists

TABLE 8–1 Comparison of Domains of Diagnostic Criteria for Pervasive Developmental Disorders

	Autistic Disorder	Rett's Disorder	Childhood Disintegrative Disorder	Asperger's Disorder	Pervasive Developmental Disorder NOS
Age at onset	Delays or abnormal functioning in social interaction, language, or play by age 3 y	Apparently normal prenatal development Apparently normal motor development for first 5 mo Deceleration of head growth between ages 5 and 48 mo	Apparently normal development for at least the first 2 y Clinically significant loss of previously acquired skills before age 10 y	No clinically significant delay in language, cognitive development, or development of age-appropriate self-help skills, adaptive behavior, and curiosity about the environment in childhood	Category used in cases of pervasive impairment in social interaction and communication, with presence of stereotyped behaviors or interests when criteria are not met for a specific disorder

Social interaction	Qualitative impairment in social interaction, as manifested by at least two of the following: • Marked impairment in the use of multiple nonverbal behaviors, e.g., eye-to-eye gaze • Failure to develop peer relationships appropriate to developmental level • Lack of spontaneous seeking to share enjoyment with other people • Lack of social or emotional reciprocity	Loss of social engagement early in the course (although often social interaction develops later)	Same as autistic disorder along with loss of social skills (previously acquired)	Same as autistic disorder

Table continued on following page

TABLE 8–1 Comparison of Domains of Diagnostic Criteria for Pervasive Developmental Disorders (*Continued*)

	Autistic Disorder	Rett's Disorder	Childhood Disintegrative Disorder	Asperger's Disorder	Pervasive Developmental Disorder NOS
Communication	Qualitative impairments of communication as manifested by at least one of the following: • Delay in, or total lack of, the development of spoken language • Marked impairment in initiating or sustaining a conversation with others, in individuals with adequate speech • Stereotyped and repetitive use of language or idiosyncratic language • Lack of varied, spontaneous make-believe or imitative play	Severely impaired expressive and receptive language development and severe psychomotor retardation	Same as autistic disorder along with loss of expressive or receptive language previously acquired	No clinically significant delay in language	

Behavior	Restricted, repetitive, and stereotyped patterns of behavior, as manifested by one of the following: • Preoccupation with one or more stereotyped or restricted patterns of interest • Adherence to nonfunctional routines or rituals • Stereotyped and repetitive motor mannerisms • Persistent preoccupation with parts of objects	Loss of previously acquired purposeful hand movement Appearance of poorly coordinated gait or trunk movements	Same as autistic disorder along with loss of bowel or bladder control, play, motor skills previously acquired	Same as autistic disorder
Exclusions	Disturbance not better accounted for by Rett's disorder or childhood disintegrative disorder	Disturbance not better accounted for by another PDD or schizophrenia		Criteria are not met for another PDD or schizophrenia

Data from American Psychiatric Association: Diagnostic and Statistical Manual of Mental Disorders, 4th ed. Washington, DC: American Psychiatric Association, 1994.

from the time of diagnosis onward. IQs tend to be stable over time and are thought to be one of the most important predictors of outcome in autism. The fundamental cognitive deficits observed consist of deficiencies in language, abstraction, sequencing, and coding operations. Relative strengths lie in visuospatial skills. A small number of autistic individuals have phenomenal abilities in particular areas, such as memory, calendar calculation, or artistic endeavors. These so-called savant talents are seen also in individuals with other developmental disorders.

ETIOLOGY

The most contemporary etiological theories suggest either a genetic or another early disruption in the development of brain functioning with overt clinical manifestations potentially modified by social or environmental experiences.

Chromosomal abnormalities associated with PPDs are listed in Table 8–2. Twin and family studies have yielded some useful information about genetic aspects of autism. A study in the Nordic countries involving 21 pairs of twins and a set of identical triplets reported a concordance for autism of 91% in monozygotic twin pairs versus 0% in dizygotic twin pairs.

Between 30% to 75% of autistic individuals have nonspecific neurological abnormalities including poor coordination, hypotonicity or hypertonicity, choreiform movements, abnormal posture and gait, tremor, and myoclonic jerking. About 25% of autistic individuals have seizures by the end of adolescence or electroencephalographical abnormalities. Seizures have been highly correlated with mental retardation and may be correlated more with mental impairment than with the presence of PDD or autism.

TABLE 8–2	Chromosomal Abnormalities Associated with Autistic Disorder or Other Pervasive Developmental Disorders

Fragile X syndrome (trinucleotide expansion at Xq27.3)

Down's syndrome (trisomy 21)

Prader-Willi syndrome (deletion or maternal isodisomy of chromosome 15)

Marker chromosome

Duplication of 15q11–q13

TABLE 8–3	Suggested Work-up for Children and Adults with Autistic Disorder or Other Pervasive Developmental Disorders

History
  Particular attention to
    Developmental phases of language, social interactions, play
    Family history of psychiatric and neurological disease
Physical examination
  Thorough physical examination including a search for
    Neurological problems
    Cardiac problems
    Congenital anomalies
    Skin lesions or abnormalities
    Dysmorphology
Psychological evaluation
  Autism Diagnostic Interview—Revised
  Autism Diagnostic Observation Schedule
  Cognitive testing (e.g., Differential Abilities Scales)
  Vineland Adaptive Behavior Scales
Speech and language evaluation
Audiological evaluation
Visual acuity evaluation

EVALUATION

The diagnosis of autism is carried out by gathering information about the child's historical background, behavior, and cognitive abilities (Table 8–3).

An essential piece of the comprehensive evaluation is gained through direct observation of the child. Ideally, this should be done in a variety of settings to obtain an overall view of the child's behaviors and functioning under differing environmental conditions.

The child's overall physical health should be assessed, and particular attention should be paid to findings that could be related to PDDs. For instance, cardiac and other congenital physical anomalies should be noted, and a skin and dysmorphology examination should be done to search for lesions consistent with genetic, metabolic, or structural disorders. All children with speech delay or articulation problems should have audiological testing, because even subtle hearing loss can affect development. Vision testing should be performed if there is any consideration of visual deficit. A high index of suspicion should be maintained for seizure disorder since there are no specific, diagnostic laboratory tests.

Chromosomal studies are indicated for children with history and

TABLE 8–4	Differential Diagnosis of Autistic Disorder and Other Pervasive Developmental Disorders

Developmental language disorder
Mental retardation
Acquired epileptic aphasia (Landau-Kleffner syndrome)
Fragile X syndrome
Schizophrenia
Selective mutism
Psychosocial deprivation
Hearing impairment
Visual impairment
Traumatic brain injury
Dementia
Metabolic disorders (inborn errors of metabolism, e.g., phenylketonuria)

physical examination findings suggestive of fragile X syndrome or other specific chromosomal abnormalities.

DIFFERENTIAL DIAGNOSIS

Diagnosis of autistic disorder and other PDDs requires distinguishing among several disorders that consist of deviations in socialization, language, and play as illustrated in Table 8–4.

COURSE AND NATURAL HISTORY

Follow-up studies of autistic children into adulthood show that approximately two thirds remain seriously impaired and are incapable of caring for their own needs. In fact, the majority of these individuals live in long-term institutional settings during their adult years. Between 5% and 17% of autistic adults are able to work and hold some kind of a social life in their community. Despite social improvement in about half of autistic children for

TABLE 8–5	Goals for Treatment

Advancement of normal development, particularly regarding cognitive, language, and socialization
Promotion of learning and problem solving
Reduction of behaviors that impede learning
Assistance of families coping with autistic disorder
Treatment of comorbid psychiatric disorders

periods of years, most autistic individuals have abnormal social relationships. It is rare for an autistic adult to marry or sustain a long-term sexual relationship. Outcome in autism is overwhelmingly determined by IQ and language abilities, with IQ being the most powerful predictor.

GOALS OF TREATMENT

Goals in treating autistic disorder and PDDs are summarized in Table 8–5.

TABLE 8–6	Psychopharmacological Approach to Presenting Symptoms in Pervasive Developmental Disorders

Rituals, Compulsions, Irritability

Potent serotonin transporter inhibitors
  Selective serotonin reuptake inhibitor
    Fluoxetine 5–80 mg/d in a single dose
    Paroxetine 2.5–50 mg/d in one or two divided doses
    Sertraline 25–200 mg/d in one or two divided doses
    Fluvoxamine 25–300 mg/d in two or three divided doses
  Tricyclic antidepressants
    Clomipramine 25–250 mg/d in one or two divided doses

Hyperactivity, Distractibility, Impulsitivity

Stimulant medications
  Methylphenidate 5–60 mg/d in three to five divided doses
  Dextroamphetamine 5–40 mg/d in three to five divided doses
  Pemoline 37.5–112.5 mg/d in a single dose
Clonidine 0.025–0.3 mg/d in one to three divided doses or by transdermal skin patch
Naltrexone 0.5–2.0 mg/kg/d in a single dose

Aggression, Irritability

Sympatholytics
  Propranolol 20–400 mg/d in three to four divided doses
  Nadolol 40–400 mg/d in a single dose
Anticonvulsants
  Carbamazepine to a blood level of 4–12 ng/mL
  Valproate to a blood level of 50–100 ng/mL
Lithium to a serum level of 0.8–1.2 mEq/L
Neuroleptics
Naltrexone 0.5–2.0 mg/kg in a single daily dose

TABLE 8–7	Summary of Pharmacotherapy Principles

Psychosocial interventions should accompany medication treatment.

The individual's living arrangement must ensure safe, consistent administration of medications.

Maintain a high index of suspicion for comorbid disorders, and treat these appropriately.

Establish a means of monitoring effects of medications on symptoms over time.

Assess the risk/benefit ratio of starting medications and educate the patient and family about these.

PHARMACOTHERAPY

Table 8–6 summarizes pharmacotherapy of autistic disorders and PDDs. It is a reasonable goal for psychiatrists to adopt the judicious use of psychopharmacological agents to assist in adaptation. Of necessity, this focus on facilitating adaptation requires attention to five important principles listed in Table 8–7.

Attention-Deficit and Disruptive Behavior Disorders

Attention-deficit/hyperactivity disorder (ADHD), conduct disorder (CD), and oppositional defiant disorder (ODD) form the attention-deficit and disruptive behavior disorders (AD-DBDs) in the *Diagnostic and Statistical Manual of Mental Disorders,* Fourth Edition (DSM-IV). As a group, the AD-DBDs are the most common disorders of childhood and among the most researched areas of childhood psychopathology.

DSM-IV Criteria

Attention-Deficit/Hyperactivity Disorder

A. Either (1) or (2):

(1) six (or more) of the following symptoms of **inattention** have persisted for at least 6 months to a degree that is maladaptive and inconsistent with developmental level:

Inattention

(a) often fails to give close attention to details or makes careless mistakes in schoolwork, work, or other activities

(b) often has difficulty sustaining attention in tasks or play activities

(c) often does not seem to listen when spoken to directly

(d) often does not follow through on instructions and fails to finish schoolwork, chores, or duties in the workplace

(e) often has difficulty organizing tasks and activities

(f) often avoids, dislikes, or is reluctant to engage in tasks that require sustained mental effort

(g) often loses things necessary for tasks or activities

Box continued on following page

DSM-IV Criteria

Attention-Deficit/Hyperactivity Disorder *Continued*

Inattention Continued

  (h) is often easily distracted by extraneous stimuli

  (i) is often forgetful in daily activities

(2) six (or more) of the following symptoms of **hyperactivity-impulsivity** have persisted for at least 6 months to a degree that is maladaptive and inconsistent with developmental level:

Hyperactivity

  (a) often fidgets with hands or feet or squirms in seat

  (b) often leaves seat in classroom or in other situations in which remaining seated is expected

  (c) often runs about or climbs excessively in situations in which it is inappropriate (in adolescents or adults, may be limited to subjective feelings of restlessness)

  (d) often has difficulty playing or engaging in leisure activities quietly

  (e) is often "on the go" or often acts as if "driven by a motor"

  (f) often talks excessively

Impulsivity

  (g) often blurts out answers before questions have been completed

  (h) often has difficulty awaiting turn

  (i) often interrupts or intrudes on others

B. Some hyperactive-impulsive or inattentive symptoms that caused impairment were present before age 7 years.

C. Some impairment from the symptoms is present in two or more settings (e.g., at school [or work] and at home).

D. There must be clear evidence of clinically significant impairment in social, academic, or occupational functioning.

E. The symptoms do not occur exclusively during the course of a Pervasive Developmental Disorder, Schizophrenia, or other Psychotic Disorder and are not better accounted for by another mental disorder (e.g., Mood Disorder, Anxiety Disorder, Dissociative Disorder, or a Personality Disorder).

DSM-IV Criteria 312.8

Conduct Disorder

A. A repetitive and persistent pattern of behavior in which the basic rights of others or major age-appropriate societal norms or rules are violated, as manifested by the presence of three (or more) of the following criteria in the past 12 months, with at least one criterion present in the past 6 months:

Aggression to people and animals

   (1) often bullies, threatens, or intimidates others

   (2) often initiates physical fights

   (3) has used a weapon that can cause serious physical harm to others

   (4) has been physically cruel to people

   (5) has been physically cruel to animals

   (6) has stolen while confronting a victim

   (7) has forced someone into sexual activity

Destruction of Property

   (8) has deliberately engaged in fire setting with the intention of causing serious damage

   (9) has deliberately destroyed others' property

Deceitfulness or Theft

   (10) has broken into someone else's house, building, or car

   (11) often lies to obtain goods or favors or to avoid obligations

   (12) has stolen items of nontrivial value without confronting a victim

Serious Violations of Rules

   (13) often stays out at night despite parental prohibitions, beginning before age 13 years

   (14) has run away from home overnight at least twice while living in parental or parental surrogate home

   (15) is often truant from school, beginning before age 13 years

B. The disturbance in behavior causes clinically significant impairment in social, academic, or occupational functioning.

C. If the individual is age 18 years or older, criteria are not met for Antisocial Personality Disorder.

DSM-IV Criteria 313.81

Oppositional Defiant Disorder

A. A pattern of negativistic, hostile, and defiant behavior lasting at least 6 months, during which four (or more) of the following are present:

(1) often loses temper

(2) often argues with adults

(3) often actively defies or refuses to comply with adults' requests or rules

(4) often deliberately annoys people

(5) often blames others for his or her mistakes or misbehavior

(6) is often touchy or easily annoyed by others

(7) is often angry and resentful

(8) is often spiteful or vindictive

Note: Consider a criterion met only if the behavior occurs more frequently than is typically observed in individuals of comparable age and developmental level.

B. The disturbance in behavior causes clinically significant impairment in social, academic, or occupational functioning.

C. The behaviors do not occur exclusively during the course of a Psychotic or Mood Disorder.

D. Criteria are not met for Conduct Disorder, and, if the individual is age 18 years or older, criteria are not met for Antisocial Personality Disorder.

EPIDEMIOLOGY

Prevalence rates for ADHD range from 2.0% to 6.3%. Rates for CD have been estimated to be as low as 0.9% for school-age children but as high as 8.7% for adolescents. The overall prevalence of ODD varies across studies from 5.7% to 9.9%. In school-age children, boys have higher rates than girls for all three disorders, but only in the case of CD and in the hyperactive subtype of ADHD do these higher rates persist into adolescence.

Among the three disorders that compose the AD-DBD group, there is a high rate of comorbidity. ODD and CD are present in 40% to 70% of children with ADHD. Conversely, among children with ODD and CD 40% to 60% are estimated to have ADHD. In clinical settings, the prevalence of comorbid ODD and CD among children with ADHD is presumed to be even higher than in epidemiological samples, because the occurrence of these conditions together is likely to generate substantial impairment and lead to increased referrals for treatment.

Among children with ADHD, 15% to 20% have comorbid mood disorders, 20% to 25% have anxiety disorders, and 6% to 20% have learning disabilities. However, when a broader definition of academic underachievement is used, the rates show a wide variability from a low of 10% to as high as 90%.

NEUROBIOLOGY

The principal neurotransmitter system implicated in the pathogenesis of the AD-DBD group is the catecholaminergic system, which includes the noradrenergic and dopaminergic systems. A role for the serotoninergic (5-hydroxytryptamine [5-HT]) system has more recently been elucidated (Table 9–1).

Positron emission tomography has shown areas of hypoperfusion in the frontal lobe and basal ganglia regions during an object-naming task as well as hypoperfusion of striatal brain regions along with hyperperfusion of cerebral sensory and somatosensory areas. Similarly, reduced rates of cerebral glucose metabolism have been reported in adults who met criteria for ADHD as children in comparison with normal adult controls subjects.

GENETICS

The preponderance of evidence suggests that biological relatives of children with ADHD represent a population at risk for ADHD and

TABLE 9–1 Neurochemical Findings
Catecholaminergic Findings
Decreased norepinephrine activity with low dopamine β-hydroxylase activity implicated in aggressive behaviors
Plasma 3-methoxy-4-hydroxyphenylglycol concentration correlated with conduct problems
Cerebrospinal fluid 3-methoxy-4-hydroxyphenylglycol concentration correlated with a measure of aggression
Indication of dysfunction in dopamine-rich striatal and caudate regions of brain
Serotoninergic Findings
Negative correlations between cerebrospinal fluid concentration of 5-hydroxy-indoleacetic acid and ratings of aggression
Reduced number of ^{3}H-imipramine binding sites found in children with comorbid CD and ADHD
Enhanced prolactin response in aggressive boys compared with nonaggressive boys

supports the notion that transmission in families may be partly mediated by genetic factors.

COURSE AND NATURAL HISTORY

Behaviors characteristic of the AD-DBDs are observable from the preschool years onward. As early as age 1.5 years, hyperactive behaviors such as "moves too much during sleep" have been reported, followed by the appearance of "difficulty playing quietly" and "excessive climbing/running" by age 3 years. Attentional problems are usually reported after hyperactivity. However, it is likely that these problems are present early but are not reported until the child enters school, when there are increased environmental and cognitive demands placed upon him or her.

The presentation of oppositional behaviors shows greater variability. During the preschool years, transient oppositional behavior is common. However, when the oppositionality is of a persistent nature and lasts beyond the preschool years, the escalation to more disruptive behaviors is likely.

In general, conduct problems first appear in middle childhood. The progression of conduct problems is from rule violations, such as school attendance, to aggression toward animals and people. In males, the more serious forms of conduct problems, such as rape or mugging, generally emerge after age 13 years.

A different group of children show conduct problems for the first time during adolescence, without preexisting oppositional or aggressive behaviors. This group tends to have disorders that are transient and nonaggressive in nature.

When conduct disorder is seen in adolescence for the first time, the problems tend to diminish by adulthood. However, if conduct disorder is present from middle childhood, there is much greater persistence of aggression through adulthood and often a history of arrests or incarceration.

Considerable data indicate that a subgroup of hyperactive children shows higher rates of delinquency and substance abuse during adolescence, and this continues into adulthood. Families of these children tend to be less stable, have higher divorce rates, and move more frequently. The difficulties experienced by these adolescents and adults include poor self-esteem, problems in interpersonal relationships, and difficulties in keeping jobs as well as assault and armed robbery in a minority of cases. Children with childhood symptoms representing both ADHD and CD are over-represented in this group.

ASSESSMENT

The clinical evaluation of a child with AD-DBD requires a multisource, multimethod approach. In addition to the clinical interview, supplemental information may be obtained from school reports, rating scales completed by teachers and parents, psychometric data, and direct observations of the child.

Rating Scales

Rating scales like the Connors and Achenbach scales are among the most commonly used assessment instruments and are a helpful aid for the psychiatrist. They provide a view of the child's behavior that may be different from that observed by the psychiatrist because children with AD-DBDs often do not evidence symptoms in the office. Teacher and parent rating scales are complementary because they yield data from different situations. Rating scales have several limitations, and diagnoses should not be made on the bases of these data alone.

Interviews

Interviews with children and their parents are an essential step in the clinical evaluation. In clinical practice, interviews usually follow a loosely structured format with a flexible approach that allows the in-depth exploration of relevant clinical information.

Psychological and Psychometric Evaluation

Psychological and cognitive test performance is generally not required to determine the presence of an AD-DBD. Yet, such evaluations may be indicated as part of a comprehensive assessment, particularly when assessment of cognitive functioning is required and is crucial for determining school placement.

Many children with AD-DBDs have impaired social skills and consequently experience difficulties with peer relationships. Data suggest that both hyperactivity and aggression are related to peer rejection, which may occur as early as the preschool years. The level of hyperactivity, the age at onset of aggression, and the developmental level of the child all affect the extent of peer rejection experienced.

DIFFERENTIAL DIAGNOSIS

Proper differential diagnosis of the AD-DBDs requires discrimination not only among ADHD, ODD, and CD but also from a wide range of other psychiatric, developmental, and medical conditions. Mood and anxiety disorders, learning disorders, mental retardation, pervasive developmental disorders, cognitive disorders, and psychotic disorders may all present with impairment of attention as well as hyperactive-impulsive behaviors. The diagnosis of ADHD in DSM-IV requires that the symptoms of inattention–cognitive disorganization and impulsivity-hyperactivity are not better accounted for by one of these conditions. In addition, a variety of medical conditions such as epilepsy, Tourette's disorder, thyroid disease, postinfectious or posttraumatic encephalopathy, and sensory impairments must be considered. Finally, many medications prescribed for children can mimic ADHD symptoms. Examples include anticonvulsants (e.g., phenobarbital), antihistamines, decongestants, bronchodilators (e.g., theophylline), and systemic steroids.

TABLE 9–2	Agents Effective in Treating ADHD
Drug	**Upper Dose Limit**
Methylphenidate*	60 mg
Dextroamphetamine*	40 mg
Pemoline**	112.5 mg
Desipramine†‡	2.5–5 mg/kg/d
Clonidine†	0.025–0.3 mg/d

*Before a trial of any stimulant, height/weight, CBC, BP should be obtained
**Requires baseline liver function tests
†Has not been approved by the FDA for the treatment of ADHD
‡Requires pretreatment ECG

TREATMENT

Successful treatment planning in children with AD-DBDs requires consideration not only of the core symptoms but also of family and social factors and comorbidity with other disorders. Multimodal treatments are frequently necessary. Optimal planning for most children with ADHD should involve a combination of psychopharmacological and psychosocial treatments. A diagnosis of ODD without any comorbid condition requires behavioral interventions and not medication. In children with CD only, treatment usually entails a variety of psychosocial interventions with the possibility of augmenting treatment with one of several pharmacological agents.

Psychopharmacology

The agents listed in Table 9–2 are effective in treating ADHD.

Psychosocial Interventions

A variety of psychosocial therapies have been found useful for treating children with AD-DBDs. These can be broadly grouped into behavioral therapy and cognitive-behavioral therapy. Because family, peer, and school interactions are important in the morbidity and maintenance of these disorders, effective psychosocial treatments target each of these areas.

Despite their potential benefits, a problem with psychosocial interventions is that short-term gains are limited to the period that the programs are actually in effect. Furthermore, a substantial number of children, particularly those with the most severe presentation and greatest psychosocial adversity, fail to show improvement. Additional problems in implementation include the unwillingness of many teachers to use behavioral programs and the fact that as many as half the parents discontinue parent training. Finally, these interventions are labor-intensive, and long-term improvements have not been reported, which makes these therapies of limited value when used alone.

Feeding and Other Disorders of Infancy or Early Childhood

DEFINITION

In the literature, the term *feeding disorder* generally encompasses a variety of conditions ranging from problem behaviors during feeding, poor appetite, food refusal, food selectivity, food avoidance, and pica to rumination and vomiting. The term feeding disorder is generally used to emphasize the dyadic nature of eating problems in infants and young children.

DSM-IV Criteria 307.59

Feeding Disorder of Infancy or Early Childhood

A. Feeding disturbance as manifested by persistent failure to eat adequately with significant failure to gain weight or significant loss of weight over at least 1 month.

B. The disturbance is not due to an associated gastrointestinal or other general medical condition (e.g., esophageal reflux).

C. The disturbance is not better accounted for by another mental disorder (e.g., rumination disorder) or by lack of available food.

D. The onset is before age 6 years.

This general definition of feeding disorder in the *Diagnostic and Statistical Manual of Mental Disorders,* Fourth Edition (DSM-IV) does not take into account the heterogeneity of feeding and growth problems in infants and its implication for treatment. Some authors have used various diagnostic methods and assigned different labels to address the heterogeneity of feeding problems associated with failure to thrive.

EPIDEMIOLOGY

It is estimated that up to 35% of infants and young children have feeding problems. These common feeding difficulties include the infant's eating "too much" or "too little," restricted food preferences, delay in self-feeding, objectionable mealtime behaviors, and bizarre food habits. Severe feeding problems, such as refusal to eat or vomiting, which are associated with poor weight gain, have been reported to occur in 1% to 2% of infants younger than 1 year of age.

DIAGNOSIS

The diagnostic assessment of feeding disorders should include assessment of the infant's relationship with his or her primary caretakers; the infant's temperamental characteristics; the infant's medical, developmental, and feeding history; the caretakers' psychological functioning and past history; and the family's socioeconomic background, stressors, and social support system.

TREATMENT

Treatment begins with the first contact with the infant and her or his caregivers. The establishment of a therapeutic alliance with the caregivers is critical to any successful treatment. The diagnostic evaluation needs to identify the specific dynamics of each feeding disorder for development of a specific treatment plan.

RUMINATION DISORDER

DSM-IV Criteria 307.53

Rumination Disorder

A. Repeated regurgitation and rechewing of food for a period of at least 1 month following a period of normal functioning.

B. The behavior is not due to an associated gastrointestinal or other general medical condition (e.g., esophageal reflux).

C. The behavior does not occur exclusively during the course of anorexia nervosa or bulimia nervosa. If the symptoms occur exclusively during the course of mental retardation or a pervasive developmental disorder, they are sufficiently severe to warrant independent clinical attention.

ETIOLOGY

Rumination can be seen along a continuum: a patient may have gastrointestinal disease, such as hiatal hernia or reflux, and little psychiatric illness at one end of the spectrum; or conversely, a patient might have no reflux and severe psychiatric illness in the mother-infant relationship at the other end of the spectrum. Reflux or a temporary illness associated with vomiting frequently precedes the rumination. At some point, the infant seems to learn to initiate vomiting and turn it into rumination to achieve self-regulation. It appears that in circumstances in which the infant fails to elicit or loses either caring attention or tension-relieving responses from the caretaker, the infant resorts to rumination as a means of self-soothing and relief of tension. Once the infant has discovered rumination as a means of self-regulation, the rumination appears to develop into a habit that is difficult to break, like other habit disorders (e.g., head banging and hair pulling).

DIAGNOSIS

Most frequently, infants who ruminate come to the attention of professionals because of "frequent vomiting" and weight loss. A medical illness or a stressor in the parents' life is frequently associated with the onset of vomiting.

In addition to assessing the rumination in the infant, the mother-infant relationship and the mother's life circumstances need to be evaluated because the mother's ability to soothe and to stimulate her infant is critical for successful intervention.

TREATMENT

Diverse theories of etiology have resulted in various proposed methods of treatment. Besides surgical interventions to prevent reflux and the early use of mechanical restraints, treatment has been primarily behavioral or psychodynamic or a combination of both.

Before treatment is initiated, the diagnostic evaluation needs to determine whether the infant's rumination is situational or pervasive, whether the infant has learned to ruminate because of little stimulation and gratification from the mother, or whether the rumination serves the infant as a way of relieving tension in a stressed mother-infant relationship. After an understanding of the mother's situation has been gained, treatment is best individualized by a combination of psychodynamic and behavioral interventions to enhance the mother-infant relationship in general and to address the symptom of rumination in particular.

PICA

DEFINITION

Young children with this disorder typically eat plaster, paper, paint, cloth, hair, insects, animal droppings, sand, pebbles, and dirt.

DSM-IV Criteria 307.52

A. Persistent eating of nonnutritive substances for a period of at least 1 month.

B. The eating of nonnutritive substances is inappropriate to the developmental level.

C. The eating behavior is not part of a culturally sanctioned practice.

D. If the eating behavior occurs exclusively during the course of another mental disorder (e.g., mental retardation, pervasive developmental disorder, schizophrenia), it is sufficiently severe to warrant independent clinical attention.

EPIDEMIOLOGY

The onset of pica is usually during the toddler age between 12 and 24 months. Because infants commonly mouth objects, it is difficult to make the diagnosis in young infants.

The clinical profile of 108 children ages 1.5 to 10 years who practiced pica is as follows: 85% were younger than 5 years; 29% were 1.5 to 2 years of age; the male/female ratio was 1 : 1.4; the most common form of pica was geophagia (eating of clay, dirt, or sand); and the family history for pica was positive in 41% of the patients. Children with pica are more susceptible to malnutrition, anemia, diarrhea or constipation, and worm infestation.

DIAGNOSIS

Because mouthing of objects is still common in toddlers between 1 and 2 years of age, the diagnosis of pica should be made only if the behavior is persistent and inappropriate for the child's developmental level. The diagnosis of pica should be explored in children with accidental poisoning, lead intoxication, or worm infestation. Young children with signs of malnutrition or iron deficiency should also be considered for the diagnosis of pica.

The home environment and the parents' relationship with each other and with the child need to be explored to assess the parents' availability to nurture and supervise the child. Above all, mother and child should be observed during a meal and during play to gain a better understanding of their relationship and how the symptoms of pica can be understood in the context of that relationship.

TREATMENT

Mothers need to be made aware of the dangers of pica and should be enlisted in providing a childproof environment. This might include removing lead paint in old substandard housing units or instituting anthelmintic therapy for family pets.

Tic Disorders

PHENOMENOLOGY AND DIAGNOSTIC CRITERIA

Tics

Tourette's disorder is the most notable of the tic disorders. The cardinal features of Tourette's disorder and the other tic disorders are motor and vocal tics.

Motor tics are usually brief, rapid, and stereotyped movements but can also be slower, more rhythmical, or dystonic in nature. Simple motor tics are movements of individual muscle groups and include brief movements such as eye blinking, head shaking, and shoulder shrugging. Complex motor tics involve multiple muscle groups, such as a simultaneous eye deviation, head turn, and shoulder shrug. Some complex tics appear more purposeful, such as stereotyped hopping, touching, rubbing, or making obscene gestures (copropraxia).

Vocal tics are usually brief, staccato-like sounds but can also be words or phrases. Simple vocal tics, often caused by the forceful movement of air through the nose and mouth, include sniffing, throat clearing, grunting, or barking-type sounds. Complex vocal tics usually include words, phrases, or the repetition of one's own words or the words of others. Coprolalia, although often incorrectly considered essential for the diagnosis of Tourette's disorder, is infrequent; only 2% to 6% of cases are affected.

Tics most often begin in childhood, wax and wane in severity, and change in character and quality over time. Tics are exacerbated by excitement and tension and can attenuate during periods of focused, productive activity and sleep. Tics are involuntary, yet because they are briefly suppressible or can be triggered by an environmental stimulus (e.g., mimicking another person's movement, speech, or behavior), they may appear as volitional acts. If the tic is resisted, tension can develop until it is released by completion of the tic. In some individuals, tics are preceded or provoked by a thought or physical sensation referred to as a premonitory urge.

Diagnostic Criteria for the Tic Disorders

There are four diagnostic categories included in the tic disorders section of the *Diagnostic and Statistical Manual of Mental Disorders,* Fourth Edition (DSM-IV).

DSM-IV Criteria 307.23

Tourette's Disorder

A. Both multiple motor and one or more vocal tics have been present at some time during the illness, although not necessarily concurrently. (A *tic* is a sudden, rapid, recurrent, nonrhythmic, stereotyped motor movement or vocalization.)

B. The tics occur many times a day (usually in bouts) nearly every day or intermittently throughout a period of more than 1 year, and during this period there was never a tic-free period of more than 3 consecutive months.

C. The disturbance causes marked distress or significant impairment in social. occupational, or other important areas of functioning.

D. The onset is before age 18 years.

E. The disturbance is not due to the direct physiological effects of a substance (e.g., stimulants) or a general medical condition (e.g., Huntington's disease or postviral encephalitis).

DSM-IV Criteria 307.22

Chronic Motor or Vocal Tic Disorder

A. Single or multiple motor or vocal tics (i.e., sudden, rapid, recurrent, nonrhythmic, stereotyped motor movements or vocalizations), but not both, have been present at some time during the illness.

B. The tics occur many times a day nearly every day or intermittently throughout a period of more than 1 year, and during this period there was never a tic-free period of more than 3 consecutive months.

C. The disturbance causes marked distress or significant impairment in social, occupational, or other important areas of functioning.

D. The onset is before age 18 years.

E. The disturbance is not due to the direct physiological effects of a substance (e.g., stimulants) or a general medical condition (e.g., Huntington's disease or postviral encephalitis).

F. Criteria have never been met for Tourette's disorder.

Transient Tic Disorder

A. Single or multiple motor and/or vocal tics (i.e., sudden, rapid, recurrent, nonrhythmic, stereotyped motor movements or vocalizations).

B. The tics occur many times a day, nearly every day for at least 4 weeks, but for no longer than 12 consecutive months.

C. The disturbance causes marked distress or significant impairment in social, occupational, or other important areas of functioning.

D. The onset is before age 18 years.

E. The disturbance is not due to the direct physiological effects of a substance (e.g., stimulants) or a general medical condition (e.g., Huntington's disease or postviral encephalitis).

F. Criteria have never been met for Tourette's disorder or chronic motor or vocal tic disorder.

Specify if:

Single episode or **recurrent**

TABLE 11–1	Obsessions and Compulsions Characteristic of Obsessive-Compulsive Disorder and Tourette's Disorder	
	Obsessive-Compulsive Disorder	**Tourette's Disorder**
Obsessions	Contamination Dirt and germs Body wastes Environmental	"Just right" phenomena Symmetry Blurting out obscenity Saying the right thing Violent images Sexual thoughts Embarrassment
Compulsions	Cleaning	Touching Blinking Repeating Self-injurious behavior Hoarding Counting Ordering

Adapted from George MS, Trimble MR, Ring HA, et al: Obsessions in obsessive-compulsive disorder with and without Gilles de la Tourette's syndrome. Am J Psychiatry 1993; 150:93-97. Copyright 1993, the American Psychiatric Assocation. Reprinted by permission.

Frequently Co-occurring Symptoms or Disorders

Whereas tic disorders are common (1:100), Tourette's disorder occurs in only 5:10,000 children. The most common co-occurring disorders are attention-deficit/hyperactivity disorder (ADHD; 50% to 60%) and obsessive-compulsive disorder (OCD; 30% to 70%). The exact relationship of these problems to Tourette's disorder is controversial and the subject of intensive research efforts.

Differences in clinical phenomenology have been noted in studies of obsessions and compulsions in patients having Tourette's disorder compared with patients having OCD (without Tourette's disorder) (Table 11–1).

ETIOLOGY

Genetics

Comparison of the concordance rates for Tourette's disorder in monozygotic and dizygotic twins identifies Tourette's disorder as an inherited condition. The twin studies, however, are unable to identify a particular mode of genetic transmission or to identify the breadth of the clinical phenotype.

PATHOPHYSIOLOGY

In Tourette's disorder, the wide variety of motor, sensory, cognitive, and affective symptoms suggest several neuroanatomical sites of disease as well as neurochemical substrates. Sites include the basal ganglia and their interconnections with the frontal cortex and limbic system.

Reports of group A β-hemolytic streptococcus–related antineuronal antibodies being associated with the development or exacerbation of tics and OCD suggest a role for infectious agents and autoimmune processes in the etiology of these complex disorders.

Psychosocial Aspects of Tourette's Disorder

Psychosocial issues do not play a large etiological role in the development of the tic disorders; however, psychosocial issues do play a major role in adaptation and impairment in Tourette's disorder and are often the focus of treatment and rehabilitative efforts. Clinical work that involves the family, friends, school, and workplace is often the bedrock of treatment in a patient with Tourette's disorder. Many of the psychosocial issues in Tourette's disorder are not unique but are shared by other neuropsychiatric disorders.

CHILDREN. For children with Tourette's disorder, the onset of symptoms occurs early in development and directly affects family life and relationships with peers and schoolmates.

YOUNG ADULTS. The transition to young adulthood often occurs when an important component of the individual's early experience and identity (i.e., Tourette's disorder) begins to show some improvement. Young adults most vulnerable during this transition are those who, as a result of their Tourette's disorder, did not develop the foundations of an adult identity as a child. These adults often face the rigors of adult life without the necessary skills to manage, but also without the presence of tic symptoms of sufficient severity to explain their impairment.

ADULTS. Most adults with Tourette's disorder were not diagnosed in childhood. Without the "protection" of the diagnosis, they often experience significant confusion, isolation, and discrimination. Many adults who appear to function well in spite of significant adversity may be doing so at an emotional cost.

DIAGNOSIS

A number of clinical features of tics are associated with impairment:

- Large, disruptive, or painful motor movements
- Vocalizations that call attention to the patient
- Premonitory sensations or cognitions that intrude into consciousness
- Tics that are socially unacceptable

Psychosocial Issues

Psychosocial issues can play a role in tic severity and in overall adaptation and impairment. Assessment of family, peer, and school support for the youngster (adequate protection) along with assessment for the presence of opportunities to be intellectually, physically, and socially challenged is important. The balance between protection and challenge in children is critical for long-term development. An environment that is too protective decreases opportunities for building skills. An environment that is too challenging can lead to frustration, anger, and maladaptive coping.

DIFFERENTIAL DIAGNOSIS

Tics have many characteristics that differentiate them from the other movement disorders. Perhaps most important to "ruling in" tics as

---

Differential Diagnosis of Tics

Simple, rapid movements
  Myoclonus
  Chorea
  Seizures
Simple, sustained movements
  Dystonia
  Athetosis
Complex or sustained movements
  Mannerisms
  Stereotypies
  Restless legs
  Seizures

From Jankovic J: Diagnosis and classification of tics and Tourette syndrome. Adv Neurol 1992; 58:7–14.

a diagnostic possibility is the childhood history of simple motor tics in the face. Other movement disorders do not have a similar pattern of movement onset or location.

COURSE AND NATURAL HISTORY

In Tourette's disorder, tic symptoms usually begin in childhood: mean age at onset is 7 years. The first tic may develop during the teenage years, but this is unusual. Motor tics of the eyes and face are the earliest and most common presenting symptoms. In many patients, the motor tics remain isolated in the face. When motor tics do progress, there is a tendency for additional tics to present sequentially from the head and face to the neck, shoulders, trunk, and extremities. Vocal tics tend to follow the development of motor tics. Complex tics of both types tend to follow the development of simple tics. Longitudinal studies suggest that tic severity is greatest in most patients during the latency and early teenage years. Most patients experience a decline in tic severity as they get older; only a small percentage of patients (10%) experience a severe or deteriorating course.

The course of ADHD symptoms in persons with Tourette's disorder is similar to that in children without it. ADHD symptoms usually begin earlier than the tic symptoms. Symptoms of hyperactivity attenuate before puberty, whereas problems with attention and concentration may continue into adulthood.

Obsessive-compulsive symptoms in persons with Tourette's disorder generally begin somewhat later than ADHD and tics and may actually progress differentially from tic symptoms. Tic symptoms tend to improve into adulthood; obsessive-compulsive symptoms may actually increase in severity. Long-term studies of the course of obsessive-compulsive symptoms in persons with Tourette's disorder have not been done.

TREATMENT

Standard approaches to treatment are shown in Table 11–2.

TABLE 11–2 Goals of Treatment
Educate the patient and family about tic disorders.
Define the co-occurring disorders.
Create a hierarchy of the clinically impairing conditions.
Treat the impairing conditions using somatic, psychological, and rehabilitative approaches.
Aid in creating a supportive yet challenging psychosocial milieu.

Treat the Impairing Conditions

TIC SUPPRESSION: PHARMACOLOGICAL

The goal of pharmacological treatment is the reduction of tic severity, not necessarily the elimination of tics. Haloperidol has been used effectively to suppress motor and phonic tics for more than 30 years. Since that time, a number of other neuroleptic agents have also been identified as useful in tic suppression, including fluphenazine and pimozide.

There are continuing efforts to identify tic-suppressing agents with tolerable side effects. Most frequently cited in this regard are the α-adrenergic agonists clonidine and guanfacine, both developed as antihypertensives. These agents do not appear to be uniformly effective in tic suppression, but they can be effective for some patients without producing significant side effects. Both clonidine and guanfacine also appear to be useful for some of the symptoms of ADHD, which makes these agents a reasonable first choice for those patients with both Tourette's disorder and ADHD.

Benzodiazepines can be useful in decreasing co-morbid anxiety in patients with Tourette's disorder. In addition, clonazepam appears also to be useful in selected patients for tic reduction.

TIC SUPPRESSION: NONPHARMACOLOGICAL

The behavioral technique shown to be most effective is habit reversal training. For Tourette's disorder, habit reversal training is the use of a competing muscle contraction or behavioral response that opposes the tic movement. This method is usually combined with relaxation training, self-monitoring, awareness training, and positive reinforcement.

Psychosocial Treatments

EDUCATION

Perhaps the most useful psychosocial and educational intervention is to make the patient aware of the Tourette Syndrome Association, both national and local chapters. This and other self-help groups can be useful as sources of support and education for patients, families, and psychiatrists.

THERAPY

Individual psychotherapy can be useful for support and development of awareness, or to address personal and interpersonal problems more effectively. Family therapy can be useful because families can have problems adjusting, functioning, and communicating.

In newly diagnosed adults, psychotherapy oriented toward adequate adjustment to the diagnosis is important but not always easy. Adult patients frequently experience a mixture of relief to be diagnosed finally and anger and resentment related to their past experiences with discrimination or inadequate medical care.

Communication Disorders

DEFINITION

The disorders of communication have traditionally been insufficiently familiar to psychiatrists despite the fact that psychiatric practice is founded on communication. A knowledge of these disorders is of especially crucial importance in the care of children because they are deeply imbricated in all aspects of normal development, psychiatric illness, and the functions of daily life.

These disorders share many common features, as noted in Table 12–1. Selective mutism is not regarded as a disorder of communication and is included among other disorders of childhood.

Significant communication problems in childhood consist of expressive and mixed receptive-expressive disorders, phonological disorder, stuttering, and communication disorder NOS. Following are the DSM-IV criteria for these disorders.

TABLE 12–1	Features Common to All Communication Disorders

Inadequate development of some aspect of communication

Absence (in developmental types) of any demonstrable causes of physical disorder, neurological disorder, global mental retardation, or severe environmental deprivation

Onset of childhood

Long duration

Clinical features resembling the functional levels of younger normal children

Impairments in adaptive functioning, especially in school

Tendency to occur in families

Predisposition toward boys

Multiple presumed etiological factors

Increased prevalence in younger age range

Diagnosis requiring a range of standardized techniques

Tendency toward certain specific associated problems, such as attention-deficit/hyperactivity disorder

Wide range of subtypes and severity

Adapted from Baker L: Specific communication disorders. In Garfinkel BD, Carlson GA, Weller EB (eds): Psychiatric Disorders in Children and Adolescents. Philadelphia: WB Saunders, 1990:257–270.

DSM-IV Criteria 315.31

Expressive Language Disorder

A. The scores obtained from standardized individually administered measures of expressive language development are substantially below those obtained from standardized measures of both nonverbal intellectual capacity and receptive language development. The disturbance may be manifest clinically by symptoms that include having a markedly limited vocabulary, making errors in tense, or having difficulty recalling words or producing sentences with developmentally appropriate length or complexity.

B. The difficulties with expressive language interfere with academic or occupational achievement or with social communication.

C. Criteria are not met for mixed receptive-expressive language disorder or a pervasive developmental disorder.

D. If mental retardation, a speech-motor or sensory deficit, or environmental deprivation is present, the language difficulties are in excess of those usually associated with these problems.

DSM-IV Criteria 315.31

Mixed Receptive-Expressive Language Disorder

A. The scores obtained from a battery of standardized individually administered measures of both receptive and expressive language development are substantially below those obtained from standardized measures of nonverbal intellectual capacity. Symptoms include those for expressive language disorder as well as difficulty understanding words, sentences, or specific types of words, such as spatial terms.

B. The difficulties with receptive and expressive language significantly interfere with academic or occupational achievement or with social communication.

C. Criteria are not met for a pervasive developmental disorder.

D. If mental retardation, a speech-motor or sensory deficit, or environmental deprivation is present, the language difficulties are in excess of those usually associated with these problems.

DSM-IV Criteria 315.39

Phonological Disorder

A. Failure to use developmentally expected speech sounds that are appropriate for age and dialect (e.g., errors in sound production, use, representation, or organization such as, but not limited to, substitutions of one sound for another [use of /t/ for target /k/ sound] or omissions of sounds such as final consonants).

B. The difficulties in speech sound production interfere with academic or occupational achievement or with social communication.

C. If mental retardation, a speech-motor or sensory deficit, or environmental deprivation is present, the speech difficulties are in excess of those usually associated with these problems.

DSM-IV Criteria 307.0

Stuttering

A. Disturbance in the normal fluency and time patterning of speech (inappropriate for the individual's age), characterized by frequent occurrences of one or more of the following:

   (1) sound and syllable repetitions

   (2) sound prolongations

   (3) interjections

   (4) broken words (e.g., pauses within a word)

   (5) audible or silent blocking (filled or unfilled pauses in speech)

   (6) circumlocutions (word substitutions to avoid problematic words)

   (7) words produced with an excess of physical tension

   (8) monosyllabic whole-word repetitions (e.g., "I-I-I-I see him")

B. The disturbance in fluency interferes with academic or occupational achievement or with social communication.

C. If a speech-motor or sensory deficit is present, the speech difficulties are in excess of those usually associated with these problems.

ASSESSMENT

In the Psychiatric Interview

It is essential that the psychiatrist seeing children be familiar with the expected milestones of speech and language development.

TREATMENT AND ITS GOALS

Speech and language therapy typically has three major goals: the development and improvement of communication skills with concurrent remediation of deficits, the development of alternative or augmentative communication strategies when required, and the social habilitation of the individual in regard to communication. Thus, a great range of approaches and components must be employed in treating children with communication disorders.

Drug therapy for this disorder remains at best controversial.

Outcome studies of communication therapy, especially for the language disorders, have often been complicated by multiple theories of language development, diagnostic and methodological variations, lack of standardization of therapeutic techniques, and comorbidity. Nonresponse to initial treatment may be common, requiring patience and persistence. Even when communication therapy does not lead to apparent improvements in language beyond developmental improvements, it may still facilitate the child's use of extant language for environmental control and self-control.

SPECIAL FEATURES

Approximately half of the children with a speech or language disorder have some other definable Axis I clinical disorder. Similarly, among children with a psychiatric diagnosis first made, there is a remarkably increased likelihood of speech and language disorders, which often go undetected.

It should come as no surprise that children with communication disorders, and especially with language disorders, are academically vulnerable. Education as we know it, especially for younger children, is largely based on language. In all, some 50% to 75% of children with language disorders will have persistent academic problems. They tend to learn less at any given time and to learn more slowly than their peers. These children need ongoing comprehensive special education services and regular reevaluation of their educational needs.

Elimination Disorders

ENURESIS

Definition

> **DSM-IV Criteria** 307.6
>
> **Enuresis (Not due to a Medical Condition)**
>
> A. Repeated voiding of urine into bed or clothes (whether involuntary or intentional).
>
> B. The behavior is clinically significant as manifested by either a frequency of twice a week for at least 3 consecutive months or the presence of clinically significant distress or impairment in social, academic (occupational), or other important areas of functioning.
>
> C. Chronological age is at least 5 years (or equivalent developmental level).
>
> D. The behavior is not due exclusively to the direct physiological effect of a substance (e.g., a diuretic) or a general medical condition (e.g., diabetes, spina bifida, a seizure disorder).
>
> *Specify* type:
>
> **Nocturnal only:** passage of urine only during nighttime sleep
>
> **Diurnal only:** passage of urine during waking hours
>
> **Nocturnal and diurnal:** a combination of the two subtypes above

Although there is no good evidence that the condition is primarily psychogenic, it is often associated with psychiatric disorder, and enuretic children are frequently referred to mental health services for treatment.

Course and Natural History

The acquisition of urinary continence at night is the end stage of a fairly consistent developmental sequence. Bowel control during sleep marks the beginning of this process and is followed by bowel control during waking hours. Bladder control during the day occurs soon after and finally, after a variable interval, nighttime bladder control is achieved. Most children achieve this final stage by the age of 36 months. With increasing age, the likelihood of spontaneous recovery from enuresis becomes less, so that, for instance, 40% of 2-year-olds with enuresis become dry in the next year and 20% of enuretic 3-year-olds become dry before age 4 years but only 6% of enuretic 4-year-olds become dry in the following year. Only 1.5% of 5-year-old bed-wetters become dry during the next 2 years.

Nocturnal enuresis is as common in boys as girls until the age of 5 years, but by age 11 years, boys outnumber girls 2:1. Not until the age of 8 years do boys achieve the same levels of nighttime continence that are seen in girls by the age of 5 years. This appears to be due to slower physiological maturation in boys. In addition, the increased incidence of secondary enuresis (occurring after an initial 1-year period of acquired continence) in boys further affects the sex ratio seen in later childhood. Daytime enuresis occurs more commonly in girls and is associated with higher rates of psychiatric disturbance.

Etiology and Pathophysiology

Biological factors described include a structural pathological condition or infection of the urinary tract (or both), low functional bladder capacity, abnormal antidiuretic hormone secretion, abnormal depth of sleep, genetic predisposition, and developmental delay.

The evidence for some genetic predisposition is strong. Approximately 70% of children with nocturnal enuresis have a first-degree relative who also has or has had nocturnal enuresis. Twin studies have shown greater monozygotic (68%) than dizygotic (36%) concordance. An association between enuresis and early delays in motor, language, and social development has been noted in both prospective community samples and a large retrospective study of clinical subjects.

Psychiatric disorder occurs more frequently in enuretic children than in other children. The relative frequency of disorder ranges from two to six times that in the general population and is more frequent in girls, in children who also have diurnal enuresis, and in children with secondary enuresis. There have been no specific types of psychiatric disorder identified in children with enuresis.

There is little evidence that enuresis is a symptom of underlying disorder because psychotherapy is ineffective in reducing enuresis, anxiolytic drugs have no antienuretic effect, tricyclic antidepressants exert their therapeutic effect independent of the child's mood, and purely symptomatic therapies such as the bell and pad are equally effective in disturbed and nondisturbed children.

A final possibility is that enuresis and psychiatric disorder are both the result of joint etiologic factors such as low socioeconomic status, institutional care, large sibships, parental delinquency, as well as early and repeated disruptions of maternal care. Shared biological factors may also be important because delayed motor, speech, and pubertal development, already shown to be associated with enuresis, have been shown to be more frequent in disturbed enuretic children than in those without psychiatric disorder.

Diagnosis and Differential Diagnosis

The presence or absence of conditions often seen in association with enuresis, such as developmental delay, UTI, constipation, and comorbid psychiatric disorder, should be assessed and ruled out as appropriate. Other causes of nocturnal incontinence should be excluded, for example, those leading to polyuria (diabetes mellitus, renal disease, diabetes insipidus) and, rarely, nocturnal epilepsy.

Assessment

HISTORY

Information on the frequency, periodicity, and duration of symptoms is needed to make the diagnosis and distinguish functional enuresis from sporadic seizure-associated enuresis. If there is diurnal enuresis, an additional treatment plan is required. A family history of enuresis increases the likelihood of a diagnosis of functional enuresis and may explain a later presentation for treatment.

Questions that are useful in obtaining information for treatment planning include "Why is this a problem?" and "Why does this need treatment now?" because these factors may influence the choice of treatment (is a rapid effect needed?) or point to other pressures or restrictions on therapy. It is important to inquire about previous management strategies—for example, fluid restriction, lifting, rewards, and punishments—used at home. If specific treatments have been prescribed, either behavioral or pharmacological, it is important to discover the reasons they may have failed, for example, parental discord, noncompliance, or relapse after an initial response. The child's views and any misconceptions that he or she may have about the enuresis, its causes, and its treatment should be fully explored.

All children should have a routine physical examination, with particular emphasis placed on detection of congenital malformations, which are possibly indicative of urogenital abnormalities. A midstream specimen of urine should be examined for the presence of infection. Radiological or further medical investigation is indicated only in the presence of infected urine, enuresis with symptoms suggestive of recurrent UTI (frequency, urgency, and dysuria), or polyuria.

Treatment

Practical management for nocturnal enuresis is presented in Table 13–1.

A number of randomized double-blind placebo-controlled trials have shown that the synthetic vasopeptide DDAVP (desmopressin) is effective in enuresis.

Assessment and Management of Diurnal Enuresis

Daytime enuresis, although it can occur together with nighttime enuresis, has a different pattern of associations and responds to

TABLE 13–1	Practical Management of Nocturnal Enuresis

Stage 1	Assessment

Obtain history: frequency, periodicity, and duration of wetting.

Why is this a problem? Why now?

Mental status: views and misconceptions (parent and child).

Discover reasons for previous failure or failures.

Perform routine physical examination (any minor congenital abnormalities?)

Midstream specimen of urine must be obtained.

Radiology and further physical investigation, is needed only if symptoms or evidence of urinary tract infection (dysuria and frequency or positive culture results) or polyuria.

Stage 2	Advice

Education that enuresis is common and not deliberate.

Aim to reduce punitive behavior.

Transmit optimism: however, anticipate disappointment at no instant cure.

Preview the stepwise recovery and warn of the possibility of relapse.

Stage 3	Baseline

Use star chart.

Focus on positive achievements (be creative).

Examine the effect of simple interventions (e.g., lifting).

Stage 4	Night Alarm

First-line management unless important to obtain rapid short-term effect.

Demonstrate night alarm equipment in the office.

Telephone follow-up within a few days commencing therapy

or

Drug Therapy

If rapid suppression of wetting is needed (e.g., before vacation or camp, to defuse aggressive or hostile situation between child and parents and siblings).

When family has *proved* incapable of using the equipment.

After failure or multiple relapses.

Medication of choice: DDAVP, 20–40 μg at night.

different methods of treatment. It is much more likely to be associated with urinary tract abnormalities, including UTI, and to be comorbid with other psychiatric disorders. As a result, a more detailed and focused medical and psychiatric evaluation is indicated. Urine should be checked repeatedly for infection, and the threshold for ordering ultrasonographical visualization of the urological system should be low. The history may make it apparent that the daytime wetting is situation specific. For example, school-based enuresis in a child who is too timid to ask to use the bathroom could be alleviated by the teacher's tactfully reminding the child to go to the bathroom at regular intervals. Treatment strategies are based on establishing a pattern of toileting before the times that diurnal enuresis is likely to occur (usually between 12 noon and 5 PM) and using positive reinforcement to promote regular use of the bathroom.

Unlike nocturnal enuresis, drug treatment with tricyclic antidepressants, such as imipramine, is ineffective, whereas the use of anticholinergic agents such as oxybutynin and terodiline shows a therapeutic impact on the frequency of daytime enuresis.

Course and Natural History

Less than one third of children in the United States have completed toilet training by the age of 2 years, with a mean age of 27.7 months. Bowel control is usually achieved before bladder

ENCOPRESIS

Definition

DSM-IV Criteria

Encopresis

A. Repeated passage of feces into inappropriate places (e.g., clothing or floor) whether involuntary or intentional.

B. At least one such event a month for at least 3 months.

C. Chronological age is at least 4 years (or equivalent developmental level).

D. The behavior is not due exclusively to the direct physiological effect of a substance (e.g., laxatives) or a general medical condition except through a mechanism involving constipation.

Code as follows:

787.6 Encopresis, with constipation and overflow incontinence: there is evidence of constipation on physical examination or by history.

307.7 Encopresis, without constipation and overflow incontinence: there is no evidence of constipation on physical examination or by history.

TABLE 13–2	Practical Management of Encopresis

Stage 1 — **Assessment**

Whether primary or secondary.
Is there physical cause?
Presence or absence of constipation.
Presence or absence of acute stress.
Presence or absence of psychiatric disorder including phobic symptoms or smearing.
ABC (antecedents, behavior, consequences), of encopresis including secondary gain.
Discover reasons for previous failure or failures.

Stage 2 — **Advice**

Education regarding diet, constipation, and toileting.
Aim to reduce punitive or coercive behavior.
Transmit optimism: however, anticipate disappointment at no instant cure.
Preview the stepwise recovery and warn of the possibility of relapse.

Stage 3 — **Toileting**

Baseline observation using star chart.
Focus on positive achievements, e.g., toileting, rather than soiling.
High-fiber diet (try bran in soup, milk shakes).
Toilet after meals, 15 minutes maximum.
Check that adequately rising intraabdominal pressure is present.
Graded exposure scheme if "pot phobic."

with

Laxatives

Indicated if physical examination or abdominal radiograph shows fecal loading.
Medication of choice: Senokot syrup (senna) up to 10 mL twice daily, lactulose syrup up to 30 mL (20 mg) twice daily.
Dosage will be reduced over time; titrate with bowel frequency.

Enemas

Microenema (e.g., bisacodyl, 30 mL) if the bowel is excessively loaded with rock-like feces.

Stage 4 — **Biofeedback**

Consider after relapse or failure to respond to toileting or laxatives.

control. The age cutoff for "normality" is set at 4 years, the age at which 95% of children have acquired fecal continence. As with urinary continence, girls achieve bowel control earlier than do boys.

Epidemiology

The overall prevalence of encopresis in 7- and 8-year-old children has been shown to be 1.5%, with boys (2.3%) affected more commonly than girls (0.7%).

Etiology and Pathophysiology

No clear single causative pathway has been established. Encopresis may occur after an acute episode of constipation following illness or a change in diet. In addition to the pain and discomfort caused by attempts to pass an extremely hard stool, a number of specific painful perianal conditions such as anal fissure can lead to stool withholding and later fecal soiling. Stressful events such as the birth of a sibling or attending a new school have been associated with up to 25% of cases of secondary encopresis. In nonretentive encopresis, the main theories center on faulty toilet training. Stress during the training period, coercive toileting leading to anxiety and "pot phobia," and failure to learn or to have been taught the appropriate behavior have all been implicated.

Associated Features

DIAGNOSIS AND DIFFERENTIAL DIAGNOSIS

There are three types of identifiable encopresis in children: 1) it is known that the child can control defecation, but she or he chooses to defecate in inappropriate places; 2) there is true failure to gain bowel control, and the child is unaware of or unable to control soiling; and 3) soiling is due to excessively fluid feces, whether from constipation and overflow, physical disease, or anxiety. In practice, there is frequently overlap among types or progression from one to another. Unlike enuresis, fecal soiling rarely occurs at night or during sleep, and if present, is indicative of a poor prognosis.

Treatment

Practical management for encopresis is presented in (Table 13–2).

Behavioral therapy is the mainstay of treatment for encopresis. In the younger child who has been toilet trained, this focuses on practical elimination skills. Parents or caretakers, or both, need to be educated in making the toilet a pleasant place to visit and should stay with the younger child, giving encouragement and praise for appropriate effort.

Generic Substance Use and Hallucinogen Use Disorders

This chapter provides an overview of substance abuse and dependence, including its definition in the *Diagnostic and Statistical Manual of Mental Disorders,* Fourth Edition (DSM-IV); the general epidemiological features of substance abuse; its pathophysiological characteristics; and the clinical issues of diagnosis and treatment, including psychotherapy and pharmacotherapy. Many of the general principles outlined in this chapter are elaborated in later chapters in regard to specific abused substances.

DEFINITION

Substance Abuse and Dependence

DSM-IV Criteria

Substance Abuse

A. A maladaptive pattern of substance use leading to clinically significant impairment or distress, as manifested by one (or more) of the following, occurring within a 12-month period:

(1) recurrent substance use resulting in a failure to fulfill major role obligations at work, school, or home (e.g., repeated absences or poor work performance related to substance use; substance-related absences, suspensions, or expulsions from school; neglect of children or household)

(2) recurrent substance use in situations in which it is physically hazardous (e.g., driving an automobile or operating a machine when impaired by substance use)

(3) recurrent substance-related legal problems (e.g., arrests for substance-related disorderly conduct)

(4) continued substance use despite having persistent or recurrent social or interpersonal problems caused or exacerbated by the effects of the substance (e.g., arguments with spouse about consequences of intoxication, physical fights)

B. The symptoms have never met the criteria for substance dependence for this class of substance.

DSM-IV Criteria

Substance Dependence

A maladaptive pattern of substance use, leading to clinically significant impairment or distress, as manifested by three (or more) of the following, occurring at any time in the same 12-month period:

(1) tolerance, as defined by either of the following:

    (a) a need for markedly increased amounts of the substance to achieve intoxication or desired effect

    (b) markedly diminished effect with continued use of the same amount of the substance

(2) withdrawal, as manifested by either of the following:

    (a) the characteristic withdrawal syndrome for the substance (refer to criteria A and B of the criteria sets for withdrawal from the specific substances)

    (b) the same (or a closely related) substance is taken to relieve or avoid withdrawal symptoms

(3) the substance is often taken in larger amounts or over a longer period than was intended

(4) there is a persistent desire or unsuccessful efforts to cut down or control substance use

(5) a great deal of time is spent in activities necessary to obtain the substance (e.g., visiting multiple doctors or driving long distances), use the substance (e.g., chain-smoking), or recover from its effects

(6) important social, occupational, or recreational activities are given up or reduced because of substance use

Box continued on following page

DSM-IV Criteria

Substance Dependence *Continued*

(7) the substance use is continued despite knowledge of having a persistent or recurrent physical or psychological problem that is likely to have been caused or exacerbated by the substance (e.g., current cocaine use despite recognition of cocaine-induced depression, or continued drinking despite recognition that an ulcer was made worse by alcohol consumption)

Specify if:

With physiological dependence: evidence of tolerance or withdrawal (i.e., either item 1 or 2 is present)

Without physiological dependence: no evidence of tolerance or withdrawal (i.e., neither item 1 nor 2 is present)

Course specifiers (see text for definitions):

Early full remission

Early partial remission

Sustained full remission

Sustained partial remission

On agonist therapy

In a controlled environment

This section reviews the application of the dependence syndrome to a variety of abused drugs and uses the number of dependence syndrome criteria met as a measure of severity. Treatment-seeking opioid abusers are likely to meet most of the dependence syndrome criteria, and therefore their use is at the high end of severity. Cannabis users, in contrast, are likely to meet relatively few dependence syndrome criteria, and therefore their use is of a lesser degree of severity. Individuals with alcoholism or cocaine abuse tend to demonstrate a much wider variability among treatment seekers, with the proportion of patients having relatively low levels of dependence approximately equal to those having extremely high levels of dependence. Thus, the severity of substance dependence is variable depending on the type of drug abused.

Substance abuse is a maladaptive pattern of substance use leading to significant adverse consequences. In the areas of psychosocial, medical, or legal problems, these consequences must recur during a 12-month period, but tolerance, withdrawal, and compulsive use are not necessary for a substance abuse diagnosis. This diagnosis does not apply to caffeine or nicotine.

Substance Intoxication

DSM-IV Criteria

Substance Intoxication

A. The development of a reversible substance-specific syndrome due to recent ingestion of (or exposure to) a substance. Note: Different substances may produce similar or identical syndromes.

B. Clinically significant maladaptive behavioral or psychological changes that are due to the effect of the substance on the central nervous system (e.g., belligerence, mood lability, cognitive impairment, impaired judgment, impaired social or occupational functioning) and develop during or shortly after use of the substance.

C. The symptoms are not due to a general medical condition and are not better accounted for by another mental disorder.

Substance intoxication is a reversible substance-specific syndrome with maladaptive, behavioral, or psychological changes developing during or shortly after use of the substance. It does not apply to nicotine. Recent use can be documented by a history or toxicological screening of body fluids (urine or blood). Different substances may produce similar or identical syndromes and, in polydrug users, intoxication may involve a complex mixture of disturbed perceptions, judgment, and behavior that can vary in severity and duration according to the setting in which the substances were taken.

Substance Withdrawal

DSM-IV Criteria

Substance Withdrawal

A. The development of a substance-specific syndrome due to the cessation of (or reduction in) substance use that has been heavy and prolonged.

B. The substance-specific syndrome causes clinically significant distress or impairment in social, occupational, or other important areas of functioning.

C. The symptoms are not due to a general medical condition and are not better accounted for by another mental disorder.

Substance withdrawal is a syndrome due to cessation of, or reduction in, heavy and prolonged substance use. It causes clinically significant impairment or distress and is usually associated with substance dependence. The withdrawal syndrome usually lasts several days to 2 weeks.

EPIDEMIOLOGY

Prevalence and Incidence

Wide cultural variations in attitudes toward substance consumption have led to widely varying patterns of substance abuse and prevalence of substance-related disorders. Relatively high prevalence rates for the use of virtually every substance occur between the ages of 18 and 24 years, with intoxication being the initial substance-related disorder, usually beginning in the teens. Tolerance and withdrawal require a sustained period of use, and these manifestations of physical dependence for most drugs of abuse typically begin in the 20s and early 30s. Although most substance-related disorders are more common in men than in women, sex ratios can vary considerably with different drugs of abuse.

Comorbidity Patterns

In both the Epidemiological Catchment Area study and the National Comorbidity Survey, substance abuse and dependence were the most common comorbid disorders, usually appearing in combination with affective and anxiety disorders. In the National Comorbidity Survey, the lifetime rate of substance abuse was 27% and the comorbid rate of depression was 19%. In the Epidemiological Catchment Area study, 75% of daily substance abusers had a comorbid psychiatric disorder. A comparison of rates for other disorders is presented in Table 14–1.

ETIOLOGY AND PATHOPHYSIOLOGY

The cause of substance abuse depends on a variety of biological, psychological, and social factors. Family genetic studies have found rates of substance abuse three to four times higher in identical twins than in dizygotic twins. Although no single biological marker or specific genetic defect has been confirmed, work has suggested that some alleles associated with variations in the dopamine receptor may be more common in substance abusers than in individuals who are not substance abusers.

The neuronal pathways underlying positive reinforcement appear to converge on the dopaminergic pathways leading from the ventral tegmental area in the brain stem to the nucleus accumbens, which is part of the basal ganglia. Most drugs of abuse appear to act through this pathway to produce positive reinforcement and reward. The reinforcing effects of alcohol and benzodiazepines may be through γ-aminobutyric acid receptors. The positive reinforcing effects of hallucinogenic drugs are less clear. For example, marijuana interacts with a specific cannabinoid receptor that is pri-

TABLE 14-1	Lifetime Diagnoses of Substance Abusers and Community Sample			
	Patients with Opioid Addiction (n = 533)	Patients with Alcoholism (n = 321)	Cocaine Abusers (n = 149)	New Haven Community (n = 3058)
Major depression	53.9	38	31.5	6.7
Bipolar disorder I (mania)	0.6	2	3.4	1.1
Schizophrenia	0.8	2	0.7	1.9
Phobia	9.6	27	11.4	7.8
Antisocial personality	25.5	41	34.9	2.1
Alcoholism	34.5	100	63.8	11.5
Drug abuse	100	43	100	5.8

marily located in the cerebellum. Other hallucinogenic drugs, such as lysergic acid diethylamide, have critical effects on serotonin-ergic systems.

The negative reinforcers involved in substance dependence include the relief of withdrawal symptoms. The neurobiological systems responsible for symptoms of withdrawal are multiply determined. Two brain systems that appear to be particularly important during withdrawal are the noradrenergic system in the locus caeruleus of the brain stem and the dopaminergic system that terminates in the nucleus accumbens.

Psychological factors related to etiology include high rates of depressive disorders and sensation seeking, which are found in substance abusers. The association of sensation seeking with substance abuse suggests not only that drugs enhance pleasant sensations, such as a high, but also that abused drugs may provide potential control of aggressive impulses. Childhood precursors of substance abuse, including shy and aggressive behaviors, can also be precursors of later depressive disorders as well as of antisocial personality disorder, the adult expression of aggressive impulsivity.

Finally, social factors, including peer and family influences, which are not dependent on genetic inheritance, are important in leading to initial drug exposure.

Adolescents who begin using gateway drugs (tobacco, alcohol, and marijuana) in their early teens are more likely to have substance dependence in their 20s than are adolescents who begin use in their late teens. Life stressors related to peers and family are also possible causative factors in substance abuse and their associated comorbid psychiatric disorders.

DIAGNOSIS

Phenomenology and Variations in Presentation

The diagnosis of substance abuse and dependence is made by eliciting an appropriate history, performing laboratory tests to confirm drug use, and observing the physiological manifestations of tolerance and withdrawal. A diagnostic decision tree is presented in Figure 14–1.

The phenomenology and variations in presentation among substance abusers are related to the wide range of substance-induced states as well as the conditions under which the patient is brought to treatment. Depending on the amount of each drug ingested and the time since ingestion, the likelihood of a serious overdose can be difficult to predict. Similarly, distinguishing substance intoxication or withdrawal from an underlying psychiatric disorder or psychosis or from chronic anxiety disorders can involve variable presentations. In most of these cases, careful observation for a period of several hours to several days, in conjunction with urine toxicological screens, may be necessary to instituting proper treatment.

Assessment

SPECIAL ISSUES IN THE PSYCHIATRIC EXAMINATION

Two special issues in the psychiatric examination of substance abusers involve 1) the source of information when obtaining the

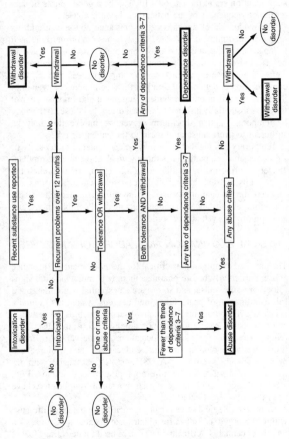

Figure 14-1 *Diagnostic decision tree.*

141

history of the substance abuse and 2) the management of aberrant behaviors.

When patients self-report the amount of substance abuse, there is a tendency to underreport the severity and duration of abuse, particularly if the patient is being referred to treatment by an outside source, such as the family, the employer, or the legal system. Tolerance and withdrawal can be assessed independently by using tests such as the naloxone challenge and the barbiturate tolerance test. In general, estimates of the amount of drug use by significant others in the patient's life can be a good source of data on the consequences of the patient's substance abuse.

The evaluation of an intoxicated substance abuser can address only a limited number of issues. These issues are primarily related to the safety of the substance abuser and other individuals who may be affected by his or her actions. Thus, a medical evaluation for signs of overdose or major cognitive impairment is critical, with consideration of detaining the patient for several hours or even days if severe complications are evident. Judgment and impulse control may be substantially affected by abused drugs, but these effects may be temporary, and a short-term preventive intervention may be sufficient to avert substantial harm to the patient or others.

Temporary suicidal behavior may be encountered in a variety of substance abusers, particularly those with alcoholism and stimulant abusers. During the evaluation session, it is important to elicit the precipitants that led the patient to seek treatment at this time and to keep the evaluation focused on specific data needed for the evaluation of substance dependence, its medical complications, and any comorbid psychiatric disorders.

PHYSICAL EXAMINATION AND LABORATORY FINDINGS

The physical examination is critical for the assessment of substance abuse, particularly before pharmacotherapy is initiated. Vital signs (blood pressure, pulse, and so on) are an essential beginning, but a full examination of heart, lungs, and nervous system is minimally necessary. Transmissible infectious diseases, such as tuberculosis and venereal diseases, are common among illicit drug abusers and require screening for adequate detection. A wide variety of infectious diseases including hepatitis, endocarditis, and acquired immunodeficiency syndrome (AIDS) are also associated with intravenous drug use, and require appropriate blood studies. With alcohol abusers, a wide range of gastrointestinal complications have been described, particularly liver dysfunction.

Urine toxicological screens can be sensitive for detecting drug use within the previous 3 days for opiates and cocaine to as long as a month for cannabis. A Breathalyzer can be used for detecting alcohol use within an 8- to 12-hour period after use. Associated medical findings on physical examination include "track marks" in intravenous drug users, nasal damage in intranasal drug users, and pulmonary damage in drug smokers.

DIFFERENCES IN DEVELOPMENTAL, GENDER, AND CULTURAL PRESENTATIONS

From a developmental perspective, the most important impact of substance abuse and dependence is in adolescence when substance abuse not only can disrupt schooling but also can have important medical consequences because of its direct hormonal effects. Another critical developmental perspective is in the children of substance abusers, who may be born with a significant neonatal withdrawal syndrome from drugs such as opioids or may have behavioral and congenital abnormalities secondary to the substance abuse by their mothers—for example, fetal alcohol syndrome in the infants of mothers who are alcohol-dependent during pregnancy and the hyperactivity that has been noted in infants born to cocaine-dependent mothers.

At the other extreme of life, in the geriatric population, substance abuse might have an important iatrogenic contribution. Many chronic debilitating diseases are associated with significant pain and may be treated with opioids. Similarly, sleep disorders in the elderly are often treated with sedatives (such as benzodiazepine and barbiturates) that produce tolerance and dependence.

Some drug abuse patterns are also more common in women than in men. For example, the phenomenon of sex for crack frequently occurs in female cocaine abusers, but men infrequently obtain cocaine using this approach. Finally, although men are more likely than women to abuse drugs generally, some drugs, such as androgenic steroids, are significantly overrepresented in male drug abusers.

Cultural differences in the presentation of drug abuse can be striking. For example, the use of hallucinogens by Native Americans in religious ceremonies shows none of the abusive characteristics of adolescent hallucinogen abuse in middle-class America.

DIFFERENTIAL DIAGNOSIS

During acute intoxication in polydrug abusers, the differential diagnosis might include psychosis, mania, organic brain syndromes, or several specific anxiety disorders.

A previous history of schizophrenia, bipolar disorder, or other major psychiatric disorder that is consistent with the presenting symptoms may also be helpful in arriving at an accurate diagnosis.

Antisocial and borderline personality disorders are commonly considered in the differential diagnosis in substance-dependent patients. If many of the antisocial or borderline characteristics are specifically tied to the patient's abuse of drugs, these characteristics will resolve with drug abstinence and should not be considered diagnostic of a personality disorder.

The symptoms of drug withdrawal frequently overlap with those of depressive disorders, and this differential diagnosis can be particularly difficult.

COURSE AND NATURAL HISTORY

The natural history of substance dependence characteristically follows the course of a chronic relapsing disorder, although a large number of individuals who experiment with potentially abusable drugs in adolescence do not go on to acquire dependence.

In contrast to most medical disorders, substance abuse differs because the substances of abuse change over time as epidemics come and go and as new drugs, such as the "designer drugs," are developed. Thus, the natural history of substance abuse and dependence is determined by the type of substance used and, for polydrug abusers, can be complicated by changing secular trends and epidemics lasting from months to decades.

TREATMENT GOALS

The most common goal of any treatment is abstinence from the abused drug. Issues of "controlled use" are debated by some psychiatrists, but this is usually not a realistic goal for dependent patients. A critical, first essential treatment goal with substance abusers is often acute treatment of overdose. After detoxification or stabilization, prevention of relapse may occur through a variety of behavioral or other psychotherapeutic approaches. For patients with psychosis, inpatient treatment or interventions with medication may be required before detoxification can occur.

Other treatment goals in longer term management include total abstinence and family involvement. Another goal is to change the role of family members from "enablers" or codependents with the substance abuser to treatment allies. These family members need to be engaged in treatment to work as active collaborators in the therapeutic plan for the patient. Although family treatment is commonly applied to many psychiatric disorders, it can have a particularly powerful impact with these behavioral disorders, especially in adolescent abusers.

STANDARD TREATMENTS

Psychiatrist-Patient Relationship

The first issue in the psychiatrist-patient relationship is approaching the substance abuser who denies a problem with abuse. This patient must be confronted in such a way that the substance abuse problem will become accessible for treatment. This confrontation may involve an "intervention," in which a variety of the significant others and social supports of the abuser are brought together to confront the potential patient about her or his substance abuse problem.

In one-to-one dealings with the patient, confidentiality must be addressed because the use of illicit drugs can be associated with a variety of illegal activities. Confidentiality must be balanced against the need to disclose enabling behaviors that can lead to a relapse of substance abuse. A psychotherapeutic issue early in treatment may be distinguishing between "slips" and a full relapse. Slips are common in substance abusers, and patients must be prepared for them and not consider them failures that will inevitably lead to full relapse and dependence.

Pharmacotherapy

A treatment decision tree presented in Figure 14–2 outlines potential roles for pharmacotherapy and psychotherapy. The general treatment approaches, along with their indications and side effects, are

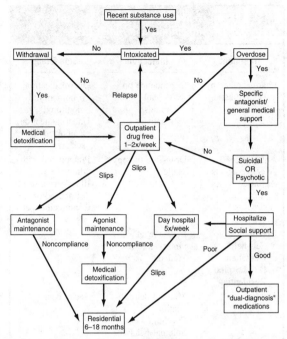

Figure 14–2 *Treatment decision tree for substance use disorders.*

seen in Table 14–2. Medications for substance abuse and dependence can be broadly classified as those for treating withdrawal symptoms (e.g., benzodiazepines for alcohol), those for discouraging use of abused drugs by blockage (e.g., naltrexone for opioids) or aversion (e.g., disulfiram for alcohol), those for counteracting overdose (e.g., naloxone for opioids), those used for substitution of the abused drug (e.g., methadone for opioids), and those for treating comorbid psychiatric disorders (e.g., desipramine for depression).

Psychosocial Treatments

A wide range of psychosocial treatments is available in substance abuse, ranging from long-term residential treatments (6 to 8 months) to relatively low-intervention outpatient drug-free treatments with once-weekly hour-long therapy.

Other treatment approaches include inpatient treatment specifically designed for detoxification and day hospital and evening programs focusing on the prevention of relapse.

Relapse prevention, a behavioral therapy for substance abusers, has articulated the distinction between slips and relapse. Slips are single, isolated episodes of substance abuse during a period of sustained abstinence. These slips can lead to relapses and dependence if the substance abuse continues.

TABLE 14–2	General Treatment Approaches: Indications and Side Effects	
Treatment	**Indication**	**Side Effects**
Pharmacotherapy Detoxifications	Dependence on Alcohol Opioids Sedatives	Overmedication, if not carefully monitored Undermedication, leading to seizures
Antagonists Aversive agents Agonists	Drug-free therapy failed	Precipitated withdrawal Illness from use of abused drugs Continued dependence
Psychotherapy Self-help Outpatient Day hospital Residential	Lower level intervention failed	
Inpatient	Medical detoxification Psychotic behavior Suicidal behavior	Social cost
Urine monitoring Breath alcohol	Outpatient treatment	None

SPECIAL TREATMENT FEATURES

Psychiatric Comorbidity

Comorbid psychiatric disorders, particularly depressive and anxiety disorders, are extremely common in substance abuse, with lifetime rates approaching 50% in individuals addicted to opioids. Although the rate of major psychotic disorders among substance abusers is relatively low (3%), the rate of substance abuse in schizophrenic and manic-depressive patients may be as high as 50%.

A prominent problem in the management of substance abusers with comorbid psychiatric disorders is medication management within a substance abuse treatment setting, because of limited psychiatric resources. Integrated dual diagnosis treatments have been developed using social skills training combined with relapse prevention behavioral therapies as well as pharmacological adjuncts to standard neuroleptic agents for patients with schizophrenia.

Another special factor in treatment is the relationship between many patients and the legal system—for example, parole, probation, work release programs, or other alternatives to incarceration—because this requires the psychiatrist to report to these agencies. Contingencies must be developed with these patients to clarify the content of this reporting as well as to obtain a specific release of confidentiality so that these reporting requirements can be fulfilled.

General Medical Comorbidity

Treatment of a comorbid medical condition is essential in substance abusers because many do not seek medical care and may be seen only by the psychiatrist. The most important current comorbid disorder in substance abusers is AIDS, which is spread primarily by intravenous drug use but increasingly is also spread through sexual activity among drug abusers. Other areas of medical comorbidity include vitamin deficiencies, infectious diseases, and gastrointestinal disorders, such as cirrhosis, gastrointestinal bleeding, and peptic and duodenal ulcers. Stimulant abusers may experience cerebrovascular accidents. Also, dementing disorders need particular consideration in conjunction with alcoholism, inhalant abuse, and sedative dependence.

Demographical and Psychosocial Variables

Substance abusers are often young but seek treatment only after a delay of 5 to 10 years; because most substance abusers are young, parenting issues are critical, specifically issues of drug use during pregnancy, which can lead to "cocaine babies," fetal alcohol syndrome, and opiate withdrawal in infants. Neonatal withdrawal requires specific attention and treatments that differ from adult treatment. Geriatric substance abuse, particularly of prescribed medications, also is not well recognized and is frequently underdiagnosed.

TREATMENT-REFRACTORY PATIENTS

A variety of escalating treatment interventions can be applied to substance abuse patients who are refractory to treatment. (See Fig. 14–2 for a treatment decision tree detailing a series of escalating treatment levels.)

Alcohol Use Disorders

The most visible group of people affected by alcohol problems includes those who have a syndrome of alcohol dependence and who are commonly referred to as alcoholics. A less prominent but far more numerous group consists of those persons who experience problems with their drinking but who are not seriously dependent on alcohol.

EPIDEMIOLOGY

Tables 15–1 and 15–2 show prevalence rates of abstention and light, moderate, and heavier drinking from the 1988 U.S. National Health Interview Survey, presented separately for men and women.

The National Institute of Mental Health Epidemiological Catchment Area (ECA) survey, a study involving more than 20,000 community and institutional respondents in the United States, showed alcohol abuse and dependence to have the highest lifetime prevalence of any mental disorder. That study estimated that nearly one person in seven (13.5% of the U.S. population) suffers from alcohol use disorder at some time in his or her life. A later community study, the National Health Interview Survey, involved a representative sample of nearly 44,000 respondents. This study found an overall 1-year prevalence rate for alcohol abuse and dependence of 8.6%. Among men, the prevalence was 13.4%; among women, it was 4.4%.

Overall, alcohol-related mortality in 1988 totaled 107,800 deaths, or about 5% of all deaths in the United States, putting it among the top four causes of death. Of alcohol-related deaths, approximately 17% were directly attributable to alcohol, 38% resulted from diseases indirectly attributable to alcohol, and 45% were attributable to alcohol-related traumatic injury.

Alcohol-related morbidity is manifested in virtually all organ systems. The primary chronic health hazard associated with heavy drinking is cirrhosis of the liver, which in 1988 was the ninth leading cause of death in the United States.

High rates of comorbid psychiatric disorders have been found in both clinical and community samples of alcohol dependent individuals. The ECA study, for example, revealed that 36.6% of those with a lifetime alcohol use disorder received at least one other psychiatric diagnosis, which is nearly double the rate for community respondents with no lifetime diagnosis of alcohol abuse and dependence.

Foremost among the psychiatric disorders that occur more frequently in individuals with an alcohol use disorder than among those without the disorder is antisocial personality disorder (ASPD).

TABLE 15–1 Prevalence of Abstinence and Drinking Levels for Men by Age, Race, and Educational Level: 1988

Characteristics	Abstainers (%)	Drinking Levels (%)		
		Light	Moderate	Heavier
Total	32	44	37	19
Age				
18–29 y	25	42	40	18
30–44 y	25	44	39	17
45–64 y	36	45	34	21
≥65 y	51	50	31	19
Race				
Black	43	45	37	18
White	30	44	37	19
Hispanic	35	48	35	17
Education				
Less than high school	46	46	33	21
High-school graduate	31	43	39	19
Greater than high school	24	44	38	18

TABLE 15-2 Prevalence of Abstinence and Drinking Levels for Women by Age, Race, and Educational Level: 1988

Characteristics	Abstainers (%)	Drinking Levels (%)		
		Light	Moderate	Heavier
Total	53	64	29	7
Age				
18–29 y	43	64	30	6
30–44 y	45	65	29	6
45–64 y	58	64	27	9
≥65 y	75	62	29	7
Race				
Black	67	68	26	6
White	50	64	29	7
Hispanic	66	70	25	6
Education				
Less than high school	74	66	27	8
High-school graduate	53	69	28	7
Greater than high school	40	62	30	7

Drug abuse and dependence are also common among individuals with an alcohol use disorder.

The ECA study showed mood disorders to be present in 13.4% of those with an alcohol disorder. Conversely, 21.8% of individuals with a mood disorder also had an alcohol disorder.

Anxiety disorders are also highly prevalent (19.4%) among individuals with an alcohol use disorder in the ECA study. Among individuals with an anxiety disorder, 17.9% have a comorbid alcohol use disorder.

Among individuals with an alcohol use disorder, the prevalence of schizophrenia is 3.8%, which is more than three times the rate of that disorder in the general population. Conversely, among individuals with schizophrenia, the prevalence of a comorbid alcohol use disorder is 33.7%.

Given a high rate of psychiatric comorbidity, it is axiomatic that a careful psychiatric assessment be conducted in patients being seen for alcohol treatment and that alcohol use and associated problems be evaluated in patients being seen primarily for other psychiatric conditions.

ETIOLOGY AND PATHOPHYSIOLOGY

It has been estimated that there is a sevenfold risk of alcoholism in first-degree relatives of alcohol-dependent individuals, with male relatives of alcohol-dependent men having the greatest risk for the disorder. However, that the majority of alcohol-dependent individuals do not have a first-degree relative who is alcohol dependent underscores that the risk for alcohol dependence is also determined by environmental factors, which may interact in complex ways with genetics.

Molecular Genetics

Although there is widespread agreement that a genetic factor is influential in the transmission of alcohol dependence, exactly how risk of the disorder is transmitted remains unknown. A number of studies have provided support for an increased risk of alcoholism, particularly severe alcoholism, as a function of the frequency of the minor allele of the D_2 dopamine receptor gene. Other investigators have begun to examine the association between alcoholism and genes coding for proteins involved in serotoninergic neurotransmission. Subsequent investigations are likely to focus on other serotoninergic candidate genes as well as those involved in other neurotransmitter (e.g., opioidergic, glutaminergic, GABAergic) systems.

The best known typology of alcoholism is the "type 1–type 2" distinction, developed by Cloninger and coworkers (1981) (Table 15–3). Type 1 alcoholic individuals are characterized by the late onset of problem drinking, rapid development of behavioral tolerance to alcohol, prominent guilt and anxiety related to drinking, and infrequent fighting and arrests when drinking.

In contrast, type 2 alcoholic individuals are characterized by early onset of an inability to abstain from alcohol, frequent fighting and arrests when drinking, and the absence of guilt and anxiety concerning drinking. Type 1 alcoholic individuals are characterized

TABLE 15–3	Cloninger's Alcoholism Typology	
	Type 1	**Type 2**
Onset of problem drinking	Late onset	Early onset
Tolerance	Rapid development of behavioral tolerance	Not specified
Mood issues	Prominent guilt and anxiety about drinking	Absence of guilt and anxiety about drinking
Personality traits	High reward dependence	Low reward dependence
	High harm avoidance	Low harm avoidance
	Low novelty seeking	High novelty seeking

by high reward dependence, high harm avoidance, and low novelty seeking. In contrast, type 2 alcoholic individuals are characterized by high novelty seeking, low harm avoidance, and low reward dependence.

DIAGNOSIS

Phenomenology and Variations in Presentation

The DSM-IV diagnosis of alcohol dependence is given when three or more of the seven criteria are present.

DSM-IV Criteria 303.90

Alcohol Dependence

A maladaptive pattern of drinking as manifested by three or more of the following during a 12-month period:

(1) tolerance, that is, either:

    (a) a need for markedly more alcohol to achieve intoxication

    (b) markedly diminished effect despite continued consumption of the same amount of alcohol

(2) withdrawal, that is, either:

    (a) two or more signs or symptoms (autonomic hyperactivity, tremor, insomnia, nausea or vomiting, transient illusions or hallucinations, psychomotor agitation, anxiety, grand mal seizures) within several hours of stopping or reducing heavy, prolonged drinking

  (b) consuming alcohol or a related substance (e.g., benzodiazepines) to relieve or avoid withdrawal symptoms

(3) alcohol is often consumed in larger amounts or over a longer period than was intended

(4) there is a persistent desire to cut down or control drinking

(5) a great deal of time is spent in drinking or recovering from drinking

(6) important social, occupational, or recreational activities are given up or reduced because of drinking

(7) drinking is continued despite knowledge of having a persistent or recurrent physical or psychological problem that is likely to have been caused or exacerbated by alcohol

Alcohol abuse is considered to be present only if the individual has never met criteria for alcohol dependence and he or she demonstrates a pattern of drinking that leads to clinically significant impairment or distress, as evidenced by one of the four criteria.

DSM-IV Criteria 305.00

Alcohol Abuse

A maladaptive pattern of drinking as manifested by one or more of the following during a 12-month period:

(1) recurrent drinking resulting in a failure to fulfill major role obligations at work, school, or home

(2) recurrent drinking in situations in which it is physically hazardous

(3) recurrent alcohol-related legal problems

(4) continued drinking despite having persistent or recurrent social or interpersonal problems caused or exacerbated by drinking

Note: The individual must never have met criteria for alcohol dependence.

Assessment

SPECIAL ISSUES IN THE PSYCHIATRIC EXAMINATION AND HISTORY

Although denial of alcohol-related problems is legendary among alcoholic individuals, there is substantial evidence that a valid alcohol history can be obtained, given adequate assessment procedures and the right conditions. A complete alcohol history should include specific questions concerning average alcohol consumption, maximal consumption per drinking occasion, frequency of heavy drinking occasions; and drinking-related social problems (e.g., objections raised by family members, friends, or people at work), legal problems (including arrests or near-arrests for driving while intoxicated), psychiatric symptoms (e.g., precipitation or exacerbation of mood or anxiety symptoms), and medical problems (e.g., alcoholic gastritis or pancreatitis).

The Alcohol Use Disorders Identification Test (AUDIT), a 10-item screening instrument, may be used to organize the alcohol use history. AUDIT covers the domains of alcohol consumption, symptoms of alcohol dependence, and alcohol-related consequences.

It is crucial that questions concerning alcohol consumption and alcohol-related symptoms and problems be asked nonjudgmentally to enhance the likelihood of accurate reporting. Specific strategies and approaches to history taking in the patient with substance abuse include reassuring the patient that information provided will be kept confidential; beginning the interview with questions that are least likely to make the patient defensive (e.g., a review of systems or psychiatric symptoms, without relating these to alcohol use); and beginning questions with *how,* rather than with *why,* to reduce the appearance of being judgmental.

RELEVANT PHYSICAL EXAMINATION AND LABORATORY FINDINGS

Medical illness is a common consequence of heavy drinking and may be present in the absence of physical dependence. The physical examination provides essential information about the presence and extent of end-organ damage and should be focused on the systems most vulnerable to alcohol-related disease: the cardiovascular system, the gastrointestinal system, and the central and peripheral nervous systems.

A variety of laboratory tests, particularly those related to hepatic function (e.g., serum transaminase activity, bilirubin level, prothrombin time, and partial thromboplastin time), can be helpful in assessing the need for medical referral.

Elevation in γ-glutamyltransferase has been found to occur in about three fourths of alcoholics before there was clinical evidence of liver disease and is often considered to be the earliest sign of heavy alcohol consumption that is widely available clinically.

Carbohydrate-deficient transferrin values may be more sensitive than routine laboratory tests for the identification of heavy alcohol consumption. In one study, the carbohydrate-deficient transferrin value was found to have a sensitivity of 91% and a specificity of 100% in distinguishing alcoholic individuals from light drinkers or abstainers.

In a clinical setting, where laboratory results are generally not immediately available, the alcohol breath test, which measures the amount of alcohol in expired air (providing an estimate of venous ethanol concentration), is invaluable.

Venous blood levels should be obtained if dangerously high levels of intoxication are suspected, if a patient is comatose, or for medical-legal purposes. A blood alcohol level greater than 150 mg/dL in a patient showing no signs of intoxication (e.g., dysarthria, motor incoordination, gait ataxia, nystagmus, impaired attention) can be interpreted to reflect physiological tolerance. In nontolerant individuals, a blood alcohol level in excess of 400 mg/dL can result in death, and 300 mg/dL indicates a need for emergency care.

The clinician should also be alert to other acute alcohol-related signs, including alcohol withdrawal or delirium, intoxication or withdrawal from other drugs, and the acute presentation of psychiatric symptoms.

Other laboratory evaluations indicated in alcoholic patients are a urine toxicology screen including opiates, cocaine, cannabis, and benzodiazepines; routine urinalysis; blood chemistry assays; hepatitis profile; complete blood count; and serological test for syphilis. For the female patient, serum testing for pregnancy should also be done.

DIFFERENCES IN PRESENTATIONS RELATED TO SEX, DEVELOPMENT, AND CULTURE

WOMEN. Although women are more likely to abstain from alcohol or, if they do drink, are more likely to drink at lower levels than men, women have consistently been shown to be more sensitive to the toxic effects of alcohol.

Heavy drinking in pregnant women may produce malnutrition in both the mother and the fetus as well as spontaneous abortion, preterm delivery, and intrauterine growth retardation. Alcohol-related birth defects are estimated to occur in as many as 1 in 100 live births. The most severe manifestation of alcohol-related birth defects, fetal alcohol syndrome, a constellation of morphological and developmental defects resulting from high-dose prenatal alcohol exposure, is estimated to occur in 1 in 1000 to 1 in 300 live births.

Because alcohol-related birth defects can be avoided, the evaluation of pregnant patients should routinely include questions about alcohol and other substance use. Those pregnant women identified as heavy drinkers or drug users should be designated high risk and provided with specialized, comprehensive perinatal care, including rehabilitation and appropriate attention to related psychosocial disabilities.

ADOLESCENTS. As might be expected, adolescents have comparatively short histories of heavy drinking. Nonetheless, abuse of alcohol and drugs contributes in important ways to morbidity and mortality in adolescents, the leading causes of which are motor vehicle accidents, homicide, and suicide.

Furthermore, adolescents are highly vulnerable to peer pressure to abuse alcohol and drugs, so that the values and behavior of the adolescent's peer group are important elements in the evaluation of alcohol use and abuse in the adolescent.

As is generally true in dealing with adolescents, given their economic and emotional dependence, a thorough family evaluation, whenever possible, is important for understanding the adolescent's substance use and related problems.

ELDERLY PERSONS. Although heavy drinking is less prevalent in the elderly, it is nonetheless an important source of morbidity in this group. Elderly alcoholic inpatients suffer from more chronic medical problems and poorer psychosocial functioning than do the nonalcoholic elderly. The increased use of prescription medications in the elderly also increases the potential for adverse pharmacokinetic interactions with alcohol. In addition, decreased cognitive functioning associated with heavy alcohol use can increase medication errors and noncompliance in this group.

Late-onset alcoholism appears to be more common among women and people of higher socioeconomic status and is less frequently associated with a family history of alcoholism.

ETHNIC AND RACIAL GROUPS. It is difficult to generalize about ethnic and racial differences in drinking practices and alcohol-related problems. In addition to substantial differences in drinking patterns and consequences among different ethnic and racial groups, there is also considerable heterogeneity among these groups.

COURSE AND NATURAL HISTORY

Symptoms of alcohol dependence appear in this relative order: evidence of heavy drinking during the patients' late 20s, interference with functioning in multiple areas of the patients' lives during their early 30s, loss of control followed by an intensification of social and work-related problems and onset of medical consequences in the middle to late 30s, and severe long-term consequences by the late 30s and early 40s. Women appear to experience many of these milestones at a later age than men do.

There is consistent evidence that early age at onset is a predictor of greater severity of alcoholism and a poorer response to treatment.

Among men, the presence of a comorbid lifetime diagnosis of ASPD, major depression, or drug abuse and dependence is associated with poorer drinking outcomes.

Additional studies are needed to clarify both the prognostic significance of patient-related variables, including comorbid psychiatric disorders, and their interaction with different kinds of treatment.

OVERALL GOALS OF TREATMENT

Interventions can be divided into three general categories: 1) secondary prevention, 2) specialized treatment programs, and 3) mutual help groups. Secondary prevention is intended to reduce alcohol-related harm and prevent alcohol dependence. Specialized treatment is designed to treat the medical and psychiatric complications of drinking and to promote the social and psychological rehabilitation of the alcoholic person. Mutual help programs, of which Alcoholics Anonymous (AA) is a prime example, are concerned with the long-term rehabilitation of alcoholic people, many of whom require continuing care and support for many years.

A number of potentially life-threatening conditions place alcoholic individuals at increased risk. The presence of any of the following requires immediate attention: acute alcohol withdrawal (with the potential for seizures and delirium tremens), serious medical or surgical disease (e.g., acute pancreatitis, bleeding esophageal varices), and serious psychiatric illness (e.g., psychosis, suicidal intent). In all of these emergent conditions, acute stabilization should be the first priority of treatment.

In the alcoholic patient whose condition is stabilized or in the patient without these complicating features, the major focus should be on the establishment of a therapeutic alliance, which provides the context within which rehabilitation can occur. In addition to participation in structured rehabilitation, the patient should be made aware of the widespread availability of AA and the wide diversity of its membership.

STANDARD APPROACHES TO TREATMENT

Secondary Prevention

With respect to alcohol-related problems, secondary prevention refers to the provision of therapeutic interventions to persons who have already manifested some alcohol-related problems. Brief interventions that promote reduced drinking among heavy-drinking individuals who are not severely alcohol dependent can be used in a variety of clinical settings and yield substantial clinical benefit.

Specialized Treatment

Specialized treatment is directed primarily at the management of alcohol withdrawal, the social and psychological rehabilitation of the problem drinker, the prevention of relapse to alcohol dependence, and the management of alcohol-related medical conditions.

ALCOHOL WITHDRAWAL

The objectives in treating alcohol withdrawal are the relief of discomfort, prevention or treatment of complications, and preparation for rehabilitation.

Careful screening for concurrent medical problems is an important element in detoxification. Administration of thiamine (50 to 100 mg orally or intramuscularly) and multivitamins is a low-cost, low-risk intervention for the prophylaxis and treatment of alcohol-related neurological disturbances.

Social detoxification, which involves the nonpharmacological treatment of alcohol withdrawal, is most appropriate for patients in mild to moderate withdrawal. It consists of frequent reassurance, reality orientation, monitoring of vital signs, personal attention, and general nursing care.

Inpatient detoxification is indicated for serious medical or surgical illness as well as for those individuals with a past history of adverse withdrawal reactions or with current evidence of more serious withdrawal (e.g., delirium tremens).

A variety of medications have been used for the treatment of alcohol withdrawal. However, owing to their favorable side effect profile, the benzodiazepines have largely supplanted all other medications. Diazepam and chlordiazepoxide are often used because they are metabolized to long-acting compounds, which in effect are self-tapering.

Although carbamazepine appears useful as a primary treatment of withdrawal, the liver dysfunction that is common in alcoholic patients may affect its metabolism, which makes careful blood level monitoring necessary. Antipsychotics are not indicated for the treatment of withdrawal except in those instances when severe agitation or hallucinations are present, in which case they should be added to a benzodiazepine. In addition to their potential to produce extrapyramidal side effects, antipsychotics lower seizure threshold, which can be a particular problem during alcohol withdrawal.

ALCOHOL REHABILITATION

Since the 19th century, alcohol rehabilitation has typically been provided in a residential setting and lasts for periods of a month or more. Residential settings include hospital-based rehabilitation programs, freestanding units, and psychiatric units.

Inpatient treatment may be indicated when motivation to continue treatment is weak; when patients are psychotic, depressed, or suicidal; and when there are medical complications. Other factors that also may influence the choice of treatment setting include patients' social stability and the number and severity of their symptoms as well as the ability of programs to respond to individual needs.

BEHAVIORAL THERAPY

Behavioral elements most frequently employed in treatment programs are relapse prevention, social skills and assertiveness training, contingency management, deep muscle relaxation, self-control training, and cognitive restructuring. Behavioral therapists stress the importance of teaching new, adaptive skills to patients who engage in dysfunctional behaviors. These skills include altering conditions that precipitate and reinforce drinking as well as developing alternative ways of coping with persons, events, and feelings that serve to maintain drinking.

With an estimated 87,000 groups in 150 countries, AA is by far the most widely used source of help for drinking problems in the United States and throughout the world. Unfortunately, psychiatrists often refer patients to self-help groups such as AA without adequate consideration of the patient's needs and without adequate monitoring of the patient's response, which amounts to inadequate treatment. Familiarity with AA may help psychiatrists to identify those patients who might reasonably be expected to benefit from this approach. Attendance at AA tends to be correlated with long-term abstinence, but this may be interpreted to reflect motivation for recovery; the type of motivated alcoholic individual who persists with AA might do just as well with other forms of supportive therapy.

Alcoholism creates major stress on the family system by threatening health, interpersonal relations, and the economic functioning of family members. Research has shown a strong association between healthy family functioning and positive outcome after alcoholism treatment.

In addition to specific treatment for alcoholic couples or families, self-help groups for family members of alcoholics have grown substantially. Al-Anon, although not formally affiliated with AA, shares the structure and many tenets of AA's 12 Steps. Al-Anon and AA meetings are often held jointly. Alateen groups, sponsored by Al-Anon for children of alcoholics, are proliferating as well.

Despite the lack of convincing evidence concerning the safety and efficacy of medications to treat alcoholism, more than 90% of physicians in private practice reported their use by their patients. Except for the central role that benzodiazepines play in the treatment of alcohol withdrawal, pharmacotherapy has not yet had a demonstrably large effect on alcoholism treatment.

AVERSIVE DRUGS. Aversive drugs cause an unpleasant reaction when combined with alcohol. Disulfiram (Antabuse) is the most extensively researched aversive medication and the only one approved for use in the United States. It is given in a single daily dose of 125 to 500 mg that binds irreversibly to aldehyde dehydrogenase. When alcohol is consumed, it is metabolized to acetaldehyde, which accumulates because of inhibition of the enzyme that metabolizes it. Elevated levels of acetaldehyde are responsible for the aversive effects associated with the disulfiram-ethanol reaction.

Adverse effects from disulfiram are common. In addition to its effects on aldehyde dehydrogenase, disulfiram inhibits a variety of other enzymes. Disulfiram also reduces clearance rates of a number of medications. Common side effects of disulfiram include drowsiness, lethargy, peripheral neuropathy, hepatotoxic effects, and hypertension.

Although disulfiram has been used in the treatment of alcoholism for many years, the few placebo-controlled studies that have been conducted have not shown the drug to have substantial efficacy. Given the paucity of data supporting the efficacy of disulfiram for the prevention of relapse, we do not generally endorse its use. Whenever disulfiram is prescribed, patients should be warned carefully about its hazards, including the need to avoid over-the-counter preparations with alcohol and drugs that interact adversely with disulfiram as well as the potential for a disulfiram-ethanol reaction to result from alcohol used in food preparation.

TREATMENT OF COMORBID PSYCHIATRIC ILLNESS. A variety of medications have been employed in an effort to improve outcomes in alcoholic patients by treating comorbid psychiatric symptoms and disorders. The use of these medications in alcoholic patients requires careful consideration of the added potential for adverse effects attributable to comorbid medical disorders and the pharmacokinetic effects of short-term and long-term alcohol consumption. With these caveats in mind, indications for the use of these medications in alcoholic patients are similar to those for nonalcoholic populations and can be arrived at only through careful psychiatric diagnosis.

Although depressive symptoms are common early in alcohol withdrawal, they frequently remit spontaneously with time. For depression that persists beyond the period of acute withdrawal, a trial of an antidepressant is probably warranted.

In general, the use of benzodiazepines in alcoholic patients is best limited to the period of detoxification.

Buspirone is a nonbenzodiazepine anxiolytic that may have several advantages: it is less sedating than diazepam or clorazepate, it does not interact with alcohol to impair psychomotor skills, and its potential for abuse is small. When combined with appropriate psychosocial treatment, buspirone appears useful in the treatment of alcoholic patients with persistent anxiety.

Antipsychotics are currently indicated only in alcoholics with a coexistent psychotic disorder or for the treatment of alcoholic hallucinosis. Because of their capacity to lower seizure threshold, antipsychotics should be used with caution in this population.

DRUGS THAT MAY DIRECTLY REDUCE ALCOHOL CONSUMPTION. The most promising agents that directly reduce alcohol consumption are the opiate antagonists (i.e., naltrexone and nalmefene) and the serotonin uptake inhibitors (SUIs) (e.g., citalopram, fluoxetine). Further research is required with naltrexone to determine the optimal dosage, duration of treatment, and concomitant psychosocial treatment strategies. Further research with nalmefene is needed to establish its efficacy in the prevention of relapse in alcoholic patients. The efficacy of the SUIs for this indication also remains to be established.

SPECIAL FEATURES INFLUENCING TREATMENT

Psychiatric Comorbidity

There is considerable evidence that links the outcome of alcoholism treatment to comorbid psychiatric illness. General measures of psychiatric illness as well as the specific diagnoses of drug abuse and dependence, ASPD, and major depressive disorder have been shown to predict poorer outcomes in alcoholic patients.

Demographical Features

ADOLESCENT

Several factors have been associated with better treatment outcome for the adolescent: later onset of problem drinking; pretreatment attendance at school; voluntary entrance into treatment; active parental input; and availability of ancillary adolescent-specific services, including those pertaining to school, recreation, vocational needs, and contraception. Treatment of the adolescent with an alcohol use disorder also requires an appreciation of the importance of modeling, imitation, and peer pressure, which are intrinsic to identity development. The use of age-appropriate support groups (e.g., Alateen) may be particularly useful in this regard.

GERIATRIC

A wide variety of treatment approaches have been shown to be beneficial for the alcoholic elderly, ranging along a continuum of intensity that includes multidisciplinary inpatient treatment programs; outpatient individual therapy, group therapy, or day treatment; and outpatient recovery support groups. Treatment programs with experience in treating the alcoholic elderly are likely to be better able to coordinate rehabilitation with medical and social service providers, including case management and home visits.

GENDER (INCLUDING PREGNANCY)

Special treatment needs of women include information about the effects of substance use on the fetus, parenting skills, couples and family therapy, sober female role models, assertiveness training, and an awareness of sexism and its consequences.

Caffeine Use Disorders

It is important for the psychiatrist to recognize the role of caffeine as a psychoactive substance capable of producing a variety of psychiatric syndromes, despite its pervasive and well-accepted use. In this chapter, five disorders associated with caffeine use are reviewed: caffeine intoxication, caffeine withdrawal, caffeine dependence, caffeine-induced anxiety disorder, and caffeine-induced sleep disorder.

CAFFEINE INTOXICATION

DSM-IV Criteria 305.90

Caffeine Intoxication

A. Recent consumption of caffeine, usually in excess of 250 mg (e.g., more than 2–3 cups of brewed coffee).

B. Five (or more) of the following signs, developing during, or shortly after, caffeine use:

    (1) restlessness

    (2) nervousness

    (3) excitement

    (4) insomnia

    (5) flushed face

    (6) diuresis

    (7) gastrointestinal disturbance

    (8) muscle twitching

    (9) rambling flow of thought and speech

    (10) tachycardia or cardiac arrhythmia

    (11) periods of inexhaustibility

    (12) psychomotor agitation

DSM-IV Criteria 305.90

Caffeine Intoxication *Continued*

C. The symptoms in criterion B cause clinically significant distress or impairment in social, occupational, or
other important areas of functioning.

D. The symptoms are not due to a general medical condition and are not better accounted for by another mental disorder (e.g., an anxiety disorder).

The *Diagnostic and Statistical Manual of Mental Disorders,*
Fourth Edition (DSM-IV) defines caffeine intoxication as a set of
symptoms that develop during or shortly after caffeine use. There
may be two kinds of presentation associated with caffeine intoxication. The first presentation is associated with the *acute* ingestion of
a large amount of caffeine and represents an acute drug overdose
condition. The second presentation is associated with the *chronic*
consumption of large amounts of caffeine and results in a more
complicated presentation.

Despite the long history of recognition of caffeine intoxication,
there is little information available about the prevalence or incidence
of caffeine intoxication either in selected populations or in the
general community.

The symptoms of caffeine intoxication can mimic those of anxiety
and mood disorders, but there has been no evidence to suggest that
patients with these disorders are more likely to have caffeine
intoxication or that patients with caffeine intoxication are more
likely to have other psychiatric disorders.

DIAGNOSIS AND DIFFERENTIAL DIAGNOSIS

In addition to the characteristics of caffeine intoxication noted in
DSM-IV, there have been reports of fever, irritability, tremors,
sensory disturbances and tachypnea, and headaches associated with
cases of caffeine intoxication. Although a wide variety of symptoms
of caffeine intoxication have been reported, the most common signs
and symptoms appear to be anxiety and nervousness, insomnia,
gastrointestinal disturbances, tremors, tachycardia, and psychomotor agitation.

The diagnosis of caffeine intoxication is based on the history and
clinical presentation of the patient, and the extent of caffeine use can
be confirmed by a serum assay of the caffeine level.

Several conditions should be included in the differential diagnosis
of caffeine intoxication (Table 16–1).

In a patient who has caffeine intoxication superimposed on
chronic caffeine use, abrupt termination of all caffeine use may lead
to caffeine withdrawal. Because symptoms of caffeine withdrawal
can partially overlap with symptoms of caffeine intoxication (e.g.,
nervousness and anxiety), the time course of symptom resolution
can be expected to be protracted, lasting several days to a week
or more.

TABLE 16–1	Differential Diagnosis of Caffeine Intoxication

Manic episode
Amphetamine or cocaine intoxication
Sedative, hypnotic or anxiolytic withdrawal
Nicotine withdrawal

Panic disorder
Generalized anxiety disorder
Medication-induced side effect (e.g., akathisia)
Sleep disorders

TREATMENT

The primary approach to the treatment of caffeine intoxication is to teach the patient about the effects of excessive caffeine consumption. In patients who are resistant to accepting the role of caffeine in their presenting symptoms, it may be useful to suggest a trial of caffeine abstinence as both a diagnostic and a potentially therapeutic probe.

CAFFEINE WITHDRAWAL

As for caffeine intoxication, there is a long history of recognition that some people can experience symptoms of caffeine withdrawal. The observation of headaches associated with the cessation of caffeine use has been repeatedly described and is now a well-established characteristic of caffeine withdrawal. Other features of caffeine withdrawal can include sleepiness (drowsiness, yawning), work difficulty (impaired concentration, lassitude, decreased motivation for work), irritability (decreased contentedness, well-being, and self-confidence), decreased sociability (reduced friendliness and talkativeness), influenza-like symptoms (including muscle aches and stiffness, hot or cold spells, nausea or vomiting), and blurred vision.

It is possible to identify certain populations that may be at increased risk for development of caffeine withdrawal or caffeine withdrawal headaches, such as patients with high daily caffeine consumption or patients with a history of frequent headaches.

ASSESSMENT AND COURSE

The key step in establishing a diagnosis of caffeine withdrawal is to determine the history of the person's caffeine consumption (from all

TABLE 16–2	Differential Diagnosis of Caffeine Withdrawal

Initiation or cessation of another medication
Amphetamine or cocaine withdrawal

Other general medical conditions (e.g., migraine headache, viral illness)
Idiopathic drug reactions

dietary sources) and then to establish whether there has been a change in the pattern of the person's caffeine intake. Caffeine withdrawal is probably more common than is generally recognized, and it seems that there is a tendency for people to attribute the symptoms of caffeine withdrawal to other causes besides caffeine. Caffeine withdrawal may be particularly common in medical settings in which patients are required to abstain from food and fluids, such as before surgical procedures and certain diagnostic tests. In addition, caffeine withdrawal may occur in settings in which the use of caffeine-containing products is restricted or banned, such as inpatient psychiatric wards. Postoperative headache has been shown to be associated with the patient's history of caffeine consumption.

Many general medical conditions can have signs and symptoms that are similar to those found in caffeine withdrawal. Differential diagnoses could include conditions as diverse as viral illnesses; sinus conditions; other types of headaches, such as migraine and tension; other drug withdrawal states, such as amphetamine or cocaine withdrawal; and idiopathic drug reactions (Table 16–2).

COURSE AND NATURAL HISTORY (PROGNOSIS)

Caffeine withdrawal generally begins within 12 to 24 hours after discontinuation of caffeine use. The peak of caffeine withdrawal generally occurs within 24 to 48 hours, and the duration of caffeine withdrawal is generally 2 days to about 1 week. There is considerable variability, both between people and within the same person across episodes, in the manifestations, time course, and severity of caffeine withdrawal. No studies have examined the possibility of a protracted caffeine withdrawal syndrome. Human and laboratory animal studies of caffeine withdrawal are reviewed elsewhere.

TREATMENT

If the medical recommendation is made to eliminate or substantially reduce caffeine consumption, it may be useful to recommend a tapering dose schedule rather than abrupt discontinuation. During caffeine tapering, it may be useful for patients to consume extra noncaffeinated fluids, to avoid herbal preparations that contain caffeine or other psychoactive drugs, to avoid the use of anxiolytics, and to maintain a diary throughout the time they are progressively decreasing their caffeine use to monitor their progress. Abrupt cessation of caffeine should be avoided to minimize withdrawal symptoms and increase the likelihood of long-term compliance with the dietary change.

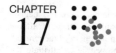

Cannabis-Related Disorders

CANNABIS-RELATED DISORDERS

As with other substances of abuse, the *Diagnostic and Statistical Manual of Mental Disorders,* Fourth Edition (DSM-IV) distinguishes a number of different cannabis-related diagnoses. These fall into two basic groups. First are disorders resulting from episodic or chronic cannabis intoxification, which include cannabis abuse and cannabis dependence. The second set includes cannabis intoxication and psychiatric syndromes presumed to be induced by cannabis. These include cannabis intoxication delirium, cannabis-induced psychotic disorder, and cannabis-induced anxiety disorder.

EPIDEMIOLOGY

Cannabis Use Disorders

Cannabis is probably the most commonly used illicit substance in the world, with an estimated 200 to 300 million regular users. In the United States, cannabis is generally thought to be the most widely used illicit drug, although some studies report that cocaine is competing with it on some measures of frequency of use.

Cannabis use disorders are frequently comorbid with other substance abuse disorders. Surveys of psychiatric populations with mixed Axis I diagnoses, but not panic disorder, have found a high prevalence of cannabis use. Cannabis use, abuse, and dependence are also commonly comorbid with conduct disorder in children and adolescents and with antisocial personality disorder in adults.

Cannabis-Induced Disorders

No formal epidemiological data exist regarding the prevalence of cannabis intoxication delirium, cannabis-induced psychotic disorder, or cannabis-induced anxiety disorder. In fact, it is not entirely certain that any of these three entities actually occur in individuals who are free of preexisting DSM-IV Axis I disorders.

DIAGNOSIS

Cannabis-Related Disorders

To diagnose any of the cannabis-related disorders, it is important to obtain a detailed history of the individual's pattern of substance abuse (including abuse not only of cannabis but of other substances) and to attempt to substantiate this report with toxicology screening for drugs of abuse. Individuals who smoke cannabis regularly can have substantial accumulations of Δ^9- or Δ^9- trans-tetrahydrocannabinol (THC) in their fat stores. Thus, for weeks after cessation of smoking, detectable levels of cannabinoids may be found in urine. However, a positive response on toxicology screening for cannabinoids cannot establish any of the cannabis-related diagnoses; it is useful only as an indicator that these diagnoses should be considered.

Cannabis Dependence

This diagnosis cannot be made without obtaining a history that the cannabis use is impairing the patient's ability to function, either physically or psychologically. Areas to inquire about include the patient's performance at work, ability to carry out social and family obligations, and physical health. It is also important to find out how much of the patient's time is spent on cannabis-related activities and whether the patient has tried unsuccessfully to stop or cut down on use in the past.

Individuals with cannabis dependence frequently report spending long periods acquiring and using the drug; frequent intoxication at times when it interferes with daily activities (driving a motor vehicle or attending classes in school); and persistence of cannabis use despite psychological impairment (i.e., impaired academic function), physical impairment (i.e., bronchitis), or adverse experiences with family members or other individuals who disapprove of use.

This diagnosis will most often be made in patients who present with other psychiatric problems, but cannabis dependence is probably underdiagnosed in both psychiatric and general medical populations because it is not considered.

The diagnosis of cannabis dependence may suggest that the individual has been abusing the drug regularly for a long enough time to result in tolerance for many effects of cannabis and to experience an unpleasant withdrawal state if use is discontinued (although neither tolerance nor withdrawal is necessary for the diagnosis). The use must be compulsive, in that the individual cannot stop using the drug even if she or he perceives that it is having negative effects and wants to stop.

Cannabis Abuse

The criteria for this diagnosis are similar to those for cannabis dependence. The individual's use of cannabis must have resulted in problems performing at school or work, interpersonal difficulties, unsafe behaviors such as driving a motor vehicle while intoxicated, health problems, or legal difficulties, and the individual must have continued to use cannabis despite these problems. The difference is that this diagnosis should be used when the individual's use of cannabis has not been regular, frequent, long-standing, or compulsive and the individual has not developed tolerance or the potential for a withdrawal state. As with cannabis dependence, it is a diagnosis unlikely to be made unless some other condition or circumstance brings the individual to medical attention.

Cannabis Intoxication

DSM-IV Criteria 292.89

Cannabis Intoxication

A. Recent use of cannabis.

B. Clinically significant maladaptive behavioral or psychological changes (e.g., impaired motor coordination, euphoria, anxiety, sensation of slowed time, impaired judgment, social withdrawal) that developed during, or shortly after, cannabis use.

C. Two (or more) of the following signs, developing within 2 hours of cannabis use:

(1) conjunctival injection

(2) increased appetite

(3) dry mouth

(4) tachycardia

D. The symptoms are not due to a general medical condition and are not better accounted for by another mental disorder.

Specify if:

With perceptual disturbances

Four criteria are necessary to make this diagnosis. First, recent use of cannabis must be established. This cannot be done with toxicology screening because the result may be negative after a single episode of smoking or, alternatively, may be positive even if the individual has not used the drug for a time much longer than the period of intoxication. Second, the patient must experience symptoms of cannabis use that are described in DSM-IV as being "clinically significant maladaptive behavioral or psychological changes" and that are temporally related to the cannabis use. Third, the patient must exhibit some physical signs of cannabis use. DSM-IV requires the patient to have at least two of four signs—conjunctival injection, increased appetite, dry mouth, and tachycardia—within 2 hours of cannabis use. Fourth, symptoms cannot be accounted for by a general medical condition or another mental disorder.

Common physiological effects of cannabis intoxication include hypertension, thirst, decreased libido, constipation, decreased intraocular pressure, irritation of the bronchial mucosa from smoking, mild bronchoconstriction followed by bronchodilation, ataxia, impaired coordination, and increased reaction time. At high doses, drowsiness, bradycardia, hypotension, peripheral vasoconstriction, hypothermia, ptosis, and pupillary constriction have been described.

Common psychological effects include impaired memory (especially short-term memory); perceptual and sensory distortions; disturbance in time perception; euphoria and dysphoria; restlessness; depersonalization; derealization; panic reactions; paranoid ideation; and impaired performance on a wide variety of cognitive, perceptual, and psychomotor tasks.

There is considerable disagreement as to how long the residual effects of intoxication last; estimates range from a few hours to more than 6 weeks. Many studies have shown that there is at least some hangover from acute intoxication, with impairment on neuropsychological testing and on tests such as driving simulators and flight simulators persisting for 24 to a maximum of 48 hours after intoxication.

Cannabis Intoxication Delirium

If cannabis intoxication delirium does occur in neurologically intact individuals, it is probably a rare complication. In a patient with delirium, even if recent cannabis use has been reported, a full diagnostic work-up should be performed to rule out a concomitant neurological condition.

Cannabis-Induced Psychotic Disorder

There are two diagnoses allocated to this entity, one featuring delusions, the other hallucinations. The diagnosis of this disorder is readily made in individuals who have psychotic symptoms (as defined in DSM-IV) that appear immediately after ingestion of cannabis. However, a careful history is required to establish whether the individual has displayed a previous psychotic disorder before cannabis use (as is often the case in such situations) or whether the symptoms arose de novo after cannabis consumption. There is little evidence that cannabis-induced psychotic disorders can arise in previously asymptomatic individuals. As with cannabis-induced psychotic disorders, there is little evidence of cannabis-induced anxiety disorders in individuals without a preexisting Axis I disorder.

A diagnostic decision tree is presented in Figure 17–1.

OVERALL GOALS OF TREATMENT

Cannabis Use Disorders

For all cannabis-related disorders, the first stage of treatment aims to achieve abstinence from cannabis use. Little systematic study of treatment of cannabis abuse or dependence exists, however, because individuals with these disorders rarely independently seek treatment.

Most of the literature on treatment is directed at substance abuse in general and not at cannabis in particular. Fortunately, however, most of the treatment models are probably applicable to cannabis use disorders. Similarities include the treatment goal of attaining abstinence and the importance of a good physician-patient relationship.

One difference is the increased importance of toxicology screening for other drugs of abuse at the initiation of cannabis abuse

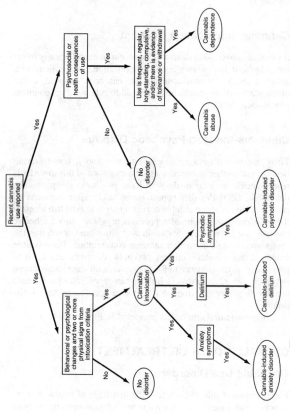

Figure 17–1 *Diagnostic decision tree for cannabis use disorders.*

treatment. This is more important with cannabis than with other drugs of abuse because cannabis is often only one of the substances used, and specific treatment may be indicated for other substances. A second difference may occur during the process of detoxification. Unlike most other substances of abuse, cannabis continues to persist in the fat stores of the body for a long time after the last use. One author has hypothesized that slow release of cannabinoids from fatty tissue may produce the phenomenon of flashbacks, during which the user experiences phenomena like those experienced during acute intoxication, such as perceptual disturbances. This persistence of cannabinoids in the body has also been suggested to cause symptoms of depression and anxiety.

There is some evidence that heavy users of cannabis may experience a withdrawal state during detoxification. This is usually mild and requires no treatment. Because the withdrawal state is not medically dangerous, like that of alcohol, or severe, like that of opioids, most patients do not require inpatient detoxification.

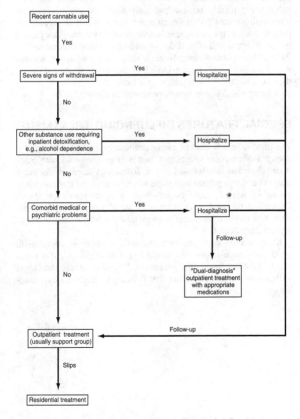

Note: Most of these patients will not be commitable and will have to voluntarily seek treatment

Figure 17–2 *Treatment decision tree for cannabis use disorders.*

For most individuals with cannabis abuse or dependence, outpatient treatment is sufficient. Several groups of patients tend to do better with an initial period of inpatient hospitalization: 1) patients who would not stop cannabis use as outpatients because they are in denial and require a radical form of intervention to help them acknowledge the severity of their problem; 2) patients addicted to other drugs besides cannabis, such as alcohol or opiates, who generally need an inpatient stay to monitor their detoxification; and 3) patients with comorbid medical or psychiatric problems, who may warrant inpatient treatment so that the comorbid conditions can be treated.

The second stage in treatment is maintenance of abstinence. The strategies used for this are essentially the same ones used for the maintenance treatment of any substance abuser and are discussed in the next section.

Cannabis-Induced Disorders

Symptoms of delirium, psychosis, or anxiety associated with cannabis use typically resolve promptly after the period of acute intoxication is past. No treatment is necessary other than keeping the patient safe and providing reassurance that the symptoms are caused by the drug and will stop. If the symptoms continue after more than 24 to 48 hours of abstinence from the drug, the possibility of another Axis I diagnosis must be considered. In such cases, treatment should then be directed at the primary Axis I disorder.

A treatment decision tree is presented in Figure 17–2.

SPECIAL FEATURES INFLUENCING TREATMENT

The most salient feature of cannabis abuse or dependence is that it does not often occur in isolation and is often comorbid with other Axis I disorders as discussed earlier. Toxicology screening for other drugs of abuse is particularly imperative, because the most common comorbid Axis I disorders are other types of substance abuse. Depending on what other substances are abused, it may be more important to direct treatment at them, treating the cannabis abuse as a secondary condition.

Many studies have shown that cannabis abuse is common in psychiatric populations with mixed Axis I disorders. Another treatment situation frequently encountered is that of an individual with a known Axis I disorder that is being exacerbated by cannabis use.

Cocaine Use Disorders

Cocaine, a central nervous system stimulant produced by the coca plant, is consumed in several preparations. Cocaine hydrochloride powder is usually sniffed through the nostrils, or it may be mixed in water and injected intravenously. Cocaine hydrochloride powder is also commonly heated ("cooked up") with baking soda and water to precipitate a gel-like substance that can be smoked ("free-basing"). "Crack" cocaine is a precooked form of cocaine alkaloid that is sold on the street as small "rocks." Abundant supplies and falling prices for cocaine have contributed greatly to the prevalence of cocaine abuse and dependence as well as other related cocaine use disorders.

Cocaine intoxication produces a state of intense euphoria that is a powerful reinforcer and can lead to the development of cocaine abuse in many individuals, although only 10% to 15% of those who try cocaine by the intranasal route of administration go on to cocaine abuse or cocaine dependence. The route of administration is strongly correlated with the development of cocaine abuse and dependence, in that the intravenous and smoked routes of administration allow rapid transport of the drug to the brain, producing intense effects that are short-lived. Rapid tolerance to euphoric effects occurs, and plasma concentrations are not correlated with peak euphoria, which produces a need for frequent dosing to regain euphoric effects (binge use) and places the cocaine abuser at risk for medical and psychiatric complications of cocaine abuse.

Cocaine abuse is characterized by a maladaptive pattern of substance use demonstrated by recurrent and significant adverse consequences related to repeated drug use. Cocaine dependence is characterized by a more pervasive pattern of frequent cocaine use and a chronic cycle of psychosocial problems.

Whereas cocaine is not physiologically addicting, the psychological addiction is powerful and can completely dominate the life of the cocaine abuser. Binge use of cocaine may be followed by what has been described as a mild withdrawal syndrome characterized by dysphoria and anhedonia, which may resemble a depressive disorder and, in some cases, may require emergent psychiatric treatment.

EPIDEMIOLOGY

The National Household Survey on Drug Abuse conducted in 1991 found that the prevalence of lifetime cocaine use in persons 12 years of age and older was 11.5%. The highest prevalence (25.8%) of cocaine use occurred in adults aged 26 to 34 years, followed by young adults aged 18 to 25 years (17.9%).

Sex Differences in Cocaine Abuse

The prevalence of substance abuse in treatment programs and in the community has been reported to be as much as four times as high in men as in women. However, substance abuse is the second most common psychiatric disorder in women aged 18 to 24 years. The risks of cocaine and other substance abuse are significant not only for women but for their unborn children, who are at risk for neuropsychological sequelae secondary to prenatal exposure. Abuse and neglect of children are common consequences of parental addiction.

Relationship of Psychiatric Disorders to Cocaine Abuse

Several studies have documented the high rate of comorbid psychiatric disorders in cocaine abusers entering treatment. These disorders include mood disorders: major depression, bipolar disorders, attention-deficit/hyperactivity disorder, anxiety disorders, and antisocial personality disorder. In general, mood disorders temporally follow the onset of cocaine abuse in patients presenting for treatment; attention-deficit/hyperactivity disorder and antisocial personality disorder precede the onset of drug abuse.[13]

COURSE AND NATURAL HISTORY

Cocaine produces a sense of intensified pleasure in most activities and a heightened sense of alertness and well-being. Anxiety and social inhibition are decreased. Energy, self-esteem, and self-perception of ability are increased. There is enhancement of emotion and sexual feeling. Pleasurable experiences, although heightened, are not distorted, and hallucinations are usually absent. The person engaging in low-dose cocaine use often receives positive feedback from others responding to the user's increased energy and enthusiasm. This, in combination with the euphoria experienced by the user, can be reinforcing, and cocaine use is perceived as free of any adverse consequences. Cocaine users quickly learn that higher doses are associated with intensified and prolonged euphoria, which results in increasing use of the drug.

The effects of cocaine are similar to those of amphetamine; the main difference in terms of abuse liability is in cocaine's much shorter duration of action. The phenomenon explains the "half-life" of cocaine-induced euphoria, which is approximately 45 minutes after intranasal use as well as characteristic binge use in which cocaine is readministered during short intervals. During binge use, the drug may be administered as frequently as every 10 minutes, resulting in rapid mood changes. Cocaine binges can last as long as 7 days, although the average length is 12 hours.

The onset of a binge pattern of cocaine use usually results in a significant level of impairment that may be manifested by neglect of personal needs, neglect of family and job responsibilities, initiation of illegal activities necessary to support the cocaine use, and engagement in irresponsible behaviors as a result of drug intoxication or acute abstinence symptoms. One or more of these issues is the usual precipitant to seeking treatment. The cocaine abuser is likely to be ambivalent about the need for treatment, and the treatment dropout rate is high (ranging from 38% to 73%); dropout usually occurs in the early phase of treatment (during the initial evaluation process).

Newly abstinent cocaine abusers can be expected to experience a triphasic abstinence pattern that includes a "crash" period lasting several hours to several days; a withdrawal period characterized by minor depressive symptoms, which lasts 2 to 10 weeks; and an extinction phase, which lasts indefinitely and is characterized by intermittent drug craving that becomes more manageable with continued abstinence.

Cocaine patients are at high risk for relapse, particularly in the first 3 months of treatment. This results from ongoing psychosocial stressors caused or exacerbated by cocaine abuse and from the lack of a good repertoire of coping skills necessary to avoid cocaine abuse, which take time to acquire in the treatment process.

Multiple treatments may be required for patients with cocaine dependence. These may include inpatient treatment for medical or psychiatric complications of the cocaine abuse, partial hospital programs, self-help groups, psychotherapy (usually group or family therapy for patients with primary cocaine use disorders), or some combination of these treatments according to the presentation of the patient.

NEUROBIOLOGICAL CHANGES RELATED TO LONG-TERM COCAINE USE

High-dose cocaine use for extended periods appears to result in sustained neurophysiological changes in brain systems that regulate psychological processes, specifically pleasure and hedonic responsivity. This has been postulated to underlie a physiological addiction to cocaine with associated withdrawal phenomena that are manifested clinically as a psychological syndrome.

DIAGNOSIS OF COCAINE USE DISORDERS

The initial evaluation period should include the collection of a complete history of all substance abuse, which is essential to accurate diagnosis and appropriate treatment. A diagnostic decision tree for cocaine use disorders is shown in Figure 18–1. The history includes the circumstances under which each drug was used, the psychoactive effects sought and obtained, the route of administration, and the frequency and amount of each drug used. Cocaine abusers frequently abuse other drugs and alcohol to enhance euphoria or to alleviate dysphoric effects associated with cocaine abuse (agitation, paranoia).

A careful psychiatric history with particular attention to onset of psychiatric symptoms in relation to drug use is essential. The determination of a premorbid psychiatric illness is critical to providing appropriate treatment. For persons in whom substance abuse is an attempt to self-medicate an underlying mental illness, the introduction of psychotropic medication in conjunction with ongoing psychotherapy may terminate illicit drug use.

A complete physical examination is necessary to determine whether medical complications of substance abuse are present.

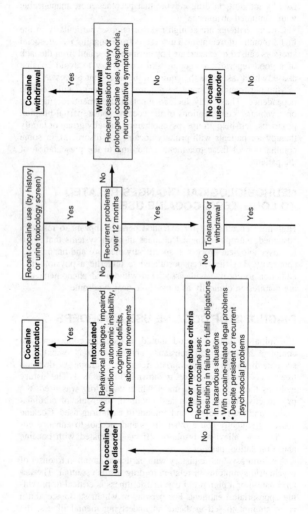

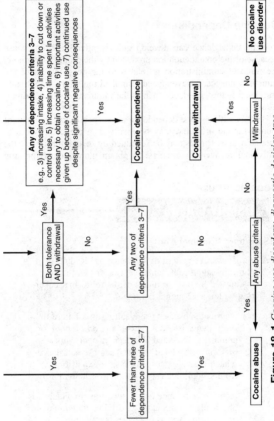

Figure 18–1 *Cocaine use disorders: diagnostic decision tree.*

177

Common medical problems seen in cocaine abusers include poor nutrition; vitamin deficiencies; anemia; human immunodeficiency virus infection; sexually transmitted diseases; and complications of intravenous drug use, including endocarditis, abscesses, cellulitis, and hepatitis. The evaluation should include blood studies to further define abnormalities and toxicological analysis of a urine specimen.

Cocaine Dependence

Cocaine dependence can develop quickly after initiation of use because of the potent euphoria produced by the drug. Furthermore, the route of administration is related to the development of cocaine dependence; intravenous and smoked routes are more highly correlated with dependence than is the intranasal route of administration.

Persons with cocaine dependence often spend large amounts of money for the drug and may be involved in illegal activities to obtain cocaine. Binges may be separated by several days while the individual recovers or attempts to obtain more money for drug

Cocaine Abuse

DSM-IV Criteria 305.60

Substance (Cocaine) Abuse

A. A maladaptive pattern of substance use leading to clinically significant impairment or distress, as manifested by one (or more) of the following, occurring within a 12-month period:

 (1) recurrent substance use resulting in a failure to fulfill major role obligations at work, school, or home (e.g., repeated absences or poor work performance related to substance use; substance-related absences, suspensions, or expulsions from school; neglect of children or household)

 (2) recurrent substance use in situations in which it is physically hazardous (e.g., driving an automobile or operating a machine when impaired by substance use)

 (3) recurrent substance-related legal problems (e.g., arrests for substance-related disorderly conduct)

 (4) continued substance use despite having persistent or recurrent social or interpersonal problems caused or exacerbated by the effects of the substance (e.g., arguments with spouse about consequences of intoxication, physical fights)

B. The symptoms have never met the criteria for substance dependence for this class of substance.

purchase. Obligations such as work and childcare may be neglected. Tolerance quickly develops, resulting in larger amounts of drug use with time. This is often associated with mental or physical complications of use including paranoia, aggressive behavior, anxiety and agitation, depression, and weight loss. Withdrawal symptoms, most prominently dysphoric mood, may be seen but are usually short-lived and clear within several days after termination of drug use. The intensity and frequency of use are less in cocaine abuse than in cocaine dependence. Episodes of abuse may occur around paydays or special occasions and may be characterized by brief periods (hours to days) of high-dose binge use followed by longer periods of abstinence or nonproblem use.

Cocaine Intoxication

DSM-IV Criteria 292.69

Cocaine Intoxication

A. Recent use of cocaine.

B. Clinically significant maladaptive behavioral or psychological changes (e.g., euphoria or affective blunting; changes in sociability; hypervigilance; interpersonal sensitivity; anxiety, tension, or anger; stereotyped behaviors; impaired judgment; or impaired social or occupational functioning) that developed during, or shortly after, use of cocaine.

C. Two (or more) of the following, developing during, or shortly after, cocaine use:

   (1) tachycardia or bradycardia

   (2) pupillary dilation

   (3) elevated or lowered blood pressure

   (4) perspiration or chills

   (5) nausea or vomiting

   (6) evidence of weight loss

   (7) psychomotor agitation or retardation

   (8) muscular weakness, respiratory depression, chest pain, or cardiac arrhythmias

   (9) confusion, seizure, dyskinesias, dystonias, or coma

D. The symptoms are not due to a general medical condition and are not better accounted for by another mental disorder.

Specify if:

With perceptual disturbances

The clinical effects of cocaine intoxication are characterized initially by euphoria (a high feeling) and also include agitation, anxiety, irritability or affective lability, grandiosity, impaired judgment, increased psychomotor activity, hypervigilance or paranoia, and hallucinations (visual, auditory, or tactile). Physical symptoms that accompany cocaine intoxication include hypertension, tachycardia, pupillary dilation, nausea, vomiting, tremor, diaphoresis, chest pain, arrhythmia, confusion, seizures, dyskinetic movements, dystonia, and, in severe cases, coma. These effects are more frequently seen in high-dose binge users of cocaine. Cardiovascular effects are probably a result of sympathomimetic properties of cocaine (i.e., release of norepinephrine and blockade of norepinephrine reuptake).

Cocaine Withdrawal

DSM-IV Criteria 292.0

Cocaine Withdrawal

A. Cessation of (or reduction in) cocaine use that has been heavy and prolonged.

B. Dysphoric mood and two (or more) of the following physiological changes, developing within a few hours to several days after criterion A:

   (1) fatigue

   (2) vivid, unpleasant dreams

   (3) insomnia or hypersomnia

   (4) increased appetite

   (5) psychomotor retardation or agitation

C. The symptoms in criterion B cause clinically significant distress or impairment in social, occupational, or other important areas of functioning.

D. The symptoms are not due to a general medical condition and are not better accounted for by another mental disorder.

Cocaine withdrawal develops within a few hours to a few days after stopping or reducing cocaine use that has been heavy and prolonged. The syndrome is characterized by dysphoria and two or more physiological changes including fatigue, vivid and unpleasant dreams, insomnia or hypersomnia, increased appetite, and psychomotor agitation or retardation. Anhedonia and craving for cocaine can be a part of the withdrawal syndrome. Depression and suicidal ideation are the most serious complications and require individualized assessment and treatment. The syndrome may last up to several days but generally resolves without treatment.

The *Diagnostic and Statistical Manual of Mental Disorders,* Fourth Edition (DSM-IV) also specifies additional cocaine-induced disorders described in other diagnostic groupings with which they share phenomenology. These include cocaine intoxication delirium, cocaine-induced psychotic disorder, cocaine-induced mood disorder, cocaine-induced anxiety disorder, cocaine-induced sleep disorder, and cocaine-induced sexual dysfunction. These disorders are diagnosed only when symptoms are in excess of those usually associated with cocaine intoxication or cocaine withdrawal and therefore warrant independent clinical attention.

Medical Complications of Cocaine Abuse

Cardiac toxicity is a leading cause of morbidity and mortality associated with cocaine use. The risk of myocardial infarct is well established in cocaine use and is not related to dose or route of administration. The risk of cocaine-related cardiac disorders is also not restricted to those with underlying coronary artery disease. However, conditions that place individuals at risk for coronary events, including hypercholesterolemia, coronary artery disease, myocarditis, or variations in coronary artery anatomy, increase the risk for coronary events during cocaine use.

Cocaine increases both heart rate and blood pressure through its ability to indirectly increase sympathetic stimulation by blocking norepinephrine reuptake at adrenergic nerve endings. Cocaine also produces vasoconstriction of small vessels, a characteristic that contributed to its popularity as a local anesthetic agent. These properties are thought to contribute to myocardial infarct and associated malignant arrhythmias by suddenly increasing myocardial oxygen demands with resultant ischemia.

Cocaine use may produce cardiac dysrhythmias through catecholaminergic effects that increase β-adrenergic stimulation of the myocardium. Cocaine-associated arrhythmias include sinus tachycardia, ventricular premature contractions, ventricular tachycardia and fibrillation, and asystole.

Cerebral infarct, subarachnoid hemorrhage, intraparenchymal hemorrhage, and intraventricular hemorrhage have been observed as acute complications of cocaine use. The physiological etiology of these events appears to be related to adrenergic stimulation resulting in a sudden surge in blood pressure. Additional risk would be encountered by a cocaine user with an arteriovenous malformation or cerebral artery aneurysm.

Seizures were one of the earliest known complications of cocaine abuse. Cocaine produces hyperpyrexia, which in combination with its effects on neurotransmitters may contribute to development of seizures. Seizures may occur as a primary effect of cocaine owing to its ability to lower the seizure threshold or may be secondary to other central nervous system or cardiac events precipitated by cocaine use.

The major medical complications of cocaine abuse are summarized in Table 18–1.

TABLE 18–1	Major Medical Complications Associated with Cocaine Abuse

Cardiac
Myocardial infarct
Arrhythmias
Cardiomyopathy

Pulmonary
Pneumonitis (associated with smoked cocaine)
Pulmonary edema

Central Nervous System
Hyperpyrexia
Seizure
Cerebral infarct
Subarachnoid hemorrhage
Intraparenchymal hemorrhage
Intraventricular hemorrhage

Additional Complications of Intravenous Use
Infectious diseases (human immunodeficiency virus infection, hepatitis)
Endocarditis
Cellulitis
Abscesses

MANAGEMENT OF COCAINE ABUSE AND DEPENDENCE

The two primary goals of cocaine treatment are 1) the initiation of abstinence through disruption of binge cycles and 2) the prevention of relapse. Treatment planning to achieve these goals must be considered in the context of the stage of the cocaine abstinence syndrome in which the patient presents. Initial assessment to determine the presenting stage is necessary to determine the level of care needed (inpatient or outpatient treatment) and other psychiatric and medical considerations important to the development of the treatment plan.

The majority of cocaine abusers are most appropriately treated in an outpatient setting. Outpatient treatment may vary by provider but generally includes multiple weekly contacts, because less frequent contact is not effective in the initiation or maintenance of abstinence. These sessions consist of some combination of individual drug counseling, peer support groups, family or couples therapy, urine monitoring, education sessions, psychotherapy, and psychiatric treatment that may include pharmacotherapy for cocaine addiction or comorbid psychiatric disorders. Inpatient treatment is reserved for those who have been refractory to outpatient treatment, whose compulsive use of cocaine represents an imminent danger, who have other comorbid psychiatric disorders, who are dependent on more than one substance and require monitored detoxification, who have severe withdrawal symptoms, or who lack social supports and resources necessary to initiate successful outpatient treatment.

Cocaine Abstinence Syndrome

The cocaine abstinence syndrome is described as consisting of three consecutive phases: crash, withdrawal, and extinction. Each phase may be characterized in part by psychiatric symptoms, which are based on individual susceptibility and the extent of drug use.

The crash is characterized by extreme exhaustion after a binge. Initial depression, agitation, and anxiety are a common experience, followed by craving for sleep. Prolonged hypersomnolence and hyperphagia are followed by a return to normal mood, although some dysphoria may remain. Clinical management consists of observation because suicidal ideation is not uncommon. Crash symptoms resemble those of major depression, which must be excluded by observation for several days of abstinence.

Cocaine withdrawal is marked by decreased energy, lack of interest, and anhedonia. These symptoms fluctuate and are not severe enough to meet diagnostic criteria for an affective disorder. However, this subjective state experienced by the cocaine abuser and contrasted with vivid memories of cocaine-induced euphoria constitutes a strong inducement to additional cocaine use. It is during this time that relapse is most likely. Withdrawal symptoms generally diminish during 2 to 10 weeks if abstinence is maintained.

The withdrawal phase is followed by extinction, an indefinite period during which evoked craving can occur, placing the individual at increased risk for relapse. Craving is evoked by moods, people, locations, or objects associated with cocaine use (money, white powder, pipes, mirrors, or syringes) that act as cues to conditioned associations with drug use and drug-induced euphoria. If these conditional cues fail to initiate cocaine use, then the cues lose their potency in time and craving becomes progressively less intense until extinction of craving occurs.

The early recovery phase of treatment varies in duration from 2 to 12 months and is characterized by multiple weekly contacts and participation in therapeutic modalities with the goal of initiation and maintenance of abstinence. The focus during early recovery should be on relapse prevention and development of new and adaptive coping skills, healthy relationships, and lifestyle changes that will facilitate abstinence. Relapses are common during early recovery.

Long-term treatment is characterized by a reduced frequency of contact (weekly group or individual therapy sessions). The focus should be on maintaining a commitment to abstinence, addressing renewed denial, and improving interpersonal skills. Participation in self-help groups should continue to be encouraged. Self-help groups based on 12-step principles encourage patients to continue viewing themselves as addicts in recovery—a cognitive structuring that many recovering drug abusers find helpful in maintaining sobriety.

PHARMACOTHERAPY FOR COCAINE ABUSE

Pharmacotherapy for the treatment of cocaine abuse is best reserved for the patient with severe dependence who has not responded to other less intensive interventions. A variety of agents have been used for treatment of cocaine addiction, but research data supporting their use are limited, and conflicting results have been obtained in some instances. Controlled trials are lacking in this area. More work is needed to determine which subgroups of cocaine abusers are most appropriate for pharmacotherapy and what agents will provide the greatest clinical benefit and least risk to patients.

Various pharmacotherapies have been used for the treatment of cocaine abuse. The following agents have been used: 1) Dopaminergic agents such as amantadine, 2) Antidepressants such as desipramine or serotoninergic drugs (i.e., fluoxetine), and 3) naltrexone. There are no agents approved by the U.S. Food and Drug Administration for the treatment of cocaine abuse. Therefore, careful consideration must be given to the risks and benefits of treatment with any pharmacological agent.

Whom to Treat

Pharmacotherapy should be considered for three categories of patients: 1) patients with other comorbid psychiatric disorders, 2) patients identified with significant general medical illnesses or medical risks from continued cocaine abuse (such as complications of intravenous drug abuse), and 3) patients in whom heavy cocaine use has resulted in neuroadaptation. In this last category are patients who use cocaine by a high-intensity route, such as intravenous injection or freebase smoking. Such patients use large amounts of cocaine at high frequency and experience rapid changes in brain cocaine concentration, which probably results in neurotransmitter deficits and alterations in receptor numbers. The reversal of such alterations is a rationale for pharmacotherapy for cocaine abuse.

When to Treat

Decisions regarding when to initiate and to discontinue pharmacotherapy should be based on four factors, which include 1) the phase of recovery; 2) the precipitant to treatment, including psychiatric comorbidity; 3) associated psychosocial problems; and 4) relapse potential. Those who have been refractory to nonpharmacological therapies in the past should also be considered candidates for pharmacotherapy.

Where to Treat

Cocaine abusers require inpatient hospitalization under some circumstances. The suicidal or psychotic patient requires inpatient treatment for stabilization. Cocaine abusers who are unable to break the cycle of heavy cocaine use often benefit from inpatient treatment, which removes them from the environment in which the heavy cocaine use was occurring. Pharmacotherapy initiated during inpatient hospitalization provides an opportunity to stabilize the patient with the medication while minimizing the risk of cocaine use, which might result in an adverse interaction between the medication and cocaine.

Relapse prevention is an outpatient treatment goal. The use of medication as part of a treatment plan is a common practice in an outpatient setting. When medications are started with outpatient cocaine abusers, it is important to educate them about possible adverse interactions between the medication and cocaine. For example, tricyclic antidepressants such as desipramine block the reuptake of catecholamines, as does cocaine. Therefore, one possible result of an interaction between desipramine and cocaine is hypertension. Clearly, inpatient hospitalization provides the safest means by which to initiate pharmacotherapy for cocaine abuse. However, outpatient medication induction is frequently practiced and has not been associated with any major medical complications to date.

PSYCHIATRIC COMORBIDITY

Treatment-seeking cocaine abusers have significant rates of psychiatric disorders. Cocaine abuse may adversely affect the psychiatric disorder, with symptoms of psychosis or suicidal ideation occurring or worsening during the course of cocaine use. The possibility that cocaine may induce or exacerbate depression has also been suggested. Patients with underlying psychotic disorders may be exquisitely sensitive to small doses of cocaine, which acutely worsens their psychiatric illness and requires pharmacological management and hospitalization. Patients with comorbid psychiatric disorders complicated by substance abuse often require increased doses of psychotropic medications to control symptoms.

A major psychiatric disorder seen in cocaine abusers is antisocial personality disorder. Identification of this disorder is important because it is associated with poor prognostic treatment outcome in cocaine abusers. There is no clear indication for use of pharmacotherapy in patients with antisocial personality disorder. In considering pharmacotherapy, it is best to stabilize such patients for several weeks and monitor symptoms carefully to determine need for medication treatment.

Cocaine abuse is widely recognized as a significant clinical problem in patients with schizophrenia. Cocaine use may hasten the onset of a psychotic disorder in a vulnerable patient and may exacerbate the course of the illness by precipitating psychotic relapse or by causing depression, anxiety, insomnia, agitation, or aggressiveness.

Phencyclidine Use Disorders

Phencyclidine (1-(1-phenylcyclohexyl)piperidine, PCP) was developed as a general anesthetic agent in the 1950s under the brand name Sernyl. The drug was considered physiologically promising because of its lack of respiratory and cardiovascular depressant effects.

Approximately 50% of patients anesthetized with PCP developed behavioral syndromes including agitation and hallucinations during emergence from anesthesia. A substantial number of subjects developed postoperative psychotic reactions, which in some cases persisted up to 10 days. As a result, after 1965, PCP was limited to veterinary applications.

Despite its well-documented aversive and disruptive behavioral effects, PCP emerged during the 1970s as a popular drug of abuse,

TABLE 19–1	Street Names for Phencyclidine and Mixtures
Phencyclidine	**Phencyclidine Mixtures and Analogues**
Angel dust	Beam me up Scottie (crack dipped in PCP)
Animal trank	
Baby doll	Blunt (marijuana and PCP in cigar wrapper)
Black whack	
Butt naked	Love boat (marijuana dipped in PCP)
Devil's dust	Peanut butter (PCP mixed in peanut butter)
Elephant tranquilizer	
Embalming fluid	Special K (ketamine)
Gorilla biscuits	Tragic magic (crack dipped in PCP)
Heaven	
Hog	
Jet fuel	
Mad dog	
Peace pill	
Rocket fuel	
Talk to the angels	
Yellow fever	
Zombie weed	

increasing in popularity to the point that in 1979, 13% of high-school seniors had tried it. Surveys of street drug samples indicate that PCP is sold under many street names (Table 19–1) and frequently combined with or misrepresented as other substances.

In recent years, indicators of PCP use have remained generally low. However, localized increases have been observed, in some cases associated with the use of new dosage forms (in particular, the use of "blunts," cigars filled with PCP-impregnated marijuana).

DIAGNOSIS AND DIFFERENTIAL DIAGNOSIS

DSM-IV Criteria 292.89

Phencyclidine Intoxication

A. Recent use of phencyclidine (or a related substance).

B. Clinically significant maladaptive behavioral changes (e.g., belligerence, assaultiveness, impulsiveness, unpredictability, psychomotor agitation, impaired judgment, or impaired social or occupational functioning) that developed during, or shortly after, phencyclidine use.

C. Within an hour (less when smoked, "snorted," or used intravenously), two (or more) of the following signs:

(1) vertical or horizontal nystagmus

(2) hypertension or tachycardia

(3) numbness or diminished responsiveness to pain

(4) ataxia

(5) dysarthria

(6) muscle rigidity

(7) seizures or coma

(8) hyperacusis

D. The symptoms are not due to a general medical condition and are not better accounted for by another mental disorder.

Specific if:
With perceptual disturbances

Phenomenology and Variations in Presentation

Psychiatrists must be alert to the wide spectrum of PCP effects on multiple organ systems. Because fluctuations in serum levels may occur unpredictably, a patient being treated for apparently selective psychiatric or behavioral complications of PCP abuse may suddenly undergo radical alterations in medical status; emergency medical intervention may become necessary to avoid permanent organ damage or death. Any patient manifesting significant cardiovascular, respiratory, neurological, or metabolic derangement subsequent to PCP use should be evaluated and treated in a medical service; the psychiatrist plays a secondary role in diagnosis and treatment until physiological stability has been reached and sustained.

PCP-intoxicated patients may come to medical attention on the basis of alterations in mental status; bizarre or violent behavior; injuries sustained while intoxicated; or medical complications, such as rhabdomyolysis, hyperthermia, or seizures.

PSYCHIATRIC PRESENTATION

The presenting symptoms may be predominantly or exclusively psychiatric, without significant alterations in level of consciousness, and may closely resemble an acute schizophrenic decompensation with concrete or illogical thinking, bizarre behavior, negativism, catatonic posturing, and echolalia. Subjective feelings and objective signs of "drunkenness" may or may not be present. Retrospective studies conducted during the period of widespread PCP abuse demonstrated that PCP psychosis could not reliably be distinguished from schizophrenia on the basis of presenting symptoms.

Studies of normal volunteers suggested that the acute psychosis induced by a single low dose of PCP usually lasts 4 to 6 hours.

In some PCP users, psychotic symptoms including hallucinations, delusions, paranoia, thought disorder, and catatonia, with intact consciousness, have been reported to persist from days to weeks after single doses. The frequency of such prolonged psychotic states after single doses has not been determined systematically. Sudden and impulsive violent and assaultive behaviors have been reported in PCP-intoxicated patients without previous histories of such conduct.

NONPSYCHIATRIC PRESENTATION

In PCP intoxication, the central nervous, cardiovascular, respiratory, and peripheral autonomic systems are affected to degrees ranging from mild to catastrophic (Table 19–2).

The level of consciousness may vary from full alertness to coma. Coma of variable duration may occur spontaneously or after an episode of bizarre or violent behavior. Prolonged coma due to continued drug absorption from ruptured ingested packages of PCP has been described.

Nystagmus (which may be horizontal, vertical, or rotatory) has been described. Consequences of PCP-induced central nervous system hyperexcitability may range from mildly increased deep tendon reflexes to grand mal seizures or status epilepticus. Seizures are usually generalized, but focal seizures or neurological deficits have been reported, probably on the basis of focal cerebral vasoconstriction. Other motor signs have been observed, such as generalized rigidity, localized dystonias, facial grimacing, and athetosis.

TABLE 19–2	Nonpsychiatric Findings in Phencyclidine Intoxication

Altered level of consciousness

Central nervous system changes including nystagmus, hyper-reflexia, and motor abnormalities

Hypertension

Cholinergic or anticholinergic signs

Hypothermia or hyperthermia

Myoglobinuria

Hypertension, one of the most frequent physical findings, was described in 57% of 1000 patients evaluated, and it was found to be usually mild and self-limiting, but 4% had severe hypertension, and some remained hypertensive for days. Autonomic signs seen in PCP intoxication may be cholinergic (diaphoresis, bronchospasm, miosis, salivation, bronchorrhea) or anticholinergic (mydriasis, urinary retention).

Hypothermia and hyperthermia have been observed. Hyperthermia may reach malignant proportions.

Rhabdomyolysis frequently results from a combination of PCP-induced muscle contractions and trauma occurring in relation to injuries sustained as a result of behavioral effects. Acute renal failure can result from myoglobinuria.

Assessment

The disruption of normal cognitive and memory function by PCP frequently renders patients unable to give an accurate history, including a history of having used PCP. Therefore, assay of urine or blood for drugs may be the only way to establish the diagnosis. PCP is frequently taken in mixtures with other drugs, typically marijuana or cocaine, which may further complicate the diagnosis.

By disrupting sensory pathways, PCP frequently renders users hypersensitive to environmental stimuli to the extent that physical examination or psychiatric interview may cause severe agitation. If PCP intoxication is suspected, measures should be taken from the outset to minimize sensory input. The patient should be evaluated in a quiet, darkened room with the minimal necessary number of medical staff present. Assessments may need to be interrupted periodically.

RELEVANT PHYSICAL EXAMINATION AND LABORATORY FINDINGS

Vital signs should be obtained immediately on presentation. Temperature, blood pressure, and respiratory rate are dose dependently increased by PCP and may be of a magnitude requiring emergency medical treatment to avoid the potentially fatal complications of malignant hyperthermia, hypertensive crisis, and respiratory arrest. In all cases, monitoring of vital signs should continue at 2- to

4-hour intervals throughout treatment, because serum PCP levels may increase spontaneously as a result of drug mobilization from lipid stores or enterohepatic recirculation.

Analgesic and behavioral changes induced by PCP not only predispose patients to physical injury but also mask these injuries, which therefore may be found only with careful physical examination.

On neurological examination, nystagmus and ataxia, although not conclusive, are strongly suggestive of PCP intoxication. Examination of deep tendon reflexes helps to establish the degree of nervous system hyperexcitability. Crossed or clonic deep tendon reflexes alert the physician to the possibility of subsequent seizures.

Because PCP is usually supplied in combination with other drugs and thus is often misrepresented, toxicological analysis of urine or blood is essential. However, there may be circumstances in which PCP may not be detected in urine even if it is present in the body, for example, when the urine is alkaline. However, in chronic PCP users, the drug may be detected in urine up to 30 days after last use. Urine should be tested for heme because of the possible complication of myoglobinuria.

Blood and urine samples should be sent for toxicological analysis. In addition, serum uric acid, creatine kinase, aspartate transaminase, and alanine transaminase elevations are common findings in PCP intoxication.

Differential Diagnosis

The presence of nystagmus and hypertension with mental status changes should raise the possibility of PCP intoxication. Because both the acute and the prolonged forms of PCP psychosis closely resemble schizophrenia, and because the sensitivity of schizophrenic patients to the psychotomimetic effects of the drug is increased, an underlying schizophrenia spectrum disorder should be considered, particularly if paranoia or thought disorder persists beyond 4 to 6 weeks after last use of PCP. PCP psychosis may also resemble mania or other mood disorders.

PCP psychosis is readily distinguishable from LSD psychosis in normal as well as in schizophrenic subjects by the lack of typical LSD effects, such as synesthesia. The cluster of psychotic symptoms, hypertension, and stereotypy may be seen in both PCP psychosis and chronic amphetamine psychosis; in such cases, accurate histories and toxicological analysis are particularly important.

In cases involving prominent PCP-induced neurological, cardiovascular, or metabolic derangement, encephalitis, head injury, post-ictal state, and primary metabolic disorders must be ruled out. Either intoxication with or withdrawal from sedative-hypnotics may be associated with nystagmus. Neuroleptic malignant syndrome should be ruled out in the differential diagnosis of PCP-induced hyperthermia and muscle rigidity.

COURSE AND NATURAL HISTORY

As drug levels decline, the clinical picture recedes in 5 to 21 days through periods of moderating neurological, autonomic, and metabolic impairments to a stage at which only psychiatric impairments are apparent. Once the physical symptoms and signs have cleared, the period of simple PCP psychosis may last 1 day to 6 weeks, whether or not neuroleptics are administered, during which the psychiatric symptoms and signs abate gradually and progressively. Even after complete recovery, flashbacks may occur if PCP sequestered in lipid stores is mobilized. Any underlying psychiatric disorders can be detected and evaluated only after complete resolution of the drug-induced psychosis.

PHYSICIAN-PATIENT RELATIONSHIP IN PSYCHIATRIC MANAGEMENT

In contrast to psychotic states induced by drugs such as LSD, in which "talking the patient down" may be highly effective, no such effort should be made in the case of PCP psychosis, particularly during the period of acute intoxication, because of the risk of sensory overload that can lead to dramatically increased agitation. The risk of sudden and unpredictable impulsive, violent behavior can also be increased by sensory stimulation.

PHARMACOTHERAPY AND SOMATIC TREATMENTS

There is no pharmacological competitive antagonist for PCP, in contrast to opiates and benzodiazepines. Oral or intramuscular benzodiazepines are recommended for agitation. Neuroleptics usually have little or no effect on acute or chronic PCP-induced psychosis or thought disorder. Because they lower the seizure threshold, neuroleptics should be used with caution. Physical restraint may be lifesaving if the patient's behavior poses an imminent threat to his or her safety or that of others; however, such restraint risks triggering or worsening rhabdomyolysis.

Because of the large volume of distribution of PCP, dialysis is ineffective as a means of clearing the drug from circulation. Administration of activated charcoal has been shown to bind PCP and to diminish toxic effects of PCP in animals.

SPECIAL FEATURES INFLUENCING TREATMENT

Psychiatric Comorbidity

PCP psychosis may be clinically indistinguishable from schizophrenia or mania. It has been suggested that some patients who remain psychotic for weeks after PCP ingestion may have an underlying predisposition to schizophrenia or mania. In some series, significant percentages of patients suffering prolonged PCP-induced psychosis are subsequently hospitalized with non-drug-induced schizophrenic disorders. In the case of a schizophrenic patient, responsiveness to neuroleptic treatment may resume after recovery from prolonged PCP psychosis.

General Medical Comorbidity

Patients with preexisting neurological, cardiovascular, respiratory, or renal disorders are at increased risk for complications of PCP intoxication, such as seizures, stroke, hypertensive crisis, respiratory arrest, or renal failure. Abusers of more than one drug may be at increased risk from the presence of other drugs exerting toxic effects on the same organ systems (e.g., cardiovascular effects of cocaine and amphetamine) or because of damage to specific organs secondary to infectious complications of parenteral drug use.

Inhalant Disorders

The term *inhalant abuse* is used to describe a variety of drug-using behaviors that cannot be classified by their pharmacology or toxicology but are grouped according to their primary mode of administration. Although other substances are inhaled (e.g., tobacco, marijuana with or without phencyclidine, and even heroin or crack), this is not the primary route of administration; therefore, they do not fall into this classification. Several subcategories of inhalants can be established according to chemical classes of products and primary abuse groups as follows: 1) industrial or household cleaning and paint-type solvents including paint thinners or solvents, degreasers or dry cleaning solvents, solvents in glues, art or office supply solvents such as correction fluids, and solvents in magic markers; 2) gases used in household or commercial products, such as butane in lighters, fluorocarbons in electronic (personal computer, office equipment) cleaners or refrigerant gases, and the aerosol refillers; 3) household aerosol products such as hair and fabric protector sprays and paint; 4) medical anesthetic gases, such as ether, chloroform, halothane, and nitrous oxide; and 5) aliphatic nitrites. Most of the foregoing compounds affect the central nervous system directly, whereas nitrites act on cardiovascular smooth muscle rather than as anesthetic agents in the central nervous system. The nitrites are also used primarily as sexual enhancers rather than as mood alterants. Therefore, discussion of inhalant abuse herein deals primarily with substances other than nitrites.

Table 20–1 enumerates the solvents (frequently noted on the labels) of the corresponding popular products currently used for recreational purposes.

An analysis of questionnaires regarding the inhalation of various products indicated that gasoline and glue are popular.

Not only are various commercial household products used for pleasure, so are many anesthetics, mostly by medical personnel.

Almost all solvents produce anesthesia if sufficient amounts are inhaled. However, the decreased ability of an agent to produce anesthesia may or may not correlate with an increased abuse of a substance and needs further exploration.

INHALANT USE DISORDERS

Inhalant Dependence

Dependence on inhalants is primarily psychological, with a less dramatic associated physical dependence occurring in some heavy users. The urgent need to continue use of inhalants has been reported among individuals with heavy use, although the nature of this phenomenon is unknown. A mild withdrawal syndrome occurs in

TABLE 20–1	Chemicals Commonly Found in Inhalants

Inhalant	Chemicals
Adhesives	
Airplane glue	Toluene, ethyl acetate
Other glues	Hexane, toluene, methyl chloride, acetone, methyl ethyl ketone, methyl butyl ketone
Special cements	Trichloroethylene, tetrachloroethylene
Aerosols	
Paint sprays	Butane, propane, fluorocarbons, toluene, hydrocarbons
Hair sprays	Butane, propane, chlorofluorocarbons (CFCs)
Deodorants, air fresheners	Butane, propane, CFCs
Analgesic spray	CFCs
Asthma spray	CFCs
Fabric spray	Butane, trichlorothane
Personal computer cleaners	Dimethyl ether, hydrofluorocarbons
Anesthetics	
Gaseous	Nitrous oxide
Liquid	Halothane, enflurane
Local	Ethyl chloride
Cleaning Agents	
Dry cleaners	Tetrachlorethylene, trichloroethane
Spot removers	Xylene, petroleum distillates, chlorohydrocarbons
Degreasers	Tetrachloroethylene, trichloroethane, trichloroethylene
Solvents and Gases	
Nail polish remover	Acetone, ethyl acetate, toluene
Paint remover	Toluene, methylene chloride, methanol, acetone, ethyl acetate
Paint thinners	Petroleum distillates, esters, acetone
Correction fluids and thinners	Trichloroethylene, trichloroethane
Fuel gas	Butane, isopropane
Cigar or cigarette lighter fluid	Butane, isopropane
Fire extinguisher propellant	Bromochlorodifluoromethane
Food Products	
Whipped cream aerosols	Nitrous oxide
Whippets	Nitrous oxide
Room Odorizers	
Poppers, fluids (Rush, Locker Room)	Isoamyl, isobutyl, isopropyl, butylnitrite (now illegal), or cyclohexyl

10 to 24 hours after cessation of use and lasts for several days. Symptoms include general disorientation, sleep disturbances, headaches, muscle spasms, irritability, nausea, and fleeting illusions. However, this is not a documented or characteristic withdrawal syndrome.

Inhalant Abuse

Abuse of inhalants may lead to harm to individuals (e.g., accidents involving automobiles, falls from buildings when in an impaired or intoxicated state [illusionary feelings], or self-inflicted harm, such as attempted or successful suicide). Frozen lips caused by rapidly expanding gases or serious burns may also occur. Chronic inhalant use is often associated with familial conflict and school problems.

INHALANT-INDUCED DISORDERS

DSM-IV Criteria 292.39

Inhalant Intoxication

A. Recent intentional use or short-term, high-dose exposure to volatile inhalants (excluding anesthetic gases and short-acting vasodilators).

B. Clinically significant maladaptive behavioral or psychological changes (e.g., belligerence, assaultiveness, apathy, impaired judgment, impaired social or occupational functioning) that developed during, or shortly after, use of or exposure to volatile inhalants.

C. Two (or more) of the following signs, developing during, or shortly after, inhalant use or exposure:

    (1) dizziness

    (2) nystagmus

    (3) incoordination

    (4) slurred speech

    (5) unsteady gait

    (6) lethargy

    (7) depressed reflexes

    (8) psychomotor retardation

    (9) tremor

    (10) generalized muscle weakness

Box continued on following page

Inhalant Intoxication *Continued*

 (11) blurred vision or diplopia

 (12) stupor or coma

 (13) euphoria

D. The symptoms are not due to a general medical condition and are not better accounted for by another mental disorder.

The primary disorder is inhalant intoxication, which is characterized by the presence of clinically significant maladaptive behavioral or psychological changes (e.g., belligerence, assaultiveness, apathy, impaired judgment, impaired social or occupational functioning) that develop during the intentional short-term, high-dose exposure to volatile inhalants (diagnostic criteria A and B in the *Diagnostic and Statistical Manual of Mental Disorders,* Fourth Edition [DSM-IV]). The maladaptive changes occurring after intentional and nonintentional exposure include disinhibition, excitedness, lightheadedness, visual disturbances (blurred vision, nystagmus), incoordination, dysarthria, an unsteady gait, and euphoria. Higher doses of inhalants may lead to depressed reflexes, stupor, coma, and death, sometimes caused by cardiac arrhythmia. Lethargy, generalized muscle weakness, and headaches may occur some hours later, depending on the dose.

TOXICOLOGY OF INHALANT ABUSE

The majority of inhalant abusers never reach a hospital or outpatient facility. Although many do not need medical attention for their inhalant habit, of those who do, many often die before reaching the hospital as a result of asphyxia, cardiac arrhythmia, or related overdose effects after inhaling fluorocarbons, low-molecular-weight hydrocarbon gases (butane, propane), nitrous oxide, or other solvents during either the first or a subsequent episode. Death may occur after inhalation of toluene-containing substances as a result of metabolic acidosis or related kidney failure if left untreated. Death may also occur accidentally when the subject is intoxicated. In most cases, inhalation does not lead to death. Some of the more common acute syndromes of the intoxicated state are listed in Table 20–2.

SEQUELAE OF CHRONIC INHALANT ABUSE

The nervous system may be affected at many levels by organic solvents as well as by other neurotoxic substances. Because of their nonfocal presentation, neurotoxic disorders may be confused with metabolic, degenerative, nutritional, or demyelinating diseases.

 Many organic solvents produce nonspecific effects (i.e., encephalopathy) after exposure to extremely high concentrations; a few produce relatively specific neurological syndromes. Two neurotoxic syndromes, a peripheral neuropathy and an ototoxicity, are well correlated with organic solvents. Less commonly, a cerebellar ataxia syndrome or a myopathy may occur alone or in combination with any of these clinical syndromes.

Neurological abnormalities vary from mild cognitive impairment to severe dementia, associated with elemental neurological signs such as cerebellar ataxia, corticospinal tract dysfunction, oculomotor abnormalities, tremor, deafness, and hyposmia.

Most of the known adverse clinical effects of inhalant abuse relate to the nervous tissue. There are, however, other significant adverse effects on other organ systems, including the kidney, liver, lung, heart, and hemopoietic systems.

Pregnancy

Clinicians especially need to be alert for pregnant women who abuse these solvents. Not only do they present to the clinic with renal tubular acidosis, but the fetuses are also affected. This condition places the mother at risk for hypokalemia and associated cardiac dysrhythmias and rhabdomyolysis. Fatty livers may also be observed in these subjects. Treatment for their metabolic imbalance needs immediate attention.

TABLE 20–2	Symptoms Related to Solvent Abuse (Not All for Gases and Nitrites)

Moderate Intoxication

Dizziness
Headache
Lethargy
Disorientation, incoherence
Ataxia, gait (uncoordinated movement)
Odoriferous, foul breath (solvent vapors)

Strong Intoxication

Blurred vision
Belligerence
Nausea, vomiting
Irritability
Delirium
Slurred speech

Severe (Rare)

Seizures
Violent actions

TREATMENT

Individuals need different treatments based on the severity of their dependence and any medical complications. Primary care should address medical concerns before dealing with the dependence on solvents and other drugs. During this period, sedatives, other depressants, neuroleptics, and other forms of pharmacotherapy are not useful in the treatment of inhalant abusers and should be avoided in most cases, as they are likely to exacerbate the depressed state.

Once it is determined that the individual is detoxified, that is, has low levels of solvent or other depressant drug, then therapy with other drugs, such as antianxiety drugs, may be useful. The determination of detoxification, even in the absence of drug (solvent) administration, is not well defined or systematic. It may take several days for the major "reversible" intoxication state to be reduced to a level at which coherent cognition can occur. Little can be done during this period other than to facilitate improvement of the basic health of these individuals, provide supportive care, and build the individual's self-esteem.

There is no accepted treatment approach for inhalant abuse. It should also be emphasized that there are various categories of solvent abusers, from those who may use only one substance (e.g., only nitrous oxide or butanes) to heavy users of a variety of solvents and gases. Many drug treatment facilities refuse to treat inhalant abusers, regarding them as resistant to treatment.

The inhalant abuser typically does not respond to usual drug rehabilitation treatment modalities. Several factors may be involved, particularly for the chronic abuser, who may have significant psychosocial problems. Treatment becomes slower and progressively more difficult when the severity of brain injury worsens as abuse progresses through transient social use (experimenting in groups) to chronic use in isolation. For these and other reasons, longer therapies are necessary than are utilized in most drug treatment facilities. Also, neurological impairment, the breadth of which still needs to be established, may be a major complication slowing the progress of rehabilitation. This problem is not as significant with other forms of drug abuse.

Drug screening would be useful in monitoring inhalant abusers. Routine urine screening for hippuric acid (the major metabolite of toluene metabolism) performed two to three times weekly can detect the high level of exposure to toluene commonly seen in inhalant abusers. Because alcohol is a common secondary drug of abuse among inhalant abusers, alcohol abuse should be monitored and considered in the approach to treatment.

Nicotine Use Disorder

Nicotine addiction from cigarette smoking and smokeless tobacco use is the most prevalent form of chemical dependence in the United States. Cigarette smoking is the primary preventable cause of morbidity and mortality in the United States, with an estimated 434,000 premature deaths occurring each year from smoking-related illnesses and 50,000 additional deaths occurring in nonsmokers from exposure to environmental tobacco smoke. Smoking causes 90% of all lung cancers and 80% to 90% of all chronic obstructive pulmonary diseases and correlates with a two times greater than average risk of death from stroke and coronary heart disease. Smoking is also associated with an increased incidence of cancer at a number of other sites, including the larynx, oral cavity, esophagus, cervix, bladder, pancreas, and kidney and with complications of pregnancy and negative effects on the fetus, including low birth weight.

Nicotine dependence and smoking are more common in individuals with comorbid psychiatric disorders than in the general population: 55% to 90% of individuals with psychiatric disorders smoke versus approximately 25% of the general population. The prevalence of smoking is especially high in persons with schizophrenia, those with affective disorders, and individuals with alcoholism or other substance use disorders.

Nicotine is the primary psychoactive agent in tobacco smoke and smokeless tobacco and has powerful addictive properties. Nicotine has a multitude of effects. It acts in two primary areas of the brain—the mesolimbic dopaminergic system, which is related to the euphoriant effects of the drug, and the locus caeruleus, which mediates stress reactions and vigilance and relates to the higher mental and cognitive functions.

Nicotine has stimulant and depressive effects on both the central and the peripheral nervous systems. It also affects the cardiovascular system (increased heart rate and blood pressure), gastrointestinal system, and skeletal motor system. Nicotine alters brain energy metabolism and stimulates the peripheral cholinergic nervous system (sympathetic and parasympathetic). Through this variety of central and peripheral actions, nicotine improves mood and decreases anxiety; decreases distress in response to stressful stimuli; decreases aggression; improves overall cognitive function and performance (improves reaction time, concentration, vigilance, and stimulus-processing capacity); and decreases the appetite for simple carbohydrates, decreases stress-induced eating, and increases resting metabolic rate.

COURSE AND NATURAL HISTORY

Smoking cessation attempts result in high relapse rates, with a relapse curve paralleling that for opiates: 65% of those who stop smoking relapse in 3 months and another 10% relapse in 3 to 6 months. The relapse rate is 80% by 1 year.

Less than 25% of the individuals who quit smoking are successful on their first attempt. Repeated failures are common before successful abstinence, with the average smoker attempting cessation two or three times before success.

Withdrawal symptoms are most severe within the first 1 to 3 days of abstinence, often continue for 3 to 4 weeks, and in some persons last for up to 6 months or longer. Current depressive symptoms and a history of depression are predictors of relapse. Weight gain may also contribute to relapse, particularly in women. In contrast, several factors have been found to predict success at smoking cessation. These predictors include individual factors, manifestations of the addiction such as severity of withdrawal, and social and environmental circumstances.

Treatment of nicotine addiction with resultant abstinence can result in highly beneficial health effects. Short-term effects (within a month) include a significant reduction in respiratory symptoms and infections such as influenza, pneumonia, and bronchitis. Excess risk of death from coronary heart disease is reduced after 1 year and continues to decline over time. In patients with coronary heart disease, smoking cessation decreases the risk of recurrent myocardial infarction and cardiovascular death by 50%. After 10 to 15 years of abstinence, the mortality rate from all causes returns to that of a person who has never smoked. Pulmonary function can also return to normal if chronic obstructive changes have not already occurred at the time of cessation.

TREATMENT

The general approach to the treatment of nicotine dependence must be viewed as having three primary components: physiological, psychological, and behavioral. The physiological dependence parallels the characteristics of other physiologically addicting substances: compulsive use, dose-related effects, rapid tolerance leading to increased intake, and the presence of a withdrawal syndrome. Psychological dependence involves the reasons a person smokes, for example, to regulate affect, to improve mood and sense of well-being, to satisfy craving, and to provide stimulation and relaxation. The behavioral component involves environmental and

TABLE 21–1	Approaches to the Pharmacological Treatment of Nicotine Addiction
Nicotine replacement or substitution (agonist administration)	
Blockade therapy (antagonist administration)	
Nonspecific attenuation therapy	
Deterrent therapy	

social cues that become associated with smoking cigarettes, for example, drinking coffee or alcohol, talking on the telephone, taking a work break, or smoking at parties or social functions. The direct beneficial effects of nicotine on, for example, mood become highly positive reinforcements, as do the associated behaviors or activities, which can act as powerful triggers for relapse during attempts at cessation.

Four different approaches with different foci have been used for the pharmacological treatment of nicotine addiction (Table 21–1). Of the four pharmacotherapeutic interventions, nicotine replacement is most widely used. Nicotine replacement is also indicated in the presence of a high degree of physiological dependence.

The substituted nicotine initially prevents significant withdrawal symptoms that may lead to relapse during the early period of smoking cessation. It is then gradually tapered and discontinued. Replacement produces a lower overall plasma level of nicotine than that experienced with smoking. Not only does replacement avoid the strongly reinforcing peaks in plasma level, but it also prevents the emergence of withdrawal symptoms by maintaining the nicotine plasma level above a threshold.

The second pharmacological approach to treating nicotine addiction involves blockade therapy or antagonist administration. The advantage of this approach over nicotine replacement is that it does not continue the reinforcing effects of nicotine nor maintain exposure to its potentially damaging effects. Several agents have been used, but mecamylamine, which has central and peripheral blockade effects, is the only agent shown presently to be effective. Although mecamylamine initially increases smoking behavior by decreasing the effective level of nicotine available from smoking, overall it mitigates the reinforcing properties of nicotine.

The third pharmacological approach involves nonspecific attenuation therapy. In this approach, a pharmacological agent is used to mitigate abstinence symptoms in a manner similar to the use of clonidine to reduce withdrawal symptoms in opioid dependence. The agent most commonly used has been clonidine in both oral and transdermal forms. Clonidine is an antihypertensive drug with central sympatholytic activity.

Antidepressants have been used in an attempt to attenuate withdrawal symptoms, to treat or prevent emergent depressive symptoms or episodes in the early phase of cessation, and to prevent relapse of depressive episodes in patients with a history of depression. Antidepressants may provide significant benefits in special populations of patients with current or prior major depression or dysthymic disorder or with current depressive symptoms when these factors predict a poor outcome. Because negative affect is the most common antecedent of a smoking relapse, this approach appears promising. If antidepressants are used, pretreatment is necessary because the benefit of the medication may not be apparent for 1 to 3 weeks.

The fourth pharmacological approach to treating nicotine dependence and withdrawal is deterrent therapy or use of a drug to produce an aversive effect if nicotine is used, similar to the use of disulfiram with alcohol dependence. The primary drug used has been silver acetate in a gum or lozenge preparation. If a cigarette is smoked, sulfite salts are produced when silver acetate contacts the

TABLE 21–2	Psychological Interventions for the Treatment of Nicotine Addiction

Self-help
Brief advice from the physician
Nicotine fading
Aversive techniques
Cognitive-behavioral therapies
Social support
Hypnosis
Acupuncture

sulfides in tobacco smoke, producing an unpleasant taste. Unfortunately, there is not an acceptable preparation because the existing gum has a short duration of action.

Combined or serial pharmacotherapeutic approaches may also be beneficial, especially in more difficult to treat cases of nicotine addiction. Examples of such combinations include the following:

- Nicotine replacement (gum and/or transdermal) combined with clonidine to cover any emergent withdrawal symptoms (no controlled studies of this approach exist presently)
- Pretreatment with an antidepressant followed by the use of nicotine replacement to cover acute withdrawal symptoms
- Pretreatment with an antidepressant, with clonidine added for acute withdrawal symptoms

In addition to pharmacological approaches, an incredible variety of psychosocial interventions has been developed to assist with the cessation of smoking. A number of the more commonly used psychosocial treatments are reviewed in Table 21–2. Psychosocial interventions, particularly behavioral therapy, have been shown to increase abstinence rates significantly.

SPECIAL CONSIDERATIONS IN TREATMENT: PSYCHIATRIC COMORBIDITY

The prevalence of smoking in psychiatric patients has been found to be much higher than in the general population. Psychiatric patients also are generally much less likely to be able to successfully stop smoking. The strongest association of smoking is with schizophrenia. Several reasons for this powerful association have been postulated, including the effect of nicotine in decreasing drug-induced side effects and in increasing dopamine in the frontal and prefrontal brain areas, which could positively influence negative symptoms or improve prefrontal cognitive function.

Both epidemiological studies and studies of clinical populations have found a strong association between smoking and depression. There is a higher lifetime prevalence of major depressive disorder in smokers than in nonsmokers. Furthermore, persons with a history of depression or those currently experiencing a major depressive disorder have a higher prevalence of cigarette smoking than do patients with no history of major depressive disorder. Finally, smokers with a history of major depressive disorder experience a much greater frequency of this disorder and increased severity of depressive symptoms occurring during cessation. The presence of depression is also associated with an increased risk of relapse and difficulty maintaining abstinence.

An 80% to 90% rate of smoking has also been found in persons with active alcoholism. Some data suggest that smokers with alcoholism may be more behaviorally, but not physically, dependent on nicotine than are other smokers. In addition, it appears that successful smoking cessation in persons with active alcoholism is much less likely than in individuals recovering from alcoholism; the cessation rate in these latter individuals is similar to that in the general population of smokers.

Opioid-Related Disorders

The term *opioids* describes a class of substances that act on opioid receptors. Numerous opioid receptors have been identified, but the physiological and pharmacological responses in humans are best understood for the μ and κ receptors. The μ receptor, for which morphine is a prototypical agonist, appears to be the one most closely related to opioid analgesic and euphorigenic effects. Opioids can be naturally occurring substances such as morphine, semisynthetics such as heroin, and synthetics with morphine-like effects such as meperidine. These drugs are prescribed as analgesics, anesthetics, antidiarrheals, and cough suppressants. In addition to morphine, heroin, and meperidine, the opioids include codeine, hydromorphone, methadone, oxycodone, and fentanyl, among others. Drugs such as buprenorphine, a partial agonist at the μ receptor, and pentazocine, an agonist-antagonist, are also included in this class because their physiological and behavioral effects are mediated through opioid receptors.

The defining features according to the *Diagnostic and Statistical Manual of Mental Disorders,* Fourth Edition (DSM-IV), of opioid dependence, abuse, intoxication, and withdrawal are similar to those for other substances. Essentially, opioid dependence is a cluster of cognitive, behavioral, and physiological symptoms indicating that the affected person is using high doses of opioids in a compulsive manner and that there is loss of control over use. Cocaine, hallucinogens, solvents, and other substances do not always produce withdrawal symptoms, but opioid dependence is almost always accompanied by significant tolerance and withdrawal.

DSM-IV Criteria 304.00

Substance (Opioid) Dependence

A maladaptive pattern of opioid use, leading to clinically significant impairment or distress, as manifested by three (or more) of the following, occurring at any time in the same 12-month period:

(1) tolerance, as defined by either of the following:

    (a) a need for markedly increased amounts of opioids to achieve intoxication or desired effect

    (b) markedly diminished effect with continued use of the same amount of opioid

(2) withdrawal, as manifested by either of the following:

    (a) the characteristic withdrawal syndrome for opioids (refer to criteria A and B of the criteria set for opioid withdrawal)

    (b) an opioid is taken to relieve or avoid withdrawal symptoms

(3) opioids are often taken in larger amounts or over a longer period than was intended

(4) there is a persistent desire or unsuccessful efforts to cut down or control opioid use

(5) a great deal of time is spent in activities necessary to obtain opioids (e.g., visiting multiple doctors or driving long distances), use opioids (e.g., chain-smoking), or recover from their effects

(6) important social, occupational, or recreational activities are given up or reduced because of opioid use

(7) opioid use is continued despite knowledge of having a persistent or recurrent physical or psychological problem that is likely to have been caused or exacerbated by opioids

Specify if:

With physiological dependence: evidence of tolerance or withdrawal (i.e., either item 1 or 2 is present)

Without physiological dependence: no evidence of tolerance or withdrawal (i.e., neither item 1 nor 2 is present)

DSM-IV Criteria 305.50

Substance (Opioid) Abuse

A. A maladaptive pattern of opioid use leading to clinically significant impairment or distress, as manifested by one (or more) of the following, occurring within a 12-month period:

    (1) recurrent opioid use resulting in a failure to fulfill major role obligations at work, school, or home (e.g., repeated absences or poor work performance related to opioid use; opioid-related absences, suspensions, or expulsions from school; neglect of children or household)

Box continued on following page

DSM-IV Criteria 305.50

Substance (Opioid) Abuse *Continued*

    (2) recurrent opioid use in situations in which it is physically hazardous (e.g., driving an automobile or operating a machine when impaired by opioid use)

    (3) recurrent opioid-related legal problems

    (4) continued opioid use despite having persistent or recurrent social or interpersonal problems caused or exacerbated by the effects of the opioids (e.g., arguments with spouse about consequences of intoxication, physical fights)

B. The symptoms have never met the criteria for opioid dependence.

DSM-IV Criteria 292.89

Opioid Intoxication

A. Recent use of an opioid.

B. Clinically significant maladaptive behavioral or psychological changes (e.g., initial euphoria followed by apathy, dysphoria, psychomotor agitation or retardation, impaired judgment, or impaired social or occupational functioning) that developed during, or shortly after, opioid use.

C. Pupillary constriction (or pupillary dilation due to anoxia from severe overdose) and one (or more) of the following signs, developing during, or shortly after, opioid use:

    (1) drowsiness or coma

    (2) slurred speech

    (3) impairment in attention or memory

D. The symptoms are not due to a general medical condition and are not better accounted for by another mental disorder.

Opioid abuse consists of intermittent use of one or more opioids in the absence of compulsive use and significant tolerance or withdrawal, or both, but resulting in recurrent social, legal, or personal problems or in use that is physically hazardous. Opioid in-

DSM-IV Criteria 292.0

Opioid Withdrawal

A. Either of the following:

 (1) cessation of (or reduction in) opioid use that has been heavy and prolonged (several weeks or longer)

 (2) administration of an opioid antagonist after a period of opioid use

B. Three (or more) of the following, developing within minutes to several days after criterion A:

 (1) dysphoric mood

 (2) nausea or vomiting

 (3) muscle aches

 (4) lacrimation or rhinorrhea

 (5) pupillary dilation, piloerection, or sweating

 (6) diarrhea

 (7) yawning

 (8) fever

 (9) insomnia

C. The symptoms in criterion B cause clinically significant distress or impairment in social, occupational, or other important areas of functioning.

D. The symptoms are not due to a general medical condition and are not better accounted for by another mental disorder.

toxication involves clinically significant maladaptive behaviors or psychological changes associated with acute opioid drug effects. Opioid withdrawal is a syndrome associated with abrupt cessation or reduction of opioid use in persons who have been taking opioids in sufficient quantities and amounts to have developed neuroadaptation to their μ or κ, or both, agonist effects. Opioid withdrawal symptoms are generally opposite those of intoxication.

EPIDEMIOLOGY

Heroin is the most commonly used drug of the opioid class.

The Epidemiological Catchment Area Study found that only 0.7% of the target population had ever met criteria for opioid dependence or abuse. This study, and other similar epidemiological surveys, may underestimate the true prevalence of opioid use disorders, as they do not often include persons in prisons or those who are homeless. More recent estimates indicate that there may be as many as 2 million opioid addicts in the United States, although exact figures are difficult to obtain.

For many people, the effect of taking an opioid for the first time is dysphoric rather than euphoric, and nausea and vomiting may result. Chronic opioid users experience mood swings ranging from sedation and euphoria when intoxicated to anxiety and dysphoria when experiencing withdrawal. Opioid users also have an increased prevalence of psychiatric and medical disorders, especially infectious diseases.

DIAGNOSIS AND DIFFERENTIAL DIAGNOSIS

Heroin is usually taken by injection, although it can be smoked, inhaled through the nose (snorted), or taken orally.

In addition to being treated in programs specifically designed for substance use disorders, patients with opioid-related disorders are seen throughout the medical treatment system, including private practices, emergency departments, and consultation and liaison settings. Physicians practicing in penal institutions see large numbers of persons with opioid use disorders because these disorders are associated with high levels of criminal activity.

Intoxication

Intoxication is characterized by maladaptive and clinically significant behavioral changes developing within minutes to a few hours after opioid use. Symptoms include an initial euphoria sometimes followed by dysphoria or apathy. Psychomotor retardation or agitation, impaired judgment, and impaired social or occupational functioning are commonly seen during intoxication.

Intoxication is accompanied by pupillary constriction unless there has been a severe overdose with consequent anoxia and pupillary dilation. Persons with intoxication are often drowsy (described as being "on the nod") or even obtunded, have slurred speech and impaired memory, and demonstrate inattention to the environment to the point of ignoring potentially harmful events. Dryness of secretions in the mouth and nose, slowing of gastrointestinal activity, and constipation are associated with both acute and chronic opioid use. Visual acuity may be impaired as a result of pupillary constriction. The magnitude of the behavioral and physiological changes resulting from opioid use depends on the dose as well as on the individual characteristics of the user, such as rate of absorption, chronicity of use, and tolerance. Symptoms of opioid intoxication usually last for several hours but are dependent on the half-life of the particular opioid ingested. Severe intoxication after an opioid overdose can lead to coma, respiratory depression, pupillary dilation, unconsciousness, and death.

Withdrawal

Withdrawal is a clinically significant, maladaptive behavioral and physiological syndrome associated with cessation or reduction of opioid use that has been heavy and prolonged. It also can be precipitated by use of an opioid antagonist such as naloxone or naltrexone.

Patients in opioid withdrawal typically demonstrate signs and symptoms that are the opposite of acute agonist effects. The first of these symptoms are subjective and consist of complaints of anxiety, restlessness, and an "achy feeling" often located in the back and legs. These symptoms are accompanied by a wish to obtain opioids (sometimes called craving) and drug-seeking behavior, along with irritability and increased sensitivity to pain. In addition, patients typically demonstrate three or more of the following: dysphoric or depressed mood, nausea or vomiting, diarrhea, muscle aches, lacrimation or rhinorrhea, increased sweating, yawning, fever, insomnia, pupillary dilation, fever, and piloerection.

For short-acting drugs such as heroin, withdrawal symptoms occur within 6 to 24 hours after the last dose in most dependent persons, peak within 1 to 3 days, and gradually subside during a period of 5 to 7 days. Symptoms may take 2 to 4 days to emerge in the case of longer acting drugs such as methadone and l-α-acetylmethadol (LAAM). Less acute withdrawal symptoms are sometimes present and can last for weeks to months. These more persistent symptoms can include anxiety, dysphoria, anhedonia, insomnia, and drug craving.

Dependence

Dependence is diagnosed by the signs and symptoms associated with compulsive, prolonged self-administration of opioid drugs used for no legitimate medical purpose or, if a medical condition exists that requires opioid treatment, the drugs are used in doses that greatly exceed the amount needed for pain relief. Persons with opioid dependence typically demonstrate continued use despite adverse physical, behavioral, and psychological consequences. Almost all persons meeting criteria for opioid dependence have significant levels of tolerance and will experience withdrawal on abrupt discontinuation of opioid drugs. Persons with opioid dependence tend to develop such regular patterns of compulsive drug use that they typically plan daily activities around obtaining and administering the drug.

Abuse

Abuse is a maladaptive pattern of intermittent use of opioids in hazardous situations (e.g., driving under the influence, being intoxicated while using heavy machinery or working in dangerous places) or periodic use resulting in adverse social, legal, or interpersonal problems. All of these signs and symptoms can also be seen in persons who are dependent. Abuse is characterized by less regular use than dependence (i.e., compulsive use not present) and by the absence of significant tolerance or withdrawal.

ASSESSMENT

A nonjudgmental and supportive yet firm approach to opioid patients is especially important. Typically, they have engaged in antisocial or other forms of problematic behavior. They are often embarrassed or afraid to describe the extent of their behavior and have extremely low self-esteem. At the same time, they are prone to be impulsive and manipulative and to act out when frustrated.

Relevant Physical Examination and Laboratory Findings

PHYSICAL EXAMINATION

Sclerosed veins (tracks) and puncture marks on the lower portions of the upper extremities are common in intravenous drug users. When these veins become unusable or otherwise unavailable, persons usually switch to veins in the legs, neck, or groin. Veins sometimes become so badly sclerosed that peripheral edema develops. When intravenous access is no longer possible, persons often inject directly into their subcutaneous tissue (skin-popping), which results in cellulitis, abscesses, and circular-appearing scars from healed skin lesions. Tetanus is a relatively rare but extremely serious consequence of injecting into the subcutaneous tissues. Infections including bacterial endocarditis, hepatitis B and C, and HIV infection also occur in other organ systems.

Persons who snort heroin or other opioids often develop irritation of the nasal mucosa. Difficulties in sexual function are common, as are a variety of sexually transmitted diseases. Men often experience premature ejaculation associated with opioid withdrawal and impotence during intoxication or chronic use. Women commonly have disturbances of reproductive function and irregular menses.

LABORATORY FINDINGS

During dependence, routine urine toxicology tests are often positive for opioid drugs. For most opioids urine tests remain positive for 12 to 36 hours. Methadone and LAAM, because they are longer acting drugs, can be identified for several days. Fentanyl is not detected by standard urine tests but can be identified by more specialized procedures.

Hepatitis screening tests are often positive, either for hepatitis B antigen (signifying active infection) or for hepatitis B or C antibody, or both (signifying past infection). Mild to moderate elevations of liver function tests are common, usually resulting from resolving hepatitis, toxic injury to the liver due to contaminants that have been mixed with the injected opioid, or concomitant use of other hepatotoxic drugs such as alcohol. Low platelet count, anemia or neutropenia, and positive HIV tests or low CD4$^+$ cell counts are often signs of HIV infection that has been acquired via injection drug use or by unprotected sexual activity that may be related to a substance use disorder.

Developmental and Sex Differences

Opioid use disorders can occur at any age, including adolescence and the geriatric years, but most affected persons are between 20 and 45 years old. Neonates whose mothers are addicted can experience opioid withdrawal, as is discussed later. Rarely, young children are affected, with some cases of heroin dependence reported in persons who are 8 to 10 years of age. Males are more commonly affected, with a typical male to female ratio being 3 : 1 or 4 : 1.

Differential Diagnosis

Individuals who are dependent on street opioids are usually easy to diagnose because of the physical signs of intravenous use, drug-seeking behavior, reports from independent observers, lack of medical justification for opioid use, urine test results, and signs and symptoms of intoxication or withdrawal.

The signs and symptoms of opioid withdrawal are fairly specific, especially lacrimation and rhinorrhea, which are not associated with withdrawal from any other abusable substances. Other psychoactive substances with sedative properties, such as alcohol, hypnotics, and anxiolytics, can cause a clinical picture that resembles opioid intoxication. A diagnosis can usually be made by the absence of pupillary constriction or by the response to a naloxone challenge. In some cases, intoxication is due to opioids along with alcohol or other sedatives. In these cases, the naloxone challenge does not reverse all of the sedative drug effects.

Opioid addicts often present with psychiatric signs and symptoms such as depression or anxiety syndromes. These symptoms can be the result of opioid intoxication or withdrawal, or they might result from the pharmacological effects of other substances that also are being abused, such as cocaine, alcohol, or benzodiazepines. They may also represent independent, non-substance-induced psychiatric disorders that require long-term treatment.

COURSE AND NATURAL HISTORY

Opioid dependence can begin at any age, but problems associated with opioid use are most commonly first observed in the late teens or early 20s. Once dependence occurs it is usually continuous for many years, even though periods of abstinence are frequent. Recurrence is common even after many years of forced abstinence, such as occurs during incarceration. Increasing age appears to be associated with a decrease in prevalence. This tendency for dependence to remit generally begins after age 40 years and has been called "maturing out." However, many persons have remained opioid dependent for 50 years or longer. Thus, although spontaneous remission can and does occur, most cases of opioid dependence follow a chronic, relapsing course.

OVERALL GOALS OF TREATMENT

Treatment for intoxication usually takes place in an emergency department, although it may also take place in the physician's office; withdrawal is usually seen in many settings, including emergency departments and treatment programs. The goal is to relieve the acute symptoms and engage the patient in long-term, specialized treatment for the substance use disorder.

All treatments for opioid dependence usually take place in three phases: acute, rehabilitation, and supportive. These phases extend for varying lengths of time depending on the response to treatment, the patient's involvement and motivation, his or her social situation, and the resources available.

PHARMACOTHERAPY

Intoxication

Acute intoxication can easily be reversed by administering naloxone (Narcan) subcutaneously or intravenously. Because naloxone is a short-acting drug, effective for only 30 to 60 minutes, it is important to observe the patient after the naloxone dose wears off to make certain that he or she does not again exhibit signs and symptoms of an overdose. Such observation is especially important in the case of an overdose with methadone or any other long-acting opioid. It is necessary to administer naloxone for a prolonged time, and in these cases, an intravenous drip can be utilized until the opioid has been metabolized and its effects are no longer life threatening.

Although treatment with 0.4 to 0.8 mg naloxone, intravenously or subcutaneously, should reverse most opioid overdoses, patients with opioid dependence could have severe precipitated withdrawal from such doses. If a patient is suspected of being dependent, it is safer to begin a slow intravenous push administration of 0.1 to 0.2 mg of naloxone and monitor the patient's respiratory status and level of consciousness; it is not necessary or desirable for the patient to have signs and symptoms of withdrawal. If the patient needs continuous naloxone administration while the opioid is being metabolized and excreted, the dose should be titrated, by adjusting the rate of the intravenous infusion, so that the patient's respiratory and cardiovascular status is stable.

Withdrawal

Withdrawal can be treated simply by administering an opioid, such as methadone, at the lowest effective dose that maintains the patient's level of dependence. Methadone (20 to 30 mg), administered orally, usually stops the signs and symptoms of withdrawal, but this dose may not be sufficient to suppress withdrawal for 24 hours. In an inpatient setting, this presents no problem because the patient may receive a second dose from 2 to 16 hours after the first, depending on when the withdrawal symptoms are observed.

If the patient is being treated in an outpatient setting, it is usually not possible to adjust the dosing schedule as easily. If higher doses are required, which they often are in cases of high levels of physiological dependence, they should be administered only if signs and symptoms of withdrawal persist for 1.5 hours or more after the first opioid dose. The patient should not be given more than 30 mg in a single dose unless the current level of physiological dependence is clearly documented. U.S. Food and Drug Administration requirements do not permit administering more than 30 mg in a single dose on the first day of methadone treatment or more than

40 mg in divided doses on the first day of treatm
day, when the initial level of tolerance is better kn
less heavily regulated and the physician has more lee
or his best judgment about the most appropriate dose
doses are not increased more rapidly than 10 to 15 mg/c

The patient's estimation of the opioid amount needed to s   .ess withdrawal should be tempered by the knowledge that persons using opioids regularly exaggerate their level of physiological dependence, usually from fear that the physician will not prescribe enough methadone. These patient reports must be very carefully assessed. It is always safest to give a lower dose (20 to 30 mg) and then to check the patient again at a later time, after the methadone has had an opportunity to work. If withdrawal symptoms persist, another 10 to 20 mg can be given. The process can be repeated until the patient is stable.

Detoxification

Unlike detoxification from alcohol and other substance use disorders in which outpatient treatment is often effective, detoxification from opioids is usually not successful unless done in an inpatient setting. Exceptions are patients who have been stably maintained with methadone for extended periods and who slowly reduce their dose over months or even years. As with all substance use disorders, if detoxification is not followed by meaningful involvement in therapy, self-help groups, or a combination of both, it is almost never successful.

Detoxification, except in a methadone-maintained outpatient setting, is most easily accomplished by using oral doses of methadone, given three to four times a day, and slowly decreasing the dose over 5 to 7 days depending on the dose needed initially to suppress withdrawal symptoms. Patients are usually started with 20 to 40 mg/d, given in divided doses; when the dose required to suppress withdrawal symptoms for 24 hours is determined, it is then lowered by 5 to 10 mg/d until it reaches zero. Optimally, one should be able to observe the patient for 1 to 2 days after the methadone has been discontinued to make certain that he or she is stable enough to enter rehabilitation; however, this is not always possible.

An alternative to using opioids for detoxification is the use of adrenergic agonists. Clonidine, an α-adrenergic agonist, has been used to depress the overactivity of the sympathetic nervous system seen in patients withdrawing from opioids. As with other pharmacotherapies, outpatient detoxification with clonidine has not been as successful as inpatient treatment. Problems identified in clonidine detoxification include hypotension, lethargy, insomnia, dizziness, and oversedation. All of these problems are more easily managed in a hospital rather than in an outpatient setting.

Opioid-dependent patients are often dependent on other drugs as well, commonly benzodiazepines, alcohol, and cocaine. Detoxification from these substances can be done along with opioid detoxification. Cocaine dependence does not usually require pharmacotherapy for detoxification, but patients should be observed for the development of acute depression that can be associated with the crash.

ders

Opioid Substitution Therapy

Methadone maintenance has been the mainstay of pharmacotherapy for opioid dependence since its introduction. Since the 1970s, LAAM, a long-acting congener of methadone, has been used experimentally for maintenance treatment. LAAM was approved by the U.S. Food and Drug Administration for maintenance therapy and is now available for general use in opioid treatment programs.

Methadone is an orally effective, long-acting agonist at the μ opioid receptor, and maintenance therapy with methadone is designed to support patients with opioid dependence for months or years while they engage in counseling and other therapy to change their lifestyles. Experience with methadone has shown it to be both safe and effective. Although patients in methadone maintenance show physiological signs of opioid tolerance, side effects are minimal and the patient's general health and nutritional status improve.

Methadone maintenance programs are licensed and regulated by the U.S. Food and Drug Administration and the Drug Enforcement Administration. For a person to be eligible for methadone maintenance, she or he must be at least 18 years of age, must be physiologically dependent on heroin or other opioids, and must have been dependent on opioids for at least 1 year. Each clinic sets its own rules within the guidelines set by state and federal agencies.

PSYCHOSOCIAL TREATMENTS

Drug Counseling and Psychotherapy

Psychosocial interventions are used in all treatments for substance-related disorders. The most extensive use of psychosocial treatments occurs in drug-free rehabilitation programs, in which a combination of education about drug effects and addiction, motivational enhancement, family therapy, individual and group counseling, and participation in self-help groups is included, often on a daily basis.

All methadone maintenance clinics must provide counseling for patients, but the amount required is up to the clinic's discretion. Data are available indicating that psychosocial treatments are necessary to maximize the efficacy of methadone maintenance and that increased levels of psychosocial treatments significantly enhance the efficacy of methadone treatment.

PSYCHIATRIC COMORBIDITY

Antisocial personality disorder is much more common in persons with opioid dependence than in the general population. Posttraumatic stress disorder is also seen with increased frequency among persons with opioid use disorders, as is the case in other types of substance use disorders.

Opioid-dependent persons are especially at risk for the development of depressive symptoms and for episodes of mild to moderate depression that meet symptomatic and duration criteria for major depressive disorder. These syndromes may represent either organic mood disorders or independent depressive illnesses. Brief periods of depression are especially common during chronic intoxication or withdrawal or in association with psychosocial stressors related to the dependence. Insomnia is common, especially during withdrawal. Delirium or brief, psychosis-like symptoms are seen occasionally during opioid intoxication.

Unlike other drugs that produce dependence (with the exception of nicotine), opioids generally reduce rather than initiate or magnify psychiatric symptoms. Opioids have antianxiety and weak antipsychotic effects. Patients maintained with methadone, even at high doses and for long periods, have not been observed to develop new psychiatric disorders.

GENERAL MEDICAL COMORBIDITY

HIV infection and acquired immunodeficiency syndrome have become some of the most common medical complications of intravenous drug use. The incidence of HIV infection is rising markedly among intravenous drug users, of whom opioid-dependent individuals constitute a large proportion. HIV infection rates have been reported to be as high as 60% among persons dependent on heroin in some areas of the United States.

The main pathways to HIV infection are through sharing of injecting equipment, including needles, "cookers," and cotton, and engaging in high-risk sexual behaviors. Sexual transmission is a more common route of HIV transmission for women than men because HIV is spread more readily from men to women than from women to men. Women who are intravenous drug users and who also engage in prostitution or other forms of high-risk sexual behavior are at extremely high risk for HIV infection. Cocaine use has also been found to be a significant risk factor across all drug-using populations, including those with opioid dependence.

Opioid dependence is associated with a high death rate of approximately 10 deaths in 1000 patients per year. Deaths among opioid-dependent persons most often result from overdose, accidents, or injuries. In addition, potentially fatal medical complications include cellulitis, hepatitis, tuberculosis, and endocarditis. All of these are more common in persons with HIV infection.

Tuberculosis has become a particularly serious problem, especially among persons who use drugs intravenously. In most cases, infection with the tubercle bacillus is asymptomatic and evident only by the presence of a positive tuberculin skin test. However, many cases of active tuberculosis have been found, especially among those infected with HIV.

HIV infection has also been seen in about one third of infants born to HIV-positive mothers, many of whom are intravenous drug users or the partners of intravenous drug users. In addition, physiological dependence on opioids is seen in about half the infants born to women who are opioid dependent. This can produce a severe withdrawal syndrome requiring medical treatment.

Sedative, Hypnotic, or Anxiolytic Use Disorders

The medications usually included in the category of sedative-hypnotics are listed in Table 23–1. The sedative-hypnotics include a chemically diverse group of medications. Although buspirone is marketed for the treatment of anxiety, its pharmacological profile is sufficiently different that it is not usually included among the sedative-hypnotics. Antidepressant medications may also have antianxiety properties, and their sedative effects are often used to assist in sleep induction, but they are usually excluded from the sedative-hypnotic classification.

Sedative-hypnotics are among the most commonly prescribed medications. They also are often misused and abused and can produce severe, life-threatening dependence. With the exception of the benzodiazepines and zolpidem, overdose with sedative-hypnotics can be lethal. The benzodiazepines are rarely lethal if taken alone, but in combination with alcohol, they too can be lethal.

Considerations of sedative-hypnotic use disorders should reflect a sensible balance between their medical utility with adverse events arising from medical treatment and their utility as intoxicants or as self-medication of symptoms resulting from abuse of other drugs.

TABLE 23–1	Medications Usually Included in the Category of Sedative-Hypnotics		
Generic Name	Trade Name	Common Therapeutic Use	Therapeutic Dose Range (mg/d)
Barbiturates			
Amobarbital	Amytal	Sedative	50–150
Butabarbital	Butisol	Sedative	45–120
Butalbital	Fiorinal, Sedapap	Sedative/ analgesic	100–300
Pentobarbital	Nembutal	Hypnotic	50–100
Secobarbital	Seconal	Hypnotic	50–100

Benzodiazepines			
Alprazolam	Xanax	Antianxiety	0.75–6
Chlordiaz-epoxide	Librium	Antianxiety	15–100
Clonazepam	Klonopin	Anticon-vulsant	0.5–4
Clorazepate	Tranxene	Antianxiety	15–60
Diazepam	Valium	Antianxiety	5–40
Estazolam	ProSom	Hypnotic	1–2
Flunitrazepam	Rohypnol*	Hypnotic	1–2
Flurazepam	Dalmane	Hypnotic	15–30
Halazepam	Paxipam	Antianxiety	60–160
Lorazepam	Ativan	Antianxiety	1–16
Midazolam	Versed	Anesthesia	—
Oxazepam	Serax	Antianxiety	10–120
Prazepam	Centrax	Antianxiety	20–60
Quazepam	Doral	Hypnotic	15
Temazepam	Restoril	Hypnotic	7.5–30
Triazolam	Halcion	Hypnotic	0.125–0.5
Others			
Chloral hydrate	Noctec, Somnos	Hypnotic	250–1000
Ethchlorvynol	Placidyl	Hypnotic	200–1000
Glutethimide	Doriden	Hypnotic	250–500
Meprobamate	Miltown, Equanil, Equagesic	Antianxiety	1200–1600
Methyprylon	Noludar	Hypnotic	200–400
Zolpidem	Ambien	Hypnotic	5–10

*Rohypnol is not marketed in the United States.

ACUTE INTOXICATION

The acute toxicity of sedative-hypnotics consists of slurred speech, incoordination, ataxia, sustained nystagmus, impaired judgment, and mood lability. In large amounts, sedative-hypnotics produce progressive respiratory depression and coma. The amount of respiratory depression produced by the benzodiazepines is much less than that produced by the barbiturates and other sedative-hypnotics.

Consistent with its general approach, the *Diagnostic and Statistical Manual of Mental Disorders,* Fourth Edition (DSM-IV) diagnosis of intoxication requires "clinically significant maladaptive behavioral or psychological changes" developing after drug use in addition to the signs and symptoms of acute toxicity.

DSM-IV Criteria 292.30

Sedative, Hypnotic, or Anxiolytic Intoxication

A. Recent use of a sedative, hypnotic, or anxiolytic

B. Clinically significant maladaptive behavioral or psychological changes (e.g., inappropriate sexual or aggressive behavior, mood lability, impaired judgment, impaired social or occupational functioning) that developed during, or shortly after, sedative, hypnotic, or anxiolytic use

C. One (or more) of the following signs, developing during, or shortly after, sedative, hypnotic, or anxiolytic use:

   (1) slurred speech

   (2) incoordination

   (3) unsteady gait

   (4) nystagmus

   (5) impairment in attention or memory

   (6) stupor or coma

D. The symptoms are not due to a general medical condition and are not better accounted for by another mental disorder.

DEPENDENCE

Barbiturates can produce tolerance and physiological dependence. Physiological dependence can be induced within several days with continuous infusion of anesthetic doses. Patients taking barbiturates daily for a month or more above the upper therapeutic range listed in Table 23–1 should be presumed to be physically dependent and in need of medically managed detoxification.

The withdrawal syndrome from short-acting sedative-hypnotics is similar to that from alcohol. Signs and symptoms of sedative-hypnotic withdrawal include anxiety, tremors, nightmares, insomnia, anorexia, nausea, vomiting, postural hypotension, seizures, delirium, and hyperpyrexia. The syndrome is qualitatively similar for all sedative-hypnotics; however, the time course of symptoms depends on the particular drug. With short-acting sedative-hypnotics (e.g., pentobarbital, secobarbital, meprobamate, oxazepam, alprazolam, and triazolam), withdrawal symptoms typically begin 12 to 24 hours after the last dose and peak in intensity between 24 and 72 hours. (Symptoms may develop more slowly in patients with liver disease or in the elderly because of decreased drug metabolism.) With long-acting drugs (e.g., phenobarbital, diazepam, and chlordiazepoxide), withdrawal symptoms peak on the fifth to eighth day.

During untreated sedative-hypnotic withdrawal, the electro-encephalogram may show paroxysmal bursts of high-voltage, slow-frequency activity that precede the development of seizures. The withdrawal delirium may include confusion and visual and auditory hallucinations. The delirium generally follows a period of insomnia. Some patients may have only delirium, others only seizures, and some may have both delirium and convulsions.

Benzodiazepines may also produce a severe, protracted withdrawal syndrome, and withdrawal symptoms may be produced in some patients after cessation of long-term therapeutic dosing.

DIAGNOSIS AND DIFFERENTIAL DIAGNOSIS

The diagnosis of sedative-hypnotic abuse and dependence is based primarily on drug use history and the DSM-IV criteria of continuing behavior dysfunction as a result of the drug abuse. With a dependence disorder developing from prescribed use, the practical difficulty is determining when the dysfunction is a result of the drug use rather than the disorder for which the medication was prescribed.

Variations in Presentations

PHYSICAL DEPENDENCE IN NON-DRUG-DEPENDENT MEDICAL PATIENTS

Long-term use of benzodiazepines can result in physical dependence in non-drug-dependent medical patients. Withdrawal symptoms or return of symptoms suppressed by the benzodiazepines may make discontinuation difficult.

Some patients who are physically dependent on or unable to discontinue a medication do not necessarily have a substance abuse disorder. Physical dependence results from neuroadaptive changes from long-term exposure to a medication. Inability to discontinue the medication may simply mean that patients are unwilling to tolerate the severity of postwithdrawal symptoms that develop. In the absence of dysfunction produced by the medication, the decision to continue taking it may be appropriate medication maintenance.

PRESENTATION IN DRUG-ABUSING PATIENTS

Abusers of alcohol and other drugs rarely present for primary treatment of sedative-hypnotic dependency. From the drug-abusing patient's point of view, sedative-hypnotic use is an effort to self-medicate anxiety or insomnia, which is often the result of alcohol or stimulant abuse. Despite their assertion that the medication is being taken for symptom relief, these patients often take the medication in larger than physician-prescribed doses, combine the medication with intoxicating amounts of alcohol or other drugs, and purchase quantities of medications from street sources. They may also use the medication as an intoxicant when other drugs are not available.

Assessment

DRUG USE HISTORY

The patient's drug use history is usually the first source of information used in assessing sedative-hypnotic abuse or dependence. If the sedative-hypnotics were being used for treatment of insomnia or anxiety, the history is often best obtained as part of the history of the disorder and its response to treatment. A detailed use of all sedative-hypnotics, including alcohol, should be elicited from the patient.

For many reasons, patients may minimize or exaggerate their drug use and not accurately report the behavioral consequences of their use. High doses of benzodiazepines, or therapeutic doses of benzodiazepines in combination with alcohol, may disrupt memory. Patients are likely to attribute impairment of function to the underlying disorder rather than to the medication use. Observations of patients' behavior by family members can be valuable information. Whenever possible, medical and pharmacy records should be obtained to help piece together as accurate a picture of drug use as possible. Pharmacy records may be helpful in establishing and verifying patients' drug use history, and urine testing can be useful in verifying recent drug use history.

PHYSICAL FINDINGS

Sustained horizontal nystagmus is a reliable indicator of sedative-hypnotic intoxication. Onset of tremor, abnormal sweating, and blood pressure or pulse increase may be produced by sedative-hypnotic withdrawal.

LABORATORY TESTS

Urine toxicology can be useful in monitoring patients' use of drugs and in confirming a history of drug or medication use. Laboratory markers can be useful in assessing alcohol use.

COURSE AND NATURAL HISTORY

Once a DSM-IV diagnosis of sedative-hypnotic dependence is established, it is unlikely that a patient will be able to return to controlled, therapeutic use of abusable sedative-hypnotics. All sedative-hypnotics, including alcohol, are cross-tolerant, and physical dependence and tolerance are quickly reestablished if a patient resumes use of sedative-hypnotics.

If after sedative-hypnotic withdrawal the patient has another primarily psychiatric disorder, such as generalized anxiety disorder, panic attacks, or insomnia, treatment strategies other than sedative-hypnotics should be used, if at all possible. Definitive diagnosis of a psychiatric disorder during early abstinence is often not possible because protracted withdrawal symptoms may mimic anxiety disorders, and disruption of sleep architecture for days to months after drug withdrawal is extremely common.

If the sedative-hypnotic dependence has developed secondary to stimulant or alcohol use, primary treatment of the chemical dependence should be a priority. Often the symptom that was driving the sedative-hypnotic use disappears after the patient is drug abstinent.

TREATMENT

Detoxification

Three general strategies are used for withdrawing patients from sedative-hypnotics, including benzodiazepines. The first strategy is to use decreasing doses of the agent of dependence. The second is to substitute phenobarbital or some other long-acting barbiturate for the addicting agent and gradually withdraw the substitute medication. The third, used for patients with a dependence on both alcohol and a benzodiazepine, is to substitute a long-acting benzodiazepine, such as chlordiazepoxide, and taper it during 1 to 2 weeks.

Detoxification Strategies for Sedative-Hypnotics

1. Use decreasing doses of the agent of dependence.
2. Substitute phenobarbital or other long-acting barbiturate and gradually withdraw.
3. Substitute a long-acting benzodiazepine and taper during 1 to 2 weeks.

The pharmacological rationale for phenobarbital substitution is that phenobarbital is long acting and little change in blood levels of phenobarbital occurs between doses. This allows the safe use of a progressively smaller daily dose. Phenobarbital is safer than the shorter acting barbiturates; lethal doses of phenobarbital are many times higher than toxic doses, and the signs of toxicity (e.g., sustained nystagmus, slurred speech, and ataxia) are easy to observe. Finally, phenobarbital intoxication usually does not produce disinhibition, so most patients view it as a medication, not as a drug of abuse.

The gradual reduction of the benzodiazepine of dependence is used primarily in medical settings for dependence arising from treatment of an underlying condition. The patient must be cooperative, must be able to adhere to dosing regimens, and must not be abusing alcohol or other drugs.

Substitution of phenobarbital can also be used to withdraw patients who have lost control of their benzodiazepine use or who are polydrug dependent. Phenobarbital substitution has the broadest use for all sedative-hypnotic drug dependencies and is widely used in drug treatment programs.

STABILIZATION PHASE

The patient's history of drug use during the month before treatment is used to compute the stabilization dose of phenobarbital. Although many addicts exaggerate the number of pills they are taking, the patient's history is the best guide to initiating pharmacotherapy for withdrawal. Patients who have overstated the amount of drug they have taken will become intoxicated during the first day or two of treatment. Intoxication is easily managed by omitting one or more doses of phenobarbital and recalculating the daily dose.

To compute the initial starting dose of phenobarbital, the patient's average daily use of each sedative-hypnotic is computed. Then, the daily dose of each drug is multiplied by the phenobarbital conversion constant, shown in Tables 23–2 and 23–3. The phenobarbital withdrawal equivalents for each drug are then added together. The maximal phenobarbital dose is 500 mg/d. The patient's average daily sedative-hypnotic dose is converted to the phenobarbital withdrawal equivalent using a conversion value such as that shown in Table 23–2. The daily amount is divided into three doses.

Before receiving each dose of phenobarbital, the patient is checked for signs of phenobarbital toxicity: sustained nystagmus, slurred speech, or ataxia. Of these, sustained nystagmus is the most reliable. If nystagmus is present, the scheduled dose of phenobarbital is withheld. If all three signs are present, the next two doses

TABLE 23–2	Phenobarbital Withdrawal Equivalents of Nonbenzodiazepines		
Generic Name	**Trade Name**	**Dose Equal to 30 mg of Phenobarbital for Withdrawal* (mg)**	**Phenobarbital Conversion Constant**
	Barbiturates		
Amobarbital	Amytal	100	0.33
Butabarbital	Butisol	100	0.33
Butalbital†	Fiorinal	100	0.33
Pentobarbital	Nembutal	100	0.33
Secobarbital	Seconal	100	0.33
	Others		
Chloral hydrate	Noctec, Somnos	500	0.06
Ethchlorvynol	Placidyl	500	0.06
Glutethimide	Doriden	250	0.12
Meprobamate	Miltown	1200	0.025
Methyprylon	Noludar	200	0.15
Zolpidem	Ambien	5	6

*Phenobarbital withdrawal conversion equivalence is not the same as therapeutic dose equivalency.

†Butalbital is in combination with opiate or nonopiate analgesics.

TABLE 23–3	Phenobarbital Withdrawal Equivalents of Benzodiazepines		
Generic Name	Trade Name	Dose Equal to 30 mg of Phenobarbital for Withdrawal* (mg)	Phenobarbital Conversion Constant
Alprazolam	Xanax	1	30
Chloridiaz-epoxide	Librium	25	1.2
Clonazepam	Klonopin	2	15
Clorazepate	Tranxene	7.5	4
Diazepam	Valium	10	3
Estazolam	ProSom	1	30
Flurazepam	Dalmane	15	2
Halazepam	Paxipam	40	.75
Lorazepam	Ativan	2	15
Oxazepam	Serax	10	3
Prazepam	Centrax	10	3
Quazepam	Doral	15	2
Temazepam	Restoril	15	2
Triazolam	Halcion	.25	120

*Phenobarbital withdrawal conversion equivalence is not the same as therapeutic dose equivalency.

of phenobarbital are withheld, and the daily dosage of phenobarbital for the next day is halved.

Signs of Phenobarbital Toxicity

- Sustained nystagmus
- Slurred speech
- Ataxia

If the patient is in acute withdrawal and has had, or is in danger of having, withdrawal seizures, the initial dose of phenobarbital is administered by intramuscular injection. If nystagmus and other signs of intoxication develop after 1 to 2 hours following the intramuscular dose, the patient is in no immediate danger from barbiturate withdrawal. Patients are maintained with the initial dosing schedule of phenobarbital for 2 days. If the patient has neither signs of withdrawal nor phenobarbital toxicity (slurred speech, nystagmus, unsteady gait), phenobarbital withdrawal is begun.

WITHDRAWAL PHASE

Unless the patient develops signs and symptoms of phenobarbital toxicity or sedative-hypnotic withdrawal, phenobarbital is decreased by 30 mg/d. Should signs of phenobarbital toxicity develop during withdrawal, the daily phenobarbital dose is decreased by 50% and the 30 mg/d withdrawal is continued from the reduced phenobarbital dose. Should the patient have objective signs of sedative-hypnotic withdrawal, the daily dose is increased by 50% and the patient is restabilized before continuing the withdrawal.

PSYCHOSOCIAL TREATMENT

Psychotherapy

Psychotherapy can have an important role in motivating a patient for primary treatment of drug dependency. Therapists can assist in breaking down patients' denial of their drug dependence by helping them see how drug use is interfering with relationships and undermining their ability to function. In some instances, it is desirable to continue the psychotherapeutic relationship while the patient is undergoing treatment for chemical dependence. With drug abusers, it is often good to separate the medication management from psychotherapy to prevent the psychotherapy from becoming bogged down in discussions of medications and medication side effects.

Twelve-Step Recovery

Alcoholics Anonymous, Narcotics Anonymous, and Cocaine Anonymous groups are important treatment adjuncts for many people recovering from alcohol and other forms of drug dependence. Although many groups are becoming more tolerant of appropriate use of pharmacotherapies, many individuals who attend 12-step recovery meetings are adamantly opposed to any form of psychotropic medication use and counsel fellow members to stop their use.

ADDITIONAL TREATMENT CONSIDERATIONS

Underlying Psychiatric Conditions

Numerous studies have documented a high prevalence of psychopathological conditions among alcohol and drug abusers. Although the abuse of drugs can induce a psychopathological condition, and there is considerable uncertainty as to the extent to which drug abuse itself contributes to estimates of psychopathology, it is clinically apparent that some drug abusers have severe underlying psychopathological conditions that must be treated if patients are to remain abstinent and functional.

HIGH-DOSE BENZODIAZEPINE WITHDRAWAL SYNDROME

Studies of humans have established that large doses of chlordiazepoxide and diazepam, taken for 1 month or more, produce a

withdrawal syndrome that is clinically similar to the withdrawal
syndrome produced by high doses of barbiturates. Other benzodiazepines have not been studied under such precise conditions, but
numerous case reports leave no doubt that they also produce a
similar withdrawal syndrome when taken in excess of the upper
therapeutic range.

Treatment of High-Dose Benzodiazepine Dependence

For high-dose benzodiazepine dependence, the pharmacological
treatment strategy is the same as that for barbiturates. The
phenobarbital conversion equivalents are shown in Table 23–3. The
dose conversions computed using Table 23–3 prevent severe
withdrawal of the classic sedative-hypnotic type. As discussed
next, some patients who take high doses of benzodiazepines, or
even therapeutic doses for months to years, may have prolonged
withdrawal symptoms. The phenobarbital dosage conversions
computed using Table 23–3 are not adequate to control these
symptoms.

LOW-DOSE BENZODIAZEPINE WITHDRAWAL SYNDROMES

Many people who have taken benzodiazepines in therapeutic doses
for months to years can abruptly discontinue the drug without
developing withdrawal symptoms. The symptoms for which the
benzodiazepine was being taken often return. The return of symptoms is called *symptom reemergence* (or recrudescence).

However, other patients, taking similar amounts of a benzodiazepine, develop symptoms ranging from mild to severe when the
benzodiazepine is stopped or when the dosage is substantially
reduced. Characteristically, patients tolerate a gradual tapering of
the benzodiazepine until they are at 10% to 20% of their peak dose.
Further reduction in benzodiazepine dose causes patients to become
increasingly symptomatic. In addiction medicine literature, the
low-dose benzodiazepine withdrawal syndrome may be called
therapeutic dose withdrawal, normal dose withdrawal, or benzodiazepine discontinuation syndrome.

Many patients experience a transient increase in symptoms for
1 to 2 weeks after benzodiazepine withdrawal. The symptoms are
an intensified return of the symptoms for which the benzodiazepine
was prescribed. The transient form of symptom intensification is
called *symptom rebound.* The term comes from sleep research in
which rebound insomnia is commonly observed after sedative-
hypnotic use. Symptom rebound lasts a few days to weeks after
discontinuation and is the most common withdrawal consequence
of prolonged benzodiazepine use.

A few patients experience a severe, protracted withdrawal
syndrome that includes symptoms (e.g., paresthesia and psychosis)
that were not present before. This withdrawal syndrome has generated much of the concern about the long-term safety of the benzodiazepines.

Dementia, Delirium, and Other Cognitive Disorders

This chapter reviews dementia, delirium, amnestic and other cognitive disorders, and the mental disorders due to a general medical condition. Delirium, dementia, and amnestic disorders are classified as cognitive because they feature impairment in such parameters as memory, language, or attention as a cardinal symptom.

In the case of delirium, the primary disturbance is in the level of consciousness with associated impairments in orientation, memory, judgment, and attention. Dementia features cognitive deficits in memory, language, and intellect. The amnestic disorder is characterized by impairment in memory in the absence of clouded consciousness or other noteworthy cognitive dysfunction. In general, the cognitive disorders should represent a decline from a previous higher level of function, of either acute (delirium) or insidious (dementia) onset, and should interfere with the patient's social or occupational functioning.

MENTAL DISORDERS DUE TO A GENERAL MEDICAL CONDITION

In most instances, there are no infallible criteria for determining whether a particular medical condition is etiologically related to an observed mental disorder. Factors that may help in establishing this association include 1) a temporal relationship between the onset, worsening, or remission of the general medical condition and that of the mental disturbance; 2) a past history of the same mental disorder during an episode of the medical condition; 3) documentation in the scientific literature of a similar mental reaction to the medical condition; and 4) the presence of features that are not typical of the primary mental disorder. In many instances, there is a significant delay between correction of the medical condition and resolution of the mental symptoms produced by it. This is especially true for elderly patients and those with previously compromised brain function. Some such medical conditions may involve structural changes in the brain (e.g., significant head injury) and are irreversible.

Diagnostic Categories

PSYCHOTIC DISORDER DUE TO A GENERAL MEDICAL CONDITION

Psychotic disorder due to a general medical condition features prominent delusions and/or hallucinations that are believed to be due to the direct physiological effects of a general medical condition. To meet the criteria for psychotic disorder due to a general medical condition, the hallucinations or delusions must not be observed only during the course of a delirious episode.

Thyroid disease, cerebral neoplasms, adrenal dysfunction, and systemic lupus erythematosus are among the more common disorders associated with psychosis. The differential diagnosis is between psychotic features associated with delirium, dementia (Alzheimer's or vascular), substance-induced psychotic disorder, a primary psychotic disorder, and an affective disorder with psychosis.

ANXIETY DISORDER DUE TO A GENERAL MEDICAL CONDITION

In anxiety disorder due to a general medical condition, the anxiety must be owing to the direct effects of a medical disturbance and can take the form of panic attacks, obsessions, or compulsions. The symptoms must not be attributable to delirium or some other condition such as adjustment disorder with anxiety.

Many medical conditions can produce anxiety. These include such endocrinological conditions as hyperthyroidism, pheochromocytoma, and Cushing's disease; insulinoma and other causes of hypoglycemia; carcinoid syndrome; acute intermittent porphyria; and certain cardiovascular conditions. Substance-induced anxiety must be excluded before the diagnosis of anxiety due to a general medical condition is made.

MOOD DISORDER DUE TO A GENERAL MEDICAL CONDITION

In mood disorder due to a general medical condition, a persistent and prominent mood disturbance is found to be due to the effects of a general medical condition. The mood can be depressed, either moderately or resembling a major depressive disorder; can have features of mania; or can be of mixed type. Medical conditions that can produce mood disturbances include cerebrovascular accidents (CVAs), degenerative disorders, multiple sclerosis, adrenal dysfunction, thyroid disease, acquired immunodeficiency syndrome (AIDS), syphilis, and carcinoma of the pancreas.

SEXUAL DYSFUNCTION DUE TO A GENERAL MEDICAL CONDITION

The sexual difficulty can include a variety of disorders such as dyspareunia, changes in libido, erectile dysfunction, and orgasmic disorders.

Medical conditions that may produce sexual dysfunction due to a general medical condition include diabetes mellitus, spinal cord abnormalities, endocrinological disorders, and various genitourinary conditions.

SLEEP DISORDER DUE TO A GENERAL MEDICAL CONDITION

The subtypes of the sleep disturbance are 1) insomnia type, 2) hypersomnia type, 3) parasomnia type, and 4) mixed.

Medical conditions that can produce a sleep disorder include degenerative disorders such as Parkinson's and Huntington's diseases, endocrine conditions, infectious states (especially viral encephalitis), and the rare Kleine-Levin syndrome.

CATATONIC DISORDER DUE TO A GENERAL MEDICAL CONDITION

Catatonia is characterized by one or more of the following: absent or excessive motor activity, negativism, mutism, unusual movements, and mimicking the words (echolalia) or actions (echopraxia) of the examiner.

Many medical conditions can produce catatonia. Various disorders of the brain (tumors, trauma, infection, inflammation, and vascular conditions) and such metabolic conditions as hypercalcemia, hepatic encephalopathy, and diabetic ketoacidosis may lead to catatonic states. Physiological consequences of catatonia such as contractures and decubitus can occur.

DSM-IV Criteria 293.89

Catatonic Disorder Due to . . . [Indicate the General Medical Condition]

A. The presence of catatonia as manifested by motoric immobility, excessive motor activity (that is apparently purposeless and not influenced by external stimuli), extreme negativism or mutism, peculiarities of voluntary movement, or echolalia or echopraxia.

B. There is evidence from the history, physical examination, or laboratory findings that the disturbance is the direct physiological consequence of a general medical condition.

C. The disturbance is not better accounted for by another mental disorder (e.g., a manic episode).

D. The disturbance does not occur exclusively during the course of a delirium.

Coding note: Include the name of the general medical condition on Axis I (e.g., 293.89, catatonic disorder due to hepatic encephalopathy); also code the general medical condition on Axis III.

PERSONALITY CHANGE DUE TO A GENERAL MEDICAL CONDITION

This personality disturbance should represent a change from a previously established personality structure or, in the case of a child, a significant deviation from normal development.

Representative features of the personality change include lability of affect, impulsivity, poor judgment, loss of social inhibitions, apathy, aggressiveness, and paranoia. Family members often describe the affected individual as "not himself." The particular manifestation of the personality disturbance is often related to the area of the brain affected. The frontal lobes are involved in the engagement of attention, the inhibition of inappropriate behavior, and the initiation and planning of complex behaviors. Thus, a disorder affecting this area may result in loss of inhibition regarding aggressive and sexual behavior; lack of interaction with the environment; and subsequent apathy, indifference, and withdrawal. Conditions that affect the temporal lobes (typically epileptic foci) may produce such features as elation, rage, verbosity, hyperreligiosity, and a strong sense of morality that may evolve into self-righteousness.

A variety of medical conditions can produce alterations in personality. Head trauma, cerebrovascular disease, epilepsy, and central nervous system neoplasms are the most common causes. Other conditions including Huntington's disease, systemic lupus erythematosus, multiple sclerosis, human immunodeficiency virus (HIV) spectrum illness, and endocrine disorders have also been implicated.

DSM-IV Criteria 310.1

Personality Change Due to ... [Indicate the General Medical Condition]

A. A persistent personality disturbance that represents a change from the individual's previous characteristic personality pattern. (In children, the disturbance involves a marked deviation from normal development or a significant change in the child's usual behavior patterns lasting at least 1 year.)

B. There is evidence from the history, physical examination, or laboratory findings that the disturbance is the direct physiological consequence of a general medical condition.

C. The disturbance is not better accounted for by another mental disorder (including other mental disorders due to a general medical condition).

D. The disturbance does not occur exclusively during the course of a delirium and does not meet criteria for a dementia.

Box continued on following page

DSM-IV Criteria 310.1

Personality Change Due to . . . *Continued*

E. The disturbance causes clinically significant distress or impairment in social, occupational, or other important areas of functioning.

Specify type:

Labile type: if the predominant feature is affective lability

Disinhibited type: if the predominant feature is poor impulse control as evidenced by sexual indiscretions, etc.

Aggressive type: if the predominant feature is marked apathy and indifference

Paranoid type: if the predominant feature is suspiciousness or paranoid ideation

Other type: if the predominant feature is not one of the above (e.g., personality change associated with a seizure disorder)

Combined type: if more than one feature predominates in the clinical picture

Unspecified type

Coding note: Include the name of the general medical condition on Axis I (e.g., 310.1, personality change due to temporal lobe epilepsy); also code the general medical condition on Axis III.

MEDICAL CONDITIONS ASSOCIATED WITH MENTAL DISORDERS

Endocrine Disorders

Hyperfunction and hypofunction of the thyroid gland have been associated with a variety of psychiatric symptoms. Hyperthyroidism features anxiety, confusion, and agitated depression.

Hypothyroidism, in its most severe form, so-called myxedema madness, can involve paranoid delusions, delirium, mania, and hallucinations.

Hyperparathyroidism produces hypercalcemia with resultant delirium, apathy, and personality changes. Cognitive impairment occurs in a minority of patients. Hypocalcemia can also result in personality changes and delirium.

Hypofunction of the adrenal glands, as in chronic adrenocortical insufficiency (Addison's disease), can produce apathy, irritability, and depression. Rarely, confusion and depression may result. Adrenocortical hyperplasia (Cushing's disease) can produce depression, amnesia, agitation, and even suicide. Sheehan's syndrome, a condition seen in postpartum women, involves hemorrhage into the pituitary gland and can present with agitation, mania, psychosis, or depression.

Infectious Disorders

Rabies encephalitis can produce agitation, restlessness, and phobia, whereas herpes simplex encephalitis may cause olfactory and gustatory hallucinations, changes in personality, and psychotic behavior. Herpes has a predilection for the frontal and temporal lobes. Neurosyphilis, Creutzfeldt-Jakob disease, subacute sclerosing panencephalitis, infections with HIV, and kuru can produce mental impairment as well.

Metabolic Disorders

Metabolic encephalopathies are serious conditions that often feature anxiety, disorientation, and memory loss. Hepatic, uremic, and hypoglycemic encephalopathies are common complications of disease states.

DEMENTIA, DELIRIUM, AND OTHER COGNITIVE DISORDERS

Dementia

Dementia is defined in the *Diagnostic and Statistical Manual of Mental Disorders* (DSM-IV) as a series of disorders characterized by the development of multiple cognitive deficits (including memory impairment) that are due to the direct physiological effects of a general medical condition, the persisting effects of a substance, or multiple etiologies (e.g., the combined effects of a metabolic and a degenerative disorder). The disorders constituting the dementias share a common symptom presentation and are identified and classified on the basis of etiology. The cognitive deficits exhibited in these disorders must be of significant severity to interfere with either occupational functioning or the individual's usual social activities or relationships. In addition, the observed deficits must represent a decline from a higher level of function and not be the consequence of a delirium. A delirium can be superimposed on a dementia, however, and both can be diagnosed if the dementia is observed when the delirium is not in evidence. Dementia typically is chronic and occurs in the presence of a clear sensorium. If clouding of consciousness occurs, the diagnosis of delirium should be considered.

CLINICAL FEATURES

Essential to the diagnosis of dementia is the presence of cognitive deficits that include memory impairment and at least one of the following abnormalities of cognition: aphasia, agnosia, apraxia, or a disturbance in executive function.

Memory function is divided into three compartments that can easily be evaluated during a Mental Status Examination. These are immediate recall (primary memory), recent (secondary) memory, and remote (tertiary) memory.

In addition to defects in memory, patients with dementia often exhibit impairments in language, recognition, object naming, and motor skills. Aphasia is an abnormality of language that often occurs in vascular dementias involving the dominant hemisphere. Patients with dementia and aphasia may exhibit paucity of speech, poor articulation, and a telegraphic pattern of speech (nonfluent, Broca's aphasia).

By contrast, dementia patients with fluent (Wernicke's) aphasia may be quite verbose and articulate, but much of the language is nonsensical and rife with such paraphasias as neologisms and clang (rhyming) associations.

Patients with dementia may also lose their ability to recognize. Agnosia is a feature of a dominant hemisphere lesion and involves altered perception in which, despite normal sensations, intellect, and language, the patient cannot recognize objects.

The two most common forms of apraxia in demented patients are ideational and gait apraxia. Ideational apraxia is the inability to perform motor activities that require sequential steps and results from a lesion involving both frontal lobes or the complete cerebrum. Gait apraxia, often seen in such conditions as normal-pressure hydrocephalus, is the inability to perform various motions of ambulation. It also results from conditions that diffusely affect the cerebrum.

Impairment of executive function is the inability to think abstractly, plan, initiate, and end complex behavior.

Obviously, aphasia, agnosia, apraxia, and impairment of executive function can seriously impede the demented patients' ability to interact with their environments. An appropriate Mental Status Examination of the patient with suspected dementia should include screening for the presence of these abnormalities.

COURSE

The course of a particular dementia is influenced by its etiology. Although historically the dementias have been considered progressive and irreversible, there is, in fact, significant variation in the course of individual dementias. The disorder can be progressive, static, or remitting.

DIFFERENTIAL DIAGNOSIS

Memory impairment occurs in a variety of conditions including delirium, amnestic disorders, and depression. In delirium, the onset of altered memory is acute, and the pattern typically fluctuates (waxing and waning) with increased proclivity for confusion during the night. Delirium is more likely to feature autonomic hyperactivity and alterations in level of consciousness.

Patients with major depression often complain of lapses in memory and judgment, poor concentration, and seemingly diminished intellectual capacity. The term *pseudodementia* has been used to denote cognitive impairment secondary to a functional psychiatric disorder, most commonly depression. In comparison with demented patients, those with depressive pseudodementia exhibit better insight regarding their cognitive dysfunction, are more likely to give "I don't know" answers, and may exhibit neurovegetative signs of depression.

An amnestic disorder also presents with a significant memory deficit but without the other associated features such as aphasia, agnosia, and apraxia. If cognitive impairment occurs only in the context of drug use, substance intoxication or substance withdrawal is the appropriate diagnosis.

Mental retardation must be considered in the differential diagnosis of dementias of childhood and adolescence along with such disorders as Wilson's disease (hepatolenticular degeneration), lead intoxication, subacute sclerosing panencephalitis, HIV spectrum disorders, and substance abuse, particularly abuse of inhalants.

The physical examination may offer clues to the etiology of the dementia; however, in the elderly, one must be aware of the normal changes associated with aging and differentiate them from signs of dementia. Often the specific physical examination findings indicate the area of the central nervous system affected by the etiological process.

Although the many and varied physical findings of dementia are too numerous to mention here, it should be obvious that the physical examination is an invaluable tool in the assessment of dementia (Table 24–1).

MENTAL STATUS EXAMINATION

The Mental Status Examination, in conjunction with a complete medical history from the patient and informants and an adequate physical examination, is essential in the evaluation and differential diagnosis of dementia (Table 24–2).

DEGENERATIVE CAUSES OF DEMENTIA

DEMENTIA OF THE ALZHEIMER TYPE. Alzheimer's disease (AD) is the most common cause of dementia, accounting for 55% to 65% of all cases. Prevalence of the disease doubles every 5 years between the ages of 65 and 85 years. Onset of symptoms occurs after the age of 40 years in 96% of cases and between the ages of 45 and 65 years in 80% of patients. Early-onset AD is associated with a more rapid course than later onset disease. Alzheimer's disease affects women three times as often as men, for unknown reasons. *Laboratory and Radiological Findings.* The role of laboratory determinations in the evaluation for AD is to exclude other causes of dementia, especially those that may prove reversible or arrestable. Before death, AD is largely a diagnosis of exclusion. Throughout the course of this disorder, laboratory values are essentially normal.

At present, in the work-up of a patient with a slowly progressive dementia, a good family history, physical examination, and laboratory and radiographic tests to rule out other causes of dementia are the most effective tools in the diagnosis of Alzheimer's disease. *Clinical Features.* The course and clinical features of AD parallel those discussed for dementia in general. Typically, the early course of AD is difficult to ascertain because the patient is usually an unreliable informant, and the early signs may be so subtle as to go unnoticed even by the patient's closest associates. These early features include impaired memory, difficulty with problem solving, preoccupation with long past events, decreased spontaneity, and an inability to respond to the environment with the patient's usual speed and accuracy.

TABLE 24–1	Physical Signs Associated with Dementia or Delirium

Physical Sign	Condition
Myoclonus	Creutzfeldt-Jakob disease
	Subacute sclerosing panencephalitis
	Postanoxia
	Alzheimer's disease (10%)
	AIDS dementia
	Uremia
	Penicillin intoxication
	Meperidine toxicity
Asterixis	Hepatic encephalopathy
	Uremia
	Hypoxia
	Carbon dioxide retention
Chorea	Huntington's disease
	Wilson's disease
	Hypocalcemia
	Hypothyroidism
	Hepatic encephalopathy
	Oral contraceptives
	Systemic lupus erythematosus
	Carbon monoxide poisoning
	Toxoplasmosis
	Pertussis, diphtheria
Peripheral neuropathy	Wernicke-Korsakoff syndrome
	Neurosyphilis
	Heavy metal intoxication
	Organic solvent exposure
	Vitamin B_{12} deficiency
	Medications: isoniazid, phenytoin

Whereas much attention has been focused on research aimed at understanding and altering the pathogenesis of AD, less work has been done regarding appropriate pharmacological agents for the varied psychological manifestations of the disease. Depression is often associated with AD. If antidepressant medication is to be used, low doses (about one third to one half of the usual initial dose) are advised, and only agents with minimal anticholinergic activity should be employed.

Anxiety and psychosis, particularly paranoid delusions, are common in AD. Benzodiazepines inhibit new memory and should be avoided if possible. Antipsychotic medications with high anticholinergic potential (thioridazine, chlorpromazine) may also affect memory, so their use must be weighed against the beneficial sedation they might produce. Haloperidol has less anticholinergic activity but may aggravate some AD symptoms such as extrapyramidal signs.

In the attempt to maintain AD patients in their homes for as long as possible, some adjustment of their environment is important. Written daily reminders can be helpful in the performance of daily activities. Prominent clocks, calendars, and windows are important, and an effort should be made to minimize changes in the patient's daily activities. Repeated demonstrations of how to lock doors and windows and operate appliances are helpful, and arranging for rapid dialing of essential telephone numbers can be important. Maintaining adequate hydration, nutrition, exercise, and cleanliness is essential.

The family of the patient with AD is also a victim of the disease. Family members must watch the gradual deterioration of the patient and accept that a significant part of their own lives must be devoted to the care of the individual. Difficult decisions about institutionalization and termination of life support are distinct possibilities, and the patients often turn their anger and paranoia toward the caregiver. Education is a valuable treatment tool for families. Information about the disease and peer support are available through Alzheimer's associations, and many such agencies provide family members with a companion for the patient to allow the family some time away.

DEMENTIA DUE TO PICK'S DISEASE. Pick's disease is a rare form of progressive dementia clinically indistinguishable from Alzheimer's disease. It is about one fifth as common as AD. Pick's disease occurs in middle adult life and has a duration that varies from 2 to 15 years. It has a strong familial tendency, but a definite genetic pattern has not been established.

DEMENTIA DUE TO PARKINSON'S DISEASE. Although dementia rarely occurs as an initial symptom of Parkinson's disease, it is found in nearly 40% of patients older than 70 years of age. Usually the patient is 50 years of age or older, and unlike Alzheimer's and Pick's dementias, this disease occurs slightly more

TABLE 24–2	Evaluation of Dementia

Medical history and physical examination

Family interview

Routine laboratory
  Chemistry (SMA 20)
  Urinalysis
  Hematology (complete blood count)

Other routine tests
  Chest radiography
  Electrocardiography

Specialized laboratory
  Thyroid functions
  VDRL (fluorescent treponemal antibody screen if indicated)
  Drug screen
  Vitamin B_{12} and folate levels
  Cerebrospinal fluid analysis (if indicated)
  HIV testing (if indicated)

Other studies
  Computed tomography or magnetic resonance imaging
  Electroencephalography

often in men. Dementia most commonly occurs in cases of Parkinson's disease in which the decline has been rapid and the response to anticholinergics has been poor.

DEMENTIA DUE TO HUNTINGTON'S DISEASE. Dementia is also a characteristic of Huntington's disease, an autosomal dominant inheritable condition localized to chromosome 4. Unfortunately, this condition does not become apparent until age 35 to 45 years, usually after childbearing has occurred.

VASCULAR DEMENTIA. Vascular dementia usually results from multiple CVAs or one significant CVA. It is generally considered the second most common cause of dementia after Alzheimer's disease, accounting for about 10% of all cases. Men are twice as likely as women to be diagnosed with this condition. Vascular dementia is characterized by a stepwise progression of cognitive deterioration with accompanying lateralizing signs. It is always associated with evidence of systemic hypertension and usually involves renal and cardiac abnormalities.

INFECTIOUS CAUSES OF DEMENTIA

DEMENTIA DUE TO SUBACUTE SCLEROSING PANEN-CEPHALITIS. Subacute sclerosing panencephalitis is an infectious cause of dementia that usually appears in childhood. The average age at onset is 10 years, and most patients are male and live in rural areas. It is diagnosed on the basis of periodic complexes on the EEG and an elevated measles titer in the cerebrospinal fluid (CSF). The CT scan shows cerebral atrophy and dilated ventricles.

DEMENTIA DUE TO CREUTZFELDT-JAKOB DISEASE. The primary features of Creutzfeldt-Jakob disease are dementia, basal ganglia and cerebellar dysfunction, myoclonus, upper motor neuron lesions, and rapid progression to stupor, coma, and death in a matter of months. The disease generally affects people 65 years of age or older, with a duration of 1 month to 6 years and an average life span after disease onset of 15 months.

DEMENTIA DUE TO HIV DISEASE. Initially, the behavioral abnormalities observed in HIV-positive patients were attributed to the emotional reaction to the disease. Subsequent investigations demonstrated that neurological complications occur in 40% to 45% of patients with AIDS, and in about 10% of cases neurological signs are the first feature of the disease.

Patients with AIDS dementia present with impairments of cognitive, behavioral, and motor systems. The cognitive disorders include memory impairment, confusion, and poor concentration. Behavioral features include apathy, reclusivity, anhedonia, depression, delusions, and hallucinations. Motor symptoms include incoordination, lower extremity paresis, unsteadiness, and difficulty with fine motor movements like handwriting and buttoning clothes. As the disease progresses, parkinsonism and myoclonus develop. Lateralizing signs such as tremors, focal seizures, abnormal reflexes, and hemiparesis can result.

Many confounding factors can increase cognitive dysfunction in AIDS, including a high incidence of drug and alcohol abuse; medications such as histamine H_2 receptor antagonists (cimetidine), corticosteroids, narcotics, and antiviral drugs (e.g., zidovudine [formerly azidothymidine, AZT]) that increase confusion; and co-existent depression (Table 24–3).

TABLE 24–3	Neuropsychiatric Effects of AIDS-Related Drugs	
Drug	**Use**	**Effect**
Ketoconazole (Nizoral)	Antifungal	Severe depression Suicidality (rare)
Foscarnet	Cytomegalovirus retinitis Herpes	Depression Confusion
Ganciclovir	Cytomegalovirus retinitis	Anxiety Psychosis
Bactrim	*Pneumocystis* pneumonia	Hallucinations Depression Apathy
Pentamidine	*Pneumocystis* pneumonia	Delirium Hallucinations
Interferon alfa	Cancer	Depression
Rifampin	Tuberculosis	Delirium Behavioral changes
Isoniazid	Tuberculosis	Memory disturbance Psychosis
Dronabinol (Marinol)	Appetite stimulant Wasting syndrome Nausea	Depression Anxiety Psychosis Euphoria
Zalcitabine (DDC)	Antiviral	Psychosis Amnesia Confusion Depersonalization Depression Mania Suicidality Mood swings
Didanosine	Antiviral	Anxiety
Zidovudine (AZT)	Antiviral	Confusion, mania Depression, anxiety

DEMENTIA DUE TO NEUROSYPHILIS. Late syphilis consists of ongoing inflammatory disease most likely in the aorta or nervous system (neurosyphilis), the latter occurring in about 10% of patients. The neurosyphilis of the late stage can consist of 1) asymptomatic neurosyphilis, 2) meningovascular syphilis, and 3) parenchymal neurosyphilis. The parenchymal neurosyphilis consists of general paresis, which occurs about 20 years after infection and includes cognitive impairment, myoclonus, dysarthria, personality changes, irritability, psychosis, grandiosity, and mania.

Dementia secondary to neurosyphilis produces various physical findings in advanced cases. These may include dysarthria, Babinski's reflux, tremor, Argyll Robertson pupils, myelitis, and optic atrophy. Although notorious, delusions of grandeur in neurosyphilis are rare. A reactive CSF VDRL result or a positive serum fluorescent treponemal antibody result in a patient with neurological symptoms who cannot document treatment should be treated with appropriate antibiotic therapy. Penicillin often improves cognitive deficits and corrects CSF abnormalities, but complete recovery is rare.

DEMENTIA DUE TO HEAD TRAUMA

The psychiatric manifestations of an acute brain injury are generally classified as a delirium or amnestic disorder; however, head trauma–induced delirious states often merge into a chronic dementia. Episodes of repeated head trauma, as in dementia pugilistica (punchdrunk syndrome), can lead to permanent changes in cognition and thus are appropriately classified as demented states.

A single head injury may result in a postconcussional syndrome with resultant memory impairment, alterations in mood and personality, hyperacusis, headaches, easy fatigability, anxiety, belligerent behavior, and dizziness.

SUBSTANCE-INDUCED PERSISTING DEMENTIA

ALCOHOL-INDUCED DEMENTIA. Chronic alcohol abuse is the third leading cause of dementia. It affects a higher proportion of women than men, and alcohol-induced dementia is a relatively late occurrence, generally after 15 to 20 years of heavy drinking. Dementia is more common in individuals with alcoholism who are malnourished.

Clinical Features. Alcohol-induced dementia secondary to the toxic effects of alcohol develops insidiously and often presents initially with changes in personality. Increasing memory loss, worsening cognitive processing, and worsening concrete thinking follow. The dementia may be affected by periodic superimposed delirious states including those caused by recurrent use of alcohol and cross-sensitive drugs, respiratory disease related to smoking, central nervous system hemorrhage secondary to trauma, chronic hypoxia related to recurrent seizure activity, folic acid deficiency, and higher rates of some neoplasms among those with alcoholism.

DEMENTIA DUE TO OTHER GENERAL MEDICAL CONDITIONS

NORMAL-PRESSURE HYDROCEPHALUS. Normal-pressure hydrocephalus is generally considered the fifth leading cause of dementia after Alzheimer's, vascular, alcohol-related, and AIDS dementias. Long considered reversible but often merely arrestible, normal-pressure hydrocephalus is a syndrome consisting of dementia, urinary incontinence, and gait apraxia.

Unlike other dementias, in the dementia caused by normal-pressure hydrocephalus, the physical effects often overshadow the mental effects.

WILSON'S DISEASE. Hepatolenticular degeneration (Wilson's disease) is an inherited autosomal recessive condition associated with dementia, hepatic dysfunction, and a movement disorder. Symptoms begin in adolescence to the early 20s, and cases are often seen in younger children. Wilson's disease should be considered along with Huntington's disease, AIDS dementia, substance abuse dementia, head trauma, and subacute sclerosing panencephalitis in the differential diagnosis of dementia that presents in adolescence and early adulthood. Personality, mood, and thought disorders are common, and physical findings include a wing-beating tremor, rigidity, akinesia, dystonia, and the pathognomonic Kayser-Fleischer ring around the cornea.

OTHER MEDICAL CONDITIONS. In addition to the conditions mentioned previously, other medical illnesses can be associated with dementia. These include endocrine disorders (hypothyroidism, hypoparathyroidism), chronic metabolic conditions (hypocalcemia, hypoglycemia), nutritional deficiencies (thiamine, niacin, vitamin B_{12}), structural lesions (brain tumors, subdural hematomas), and multiple sclerosis.

TREATMENT OF DEMENTIA

The management of dementia involves 1) identification and, if possible, correction of the underlying cause; 2) environmental manipulation to reorient the patient; 3) intervention with the family by means of education, peer support, providing access to community organizations, discussing powers of attorney, living wills, and institutionalization if appropriate, and arranging therapy if indicated; and 4) pharmacological management of psychiatric symptoms and behavior.

Tables 24–4, 24–5, and 24–6 summarize the causes of dementia.

Delirium

Delirium (acute confusional state, toxic metabolic encephalopathy) is the behavioral response to widespread disturbances in cerebral metabolism. Like dementia, delirium is not a disease but a syndrome with many possible causes that result in a similar constellation of symptoms.

The overall prevalence of delirium in the community is low, but delirium is common in hospitalized patients. The intensive care unit, geriatric psychiatry ward, emergency department, alcohol treatment units, and oncology wards have particularly high rates of delirium.

Predisposing factors in the development of delirium include old age, young age (children), previous brain damage, prior episodes of delirium, malnutrition, sensory impairment (especially vision), and alcohol dependence.

TABLE 24–4	Causes of Dementia

Vascular
  Multiinfarct
  CVA
  Binswanger's disease
Degenerative
  Alzheimer's disease
  Pick's disease
  Huntington's disease
  Parkinson's disease
Toxic
  Medications
  Alcohol
  Poisons
  Inhalants
  Heavy metals
Infectious
  HIV spectrum illness
  Neurosyphilis
  Creutzfeldt-Jakob disease
  Kuru
  Subacute sclerosing panencephalitis
Metabolic
  Chronic hypoglycemia
  Electrolyte imbalances
  Vitamin deficiencies
Endocrine
  Thyroid abnormalities
  Parathyroid abnormalities
Trauma
  Single head injury
  Dementia pugilistica
Neoplastic
  Primary brain tumor
  Metastatic brain tumor

TABLE 24–5	Causes of Dementia in Adolescents

Huntington's disease (juvenile type)
Hepatolenticular degeneration (Wilson's disease)
Subacute sclerosing panencephalitis
AIDS
Substance abuse (especially inhalants)
Head trauma

TABLE 24–6	Causes of Dementia in Children

Head injury (including child abuse)
Subacute sclerosing panencephalitis
AIDS

DSM-IV Criteria 293.0

Delirium due to ... [Indicate the General Medical Condition]

A. Disturbance of consciousness (i.e., reduced clarity of awareness of the environment) with reduced ability to focus, sustain, or shift attention.

B. A change in cognition (such as memory deficit, disorientation, language disturbance) or the development of a perceptual disturbance that is not better accounted for by a preexisting, established, or evolving dementia.

C. The disturbance develops over a short period of time (usually hours to days) and tends to fluctuate during the course of the day.

D. There is evidence from the history, physical examination, or laboratory findings that the disturbance is caused by the direct physiological consequences of a general medical condition.

Coding note: If delirium is superimposed on a preexisting dementia of the Alzheimer's type or vascular dementia, indicate the delirium by coding the appropriate subtype of the dementia (e.g., 290.3 dementia of the Alzheimer's type, with late onset, with delirium).

Coding note: Include the name of the general medical condition on Axis I (e.g., 293.0 delirium due to hepatic encephalopathy); also code the general medical condition on Axis III.

CLINICAL FEATURES

According to DSM-IV, the primary feature of delirium is a diminished clarity of awareness of the environment. Symptoms of delirium are characteristically global, of acute onset, fluctuating, and of relatively brief duration. In most cases of delirium, an often overlooked prodrome of altered sleep patterns, unexplained fatigue, fluctuating mood, sleep phobia, restlessness, anxiety, and nightmares occurs.

Several investigators have divided the clinical features of delirium into abnormalities of 1) arousal, 2) language and cognition,

3) perception, 4) orientation, 5) mood, 6) sleep and wakefulness, and 7) neurological functioning.

CAUSES OF DELIRIUM

The cause of delirium may lie in intracranial processes, extracranial ones, or a combination of the two. The most common etiologic factors are the following: 1) infection, 2) metabolic and endocrine disturbances, 3) low-perfusion states, 4) intracranial lesions, 5) postoperative states, 6) sensory and environmental changes, and 7) substance toxicity or withdrawal.

DIAGNOSIS

Appropriate work-up of delirious patients includes a complete physical, mental status, and neurological examination.

History taking from the patient, any available family, previous physicians, the old chart, and the patient's current nurse is essential. Previous delirious states, etiologies identified in the past, and interventions that proved effective should be elucidated. The appropriate evaluation of the delirious patient is reviewed in Figure 24–1.

DIFFERENTIAL DIAGNOSIS. Delirium must be differentiated from dementia, because the two conditions may have different prognoses. In contrast to the changes in dementia, those in delirium have an acute onset. The symptoms in dementia tend to be relatively stable over time, whereas clinical features of delirium display wide fluctuation with periods of relative lucidity. Clouding of consciousness is common in delirium, but demented patients are usually alert.

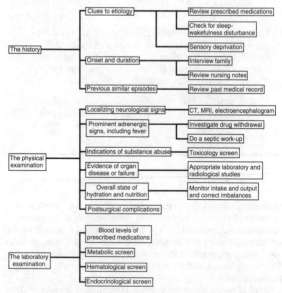

Figure 24–1 *Evaluation of delirium.*

Attention and orientation are more commonly disturbed in delirium, although the latter can become impaired in advanced dementia. Perception abnormalities, alterations in the sleep-wakefulness cycle, and abnormalities of speech are more common in delirium.

Delirium and dementia can occur simultaneously; in fact, the presence of dementia is a risk factor for delirium. Some studies suggest that about 30% of hospitalized patients with dementia have a superimposed delirium.

Delirium must often be differentiated from psychotic states related to such conditions as schizophrenia or mania and factitious disorders with psychological symptoms.

MANAGEMENT

Once delirium has been diagnosed, the etiological agent must be identified and treated. For the elderly, the first step generally involves discontinuing or reducing the dosage of potentially offending medications. Supportive therapy should include fluid and electrolyte maintenance and provision of adequate nutrition. Reorienting the patient is essential and is best accomplished in a well-lit room with a window, clock, and visible wall calendar.

Physicians must take into account that impairments of vision and hearing can produce confusional states, and the provision of appropriate prosthetic devices may be beneficial. Around-the-clock accompaniment by hospital-provided "sitters" or family members may be required.

Despite these conservative interventions, the delirious patient often requires pharmacological intervention. The drug of choice for the agitated, delirious patient is haloperidol (Haldol). It is particularly beneficial when given by the intravenous route. In general, intravenous doses in the range of 0.5 to 5.0 mg are used, with the frequency of administration depending on a variety of factors including the patient's age. Lorazepam (Ativan) has also proved effective in doses of 0.5 to 2.0 mg given intravenously.

Amnestic Disorders

The amnestic disorders are characterized by a disturbance in memory related to the direct effects of a general medical condition or the persisting effects of a substance. The impairment should interfere with social and occupational functioning and represent a significant decline from the previous level of functioning. The amnestic disorders are differentiated on the basis of the etiology of the memory loss. These disorders should not be diagnosed if the memory deficit is a feature of a dissociative disorder, is associated with dementia, or occurs in the presence of clouded sensorium, as in delirium.

The specific causes of amnestic disorders include 1) systemic medical conditions such as thiamine deficiency; 2) brain conditions, including seizures, cerebral neoplasms, head injury, hypoxia, carbon monoxide poisoning, surgical ablation of temporal lobes, electroconvulsive therapy, and multiple sclerosis; 3) altered blood flow in the vertebral vascular system, as in transient global amnesia; and 4) effects of a substance (drug or alcohol use and exposure to toxins).

DSM-IV Criteria 294.0

Amnestic Disorder Due to . . . [Indicate the General Medical Condition]

A. The development of memory impairment as manifested by impairment in the ability to learn new information or the inability to recall previously learned information.

B. The memory disturbance causes significant impairment in social or occupational functioning and represents a significant decline from a previous level of functioning.

C. The memory disturbance does not occur exclusively during the course of a delirium or a dementia.

D. There is evidence from the history, physical examination, or laboratory findings that the disturbance is the direct physiological consequence of a general medical condition (including physical trauma).

Specify if:

Transient: if memory impairment lasts for 1 month or less

Chronic: if memory impairment lasts for more than 1 month

Coding note: Include the name of the general medical condition on Axis I (e.g., 294.0 amnestic disorder due to head trauma); also code the general medical condition on Axis III.

CLINICAL FEATURES

Patients with amnestic disorder have impaired ability to learn new information (anterograde amnesia) or cannot remember material previously learned (retrograde amnesia). Memory for the event that produced the deficit (e.g., a head injury in a motor vehicle accident) may also be impaired.

Remote recall (tertiary memory) is generally good, so patients may be able to relate accurately incidents that occurred during childhood but not remember what they had for breakfast. In some instances, disorientation to time and place may occur, but disorientation to person is unusual.

The onset of the amnesia is determined by the precipitant and may be acute as in head injury or insidious as in poor nutritional states. **KORSAKOFF'S SYNDROME.** Korsakoff's syndrome is an amnestic disorder caused by thiamine deficiency. Although generally associated with alcohol abuse, it can occur in other malnourished states such as marasmus, gastric carcinoma, and HIV spectrum disease. This syndrome is usually associated with Wernicke's encephalopathy, which involves ophthalmoplegia, ataxia, and confusion.

TREATMENT

As in delirium and dementia, the primary goal for the amnestic disorders is to discover and treat the underlying cause. Because some of these conditions are associated with serious psychological states (e.g., suicide attempts by hanging, carbon monoxide poisoning, deliberate motor vehicle accidents, self-inflicted gunshot wounds to the head, and chronic alcohol abuse), some form of psychiatric involvement is often necessary.

Schizophrenia

Schizophrenia is the most severe and debilitating mental illness, and it has long been the focus of medical, scientific, and societal attention. The words used historically to describe psychotic symptoms included madness, folie, insanity, and dementia.

DSM-IV Criteria

Schizophrenia

A. *Characteristic symptoms:* Two (or more) of the following, each present for a significant portion of time during a 1-month period (or less if successfully treated):

   (1) delusions

   (2) hallucinations

   (3) disorganized speech (e.g., frequent derailment or incoherence)

   (4) grossly disorganized or catatonic behavior

   (5) negative symptoms, i.e., affective flattening, alogia, or avolition

Note: Only one criterion A symptom is required if delusions are bizarre or hallucinations consist of a voice keeping up a running commentary on the person's behavior or thoughts, or two or more voices conversing with each other.

B. *Social/occupational dysfunction:* For a significant portion of the time since the onset of the disturbance, one or more major areas of functioning such as work, interpersonal relations, or self-care are markedly below the level achieved prior to the onset (or when the onset is in childhood or adolescence, failure to achieve expected level of interpersonal, academia, or occupational achievement).

C. *Duration:* Continuous signs of the disturbance persist for at least 6 months. This 6-month period must include at least 1 month of symptoms (or less if successfully treated) that meet criterion A (i.e., active-phase symptoms) and may include periods of pro-dromal or residual symptoms. During these prodromal or residual periods, the signs of the disturbance may be manifested by only negative symptoms or two or more symptoms listed in criterion A present in an attenuated form (e.g., odd beliefs, unusual perceptual experiences).

D. *Schizoaffective and mood disorder exclusion:* Schizoaffective disorder and mood disorder with psychotic features have been ruled out because either (1) no major depressive, manic, or mixed episodes have occurred concurrently with the active-phase symptoms; or (2) if mood episodes have occurred during active-phase symptoms, their total duration has been brief relative to the duration of the active and residual periods.

E. *Substance/general medical condition exclusion:* The disturbance is not due to the direct physiological effects of a substance (e.g., a drug of abuse, a medication) or a general medical condition.

F. *Relationship to a pervasive developmental disorder:* If there is a history of autistic disorder or another pervasive developmental disorder, the additional diagnosis of schizophrenia is made only if prominent delusions or hallucinations are also present for at least a month (or less if successfully treated).

SUBTYPES OF SCHIZOPHRENIA

In the *Diagnostic and Statistical Manual of Mental Disorders* (DSM-IV), schizophrenia has been divided into clinical subtypes, based on field trials of the reliability of symptom clusters. The subtypes are divided by the most prominent symptoms, although it is acknowledged that the specific subtype may exist simultaneously with or change over the course of the illness.

DSM-IV Criteria 295.30

Paranoid Type

A type of schizophrenia in which the following criteria are met:

A. Preoccupation with one or more delusions or frequent auditory hallucinations.

B. None of the following is prominent: disorganized speech, disorganized or catatonic behavior, or flat or inappropriate affect.

In DSM-IV, *paranoid-type* schizophrenia is marked by hallucinations or delusions in the presence of a clear sensorium and unchanged cognition. Disorganized speech, disorganized behavior, and flat or inappropriate affect are not present to any significant degree. The delusions (usually of a persecutory or grandiose nature) and hallucinations most often revolve around a particular theme or themes. Because of their delusions, these patients may attempt to keep the interviewer at bay, and thus they may appear hostile or angry during an interview. This type of schizophrenia may have a later age of onset and a better prognosis than the other subtypes.

DSM-IV Criteria 295.10

Disorganized Type

A type of schizophrenia in which the following criteria are met:

A. All of the following are prominent:

    (1) disorganized speech

    (2) disorganized behavior

    (3) flat or inappropriate affect

B. The criteria are not met for catatonic type.

Disorganized-type schizophrenia, historically referred to as hebephrenic schizophrenia, presents with the hallmark symptoms of disorganized speech and/or behavior, along with flat or inappropriate (incongruent) affect. Any delusions or hallucinations, if present, also tend to be disorganized and are not related to a single theme. Patients with disorganized schizophrenia tend to have an earlier age at onset, an unremitting course, and a poor prognosis.

DSM-IV Criteria 295.20

Catatonic Type

A type of schizophrenia in which the clinical picture is dominated by at least two of the following:

    (1) motoric immobility as evidenced by catalepsy (including waxy flexibility) or stupor

    (2) excessive motor activity (that is apparently purposeless and not influenced by external stimuli)

    (3) extreme negativism (an apparently motiveless resistance to all instructions or maintenance of a rigid posture against attempts to be moved) or mutism

    (4) peculiarities of voluntary movement as evidenced by posturing (voluntary assumption of inappropriate or bizarre postures), stereotyped movements, prominent mannerisms, or prominent grimacing

    (5) echolalia or echopraxia

Catatonic-type schizophrenia has unique features that distinguish it from other subtypes of schizophrenia in DSM-IV. During the acute phase of this illness, patients may demonstrate marked negativism or mutism, profound psychomotor retardation or severe psychomotor agitation, echolalia (repetition of words or phrases in a nonsensical manner), echopraxia (mimicking the behaviors of others), or bizarreness of voluntary movements and mannerisms. Some patients demonstrate a waxy flexibility, which is seen when a limb is repositioned on examination and remains in that position as if the patient were made of wax.

DSM-IV Criteria 295.90

Undifferentiated Type

A type of schizophrenia in which symptoms that meet criterion A are present, but the criteria are not met for the paranoid, disorganized, or catatonic type.

There is no hallmark symptom of *undifferentiated-type* schizophrenia; thus, it is the subtype that meets the criteria for schizophrenia but does not fit the profile for paranoid, disorganized, or catatonic type.

DSM-IV Criteria 295.60

Residual Type

A type of schizophrenia in which the following criteria are met:

A. Absence of prominent delusions, hallucinations, disorganized speech, and grossly disorganized or catatonic behavior.

B. There is continuing evidence of the disturbance, as indicated by the presence of negative symptoms or two or more symptoms listed in criterion A for schizophrenia, present in an attenuated form (e.g., odd beliefs, unusual perceptual experiences).

The diagnosis of *residual-type* schizophrenia, according to DSM-IV, is appropriately used when there is a past history of an acute episode of schizophrenia but at the time of presentation the patient does not manifest any of the associated psychotic or positive symptoms. However, there is continued evidence of schizophrenia manifested in either negative symptoms or low-grade symptoms of criterion A. These may include odd behavior, some abnormalities of thought processes, or delusions or hallucinations that exist in a minimal form. This type of schizophrenia has an unpredictable, variable course.

EPIDEMIOLOGICAL FINDINGS: INCIDENCE AND PREVALENCE

The incidence of schizophrenia is defined as the number of new cases in a given population, usually per 1000 persons, during a specific period of time (1 year by convention). In an illness with an insidious onset, such as schizophrenia, accurate incidence rates can be difficult to determine. The incidence of schizophrenia across 13 studies representing seven countries is found to range between 0.11 (United Kingdom) and 0.54 (United States) per 1000 people per year. Small variations in these incidence rates, because they are so low, have little meaning epidemiologically.

Prevalence is defined as the number of cases present in a specified population at a given time or time interval (e.g., at a specific point in time, during a time period, or over a lifetime). Lifetime prevalence rates of schizophrenia approximate 1%.

MORBIDITY AND MORTALITY

The economic costs of schizophrenia are estimated to be six times the costs of myocardial infarction. Much of this cost is due to the high morbidity of this chronic illness. Premorbid deficits, cognitive deficits, and negative symptoms account for much of the disability. Also, schizophrenic patients with more severe courses may require repeated hospitalizations and may not be capable of maintaining independent living or stable employment.

The mortality rate of schizophrenia is estimated to be twice that of the general population. Approximately 10% of the mortality is secondary to suicide. Young male schizophrenics are most likely to complete suicide attempts, especially early in their illness. Degree of social isolation, agitation, depression, a sense of hopelessness, a history of prior suicide attempts, and recent loss may be associated with increased risk of suicide among schizophrenic patients.

COMORBIDITY WITH OTHER ILLNESSES

Schizophrenia is associated with an increased frequency of tuberculosis (not accounted for by institutionalization), celiac disease, myxedema, and arteriosclerotic heart disease. However, there is a strikingly decreased risk for rheumatoid arthritis among schizophrenia patients.

Numerous medical illnesses have symptoms similar to those of schizophrenia. The most common neurological disorder appearing with clinical similarity to schizophrenia is epilepsy, particularly of the temporal lobe. Other medical illnesses with symptoms similar to those of schizophrenia include basal ganglia calcifications and acute intermittent porphyria. Imbalances of endocrine function as well as certain infectious diseases can present with symptoms that mimic schizophrenic psychosis.

CLINICAL MANIFESTATIONS AND PHENOMENOLOGY

Positive and Negative Symptoms

In the psychiatric literature, positive symptoms have come to mean those that are actively expressed, such as hallucinations, thought disorder, delusions, and bizarre behavior, whereas negative symptoms reflect deficit states such as avolition, flattened affect, and alogia. How these distinct symptom patterns are related in schizophrenia remains unresolved.

Cognitive Impairment

It is widely accepted that schizophrenic patients experience neuropsychological deficits that can be characterized by difficulties with attention, information processing, learning, and memory.

LEARNING AND MEMORY

Although there are generally no consistent gross deficits of memory in schizophrenic patients, close examination of certain aspects of learning and memory has revealed striking abnormalities.

MENTAL STATUS EXAMINATION

There is no specific laboratory test, neuroimaging study, or clinical presentation of a patient that yields a definitive diagnosis of schizophrenia. Schizophrenia can present with a wide variety of symptoms, and a longitudinal history of symptoms and comorbid clinical variables such as medical illness and a history of substance abuse are necessary before a diagnosis can be considered. The Mental Status Examination, much like the physical examination, is an additional clinical tool that aids the psychiatrist in generating a differential diagnosis and appropriate treatment recommendations.

PHYSICAL EXAMINATION

Although there are no pathognomonic physical signs of schizophrenia, some patients have neurological "soft" signs on physical examination. The neurological deficits include nonspecific abnormalities in reflexes, coordination (as seen in gait and fingerto-nose tests), graphesthesia (recognition of patterns marked out on the palm), and stereognosis (recognition of three-dimensional pictures). Other neurological findings include odd or awkward movements (possibly correlated with thought disorder), alterations in muscle tone, an increased blink rate, a slower habituation of the blink response to repetitive glabellar tap, and an abnormal pupillary response.

The exact etiology of these abnormalities is unknown, but they historically have been associated with minimal brain dysfunction and may be more likely in patients with poor premorbid functioning and a chronic course.

OTHER CONDITIONS THAT RESEMBLE SCHIZOPHRENIA

Schizoaffective Disorder

Possibly the most difficult diagnostic dilemma in cases of patients with both psychotic and affective symptoms is in differentiating between schizophrenia and schizoaffective disorder.

DSM-IV Criteria 295.70

Schizoaffective Disorder

A. An uninterrupted period of illness during which, at some time, there is either a major depressive episode, a manic episode, or a mixed episode concurrent with symptoms that meet criterion A for schizophrenia.

Note: The major depressive episode must include criterion A1: depressed mood.

B. During the same period of illness, there have been delusions or hallucinations for at least 2 weeks in the absence of prominent mood symptoms.

C. Symptoms that meet criteria for a mood episode are present for a substantial portion of the total duration of the active and residual periods of the illness.

D. The disturbance is not due to the direct physiological effects of a substance (e.g., a drug of abuse, a medication) or a general medical condition.

Specify type:

Bipolar type: if the disturbance includes a manic or a mixed episode (or a manic or a mixed episode and major depressive episodes)

Depressive type: if the disturbance only includes major depressive episodes

Psychotic symptoms in the absence of affective disturbance confirm the diagnosis of schizophrenia. Also, if there is a mood disturbance, it must be brief in relation to the duration of the active phase of the illness. A diagnosis of schizoaffective disorder requires that psychotic symptoms be present for a minimum of 2 weeks without concurrent mood disturbance. Clinically compelling affective disturbance that is distinct from the active phase of the illness is diagnosed separately.

Brief Psychotic Disorder and Schizophreniform Disorder

DSM-IV Criteria 296.6

Brief Psychotic Disorder

A. Presence of one (or more) of the following symptoms:

   (1) delusions

   (2) hallucinations

   (3) disorganized speech (e.g., frequent derailment or incoherence)

   (4) grossly disorganized or catatonic behavior

Note: Do not include a symptom if it is a culturally sanctioned response pattern.

B. Duration of an episode of the disturbance is at least 1 day but less than 1 month, with eventual full return to premorbid level of functioning.

C. The disturbance is not better accounted for by a mood disorder with psychotic features, schizoaffective disorder, or schizophrenia and is not due to the direct physiological effects of a substance (e.g., a drug of abuse, a medication) or a general medical condition.

Specify if:

With marked stressor(s) (brief reactive psychosis): if symptoms occur shortly after and apparently in response to events that, singly or together, would be markedly stressful to almost anyone in similar circumstances in the person's culture

Without marked stressor(s): if psychotic symptoms do *not* occur shortly after, or are not apparently in response to events that, singly or together, would be markedly stressful to almost anyone in similar circumstances in the person's culture

With postpartum onset: if onset within 4 weeks postpartum

DSM-IV Criteria 295.40

Schizophreniform Disorder

A. Criteria A, D, and E of schizophrenia are met.

B. An episode of the disorder (including prodromal, active, and residual phases) lasts at least 1 month but less than 6 months. (When the diagnosis must be made without waiting for recovery, it should be qualified as "provisional.")

Specify if:

Without good prognostic features

With good prognostic features: as evidenced by two (or more) of the following:

  (1) onset of prominent psychotic symptoms within 4 weeks of the first noticeable change in usual behavior or functioning

  (2) confusion or perplexity at the height of the psychotic episode

  (3) good premorbid social and occupational functioning

  (4) absence of blunted or flat affect

The distinctions among brief psychotic disorder, schizophreniform disorder, and schizophrenia are based on duration of active symptoms. DSM-IV has maintained the requirement of 6 months of active, prodromal, and/or residual symptoms for a diagnosis of schizophrenia. Brief psychotic disorder is a transient psychotic state, not caused by medical conditions or substance use, that lasts for at least 1 day and up to a month. Schizophreniform disorder falls in between and requires symptoms for at least 1 month and not exceeding 6 months, with no requirement for loss of functioning.

Delusional Disorder

DSM-IV Criteria 297.1

Delusional Disorder

A. Nonbizarre delusions (i.e., involving situations that occur in real life, such as being followed, poisoned, infected, loved at a distance, or deceived by spouse or lover, or having a disease) of at least 1 month's duration.

B. Criterion A for schizophrenia has never been met. **Note:** Tactile and olfactory hallucinations may be present in delusional disorder if they are related to the delusional theme.

C. Apart from the impact of the delusion(s) or its ramifications, functioning is not markedly impaired and behavior is not obviously odd or bizarre.

D. If mood episodes have occurred concurrently with delusions, their total duration has been brief relative to the duration of the delusional periods.

E. The disturbance is not due to the direct physiological effects of a substance (e.g., a drug of abuse, a medication) or a general medical condition.

Specify type (the following types are assigned based on the predominant delusional theme):

Erotomanic type: delusions that another person, usually of higher status, is in love with the individual

Grandiose type: delusions of inflated worth, power, knowledge, identity, or special relationship to a deity or famous person

Jealous type: delusions that the individual's sexual partner is unfaithful

Persecutory type: delusions that the person (or someone to whom the person is close) is being malevolently treated in some way

Somatic type: delusions that the person has some physical defect or general medical condition

Mixed type: delusions characteristic of more than one of the above types but no one theme predominates

Unspecified type

If the delusions that a patient describes are not bizarre (e.g., belief that a person has taken over one's body or that radio signals are being sent through the caps in one's teeth), it is wise to consider delusional disorder in the differential diagnosis. Delusional disorder is usually characterized by specific types of false fixed beliefs, such as erotomanic, grandiose, jealous, persecutory, or somatic types. Delusional disorder, unlike schizophrenia, is not associated with a marked social impairment or odd behavior. Moreover, patients with delusional disorder do not experience hallucinations nor do they typically have negative symptoms.

Affective Disorder with Psychotic Features

If the patient experiences psychotic symptoms solely during times when affective symptoms are present, the diagnosis is more likely to be mood disorder with psychotic features. If the mood disturbance involves both manic and depressive episodes, the diagnosis is bipolar disorder.

Substance Abuse–Related Conditions

In DSM-IV psychotic disorders, delirium, and dementia caused by substance use are distinguished from schizophrenia in which there is clear-cut evidence of substance use leading to symptoms. Examples of psychotomimetic properties of substances include a PCP psychosis that clinically can resemble schizophrenia, chronic alcohol intoxication (Korsakoff's psychosis), and chronic amphetamine administration, which can lead to paranoid states.

Medical Disorders

Medical disorders ranging from vitamin B_{12} deficiency to Cushing's syndrome have been associated with a clinical presentation resembling that of schizophrenia. Because the prognosis for the associated medical condition is better than that for schizophrenia and the stigma attached to schizophrenia is significant, it is imperative that patients be provided with a thorough medical work-up before they are given a diagnosis of schizophrenia. This includes a physical examination; laboratory analyses including thyroid function tests, syphilis screening, and folate and vitamin B_{12} levels; a CT or MRI scan; and a lumbar puncture when indicated in new-onset cases.

COURSE OF ILLNESS

According to the current model, the course of schizophrenia has three phases: an early phase marked by deterioration from premorbid levels of functioning; a middle phase characterized by a prolonged period of little change termed the stabilization phase; and the last phase, which incorporates the long-term outcome data just cited, called the improving phase (Fig. 25–1).

TREATMENT

It could be argued that the successful treatment of schizophrenia requires a greater level of clinical knowledge and sophistication than the treatment of most other psychiatric and medical illnesses. It begins with the formation of a therapeutic psychiatrist-patient relationship and must combine the latest developments in pharmacological and psychosocial therapeutics and interventions.

Psychiatrist-Patient Relationship

The psychiatrist-patient relationship is the foundation for treating patients with schizophrenia. Because of the clinical manifestations of the illness, the formation of this relationship is often difficult. Paranoid delusions may lead to mistrust of the psychiatrist. Conceptual disorganization and cognitive impairment make it difficult

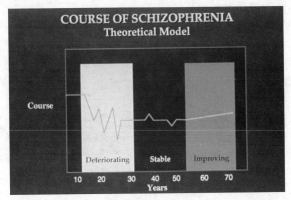

Figure 25–1 *Model of the lifelong course of illness for schizophrenia. (From Breier A, Schreiber JL, Dyer J, et al: National Institute of Mental Health longitudinal study of chronic schizophrenia: Prognosis and prediction of outcome. Arch Gen Psychiatry 1991; 48:239–246.)*

for patients to attend to what the psychiatrist is saying and to follow even the simplest directions.

Psychopharmacological Treatment

ACUTE PHARMACOLOGICAL TREATMENT

Despite increased awareness that the effective treatment of psychotic symptoms is complex, the mainstay for the psychopharmacological management of acute exacerbations or the onset of schizophrenic symptoms, both positive and negative, remains the traditional neuroleptic agents. (For a pharmacotherapy decision tree, see Fig. 25–2.) The primary goal of acute treatment is the amelioration of any behavioral disturbances that would put the patient or others at risk of harm. When treatment is initiated, improvement in clinical symptoms can be seen over hours, days, or weeks of treatment.

There is no convincing evidence that one traditional neuroleptic is more efficacious as an antipsychotic than any other. Antipsychotics should therefore be chosen based on side effect profile, history of prior response (or nonresponse) to a specific agent, or history of a family member response to a certain antipsychotic agent.

Once the decision is made to use an antipsychotic agent, an appropriate dose must be selected. Initially, higher doses or repeated dosing may be helpful in preventing grossly psychotic and agitated patients from doing harm. In general there is no clear evidence that higher doses of neuroleptics (more than 2000 mg chlorpromazine equivalents per day) have any advantage over standard doses (400 to 600 mg chlorpromazine equivalents per day). Some patients who are extremely agitated or aggressive may benefit from concomitant administration of high-potency benzodiazepines such as lorazepam,

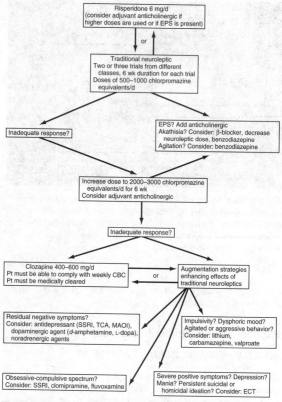

Figure 25–2 *Pharmacotherapy decision tree: schizophrenia.*

at 1 to 2 mg, until they are stable. Early adjuvant treatment with anticholinergic medication may facilitate compliance with medication by decreasing intolerable side effects.

MAINTENANCE TREATMENT

There is by now a great deal of evidence from long-term follow-up studies that patients have a higher risk of relapse and exacerbations if they are not maintained with adequate antipsychotic regimens. Noncompliance with medication, possibly because of intolerable neuroleptic side effects, may contribute to increased relapse rates.

Long-term treatment of schizophrenia is a complex issue. It is clear that the majority of patients require maintenance medication. Some patients do well with stable doses of neuroleptics for years without any exacerbations. However, many patients maintained with a stable neuroleptic dose have episodic breakthroughs of their psychotic symptoms.

It is prudent to assess patients for medication compliance when signs of relapse are suspected. Prodromal cues may be present before an exacerbation of symptoms. For example, any recent change in sleep, attention to activities of daily living, or disorganization may be a warning sign of an impending increase in psychosis.

For patients for whom compliance is a problem, long-acting, depot neuroleptics are available in the United States for both fluphenazine and haloperidol. These preparations are injected intramuscularly every 2 to 4 weeks and circumvent the need for daily oral antipsychotic medications in most cases (although some patients benefit from adjuvant oral medication). This alternative should be considered if noncompliance with oral agents has led to relapses and rehospitalization.

RISKS AND SIDE EFFECTS OF TYPICAL NEUROLEPTICS

Extrapyramidal symptoms are side effects of typical antipsychotic medications that include dystonias, pseudoparkinsonism, akinesia, and akathisia. These side effects are referred to collectively as extrapyramidal symptoms because they are mediated at least in part by dopaminergic transmission in the extrapyramidal system.

Dystonias are involuntary muscular spasms that can be brief or sustained, involving any muscle group. Pseudoparkinsonism and akinesia are characterized by muscular rigidity, tremor, and bradykinesia, much as in Parkinson's disease. Akathisia is more common, affecting more than 20% of patients taking neuroleptic medications. Treatment of these extrapyramidal symptoms can be difficult but usually involves administration of anticholinergic medications.

Nonextrapyramidal side effects of the typical antipsychotic agents include those that are secondary to blockade of muscarinic, histaminic, and α-adrenergic receptors. More commonly seen with the low-potency neuroleptics, these include sedation, tachycardia, and anticholinergic side effects such as urinary hesitancy or retention, blurred vision, or constipation.

Neuroleptic malignant syndrome (NMS) is a relatively rare but serious phenomenon seen in approximately 1% of patients taking neuroleptics. It can be fatal in 15% of cases if not properly recognized and treated. Major manifestations of NMS comprise fever, rigidity, and increased creatine kinase levels, whereas minor manifestations include tachycardia, abnormal blood pressure, tachypnea, altered consciousness, diaphoresis, and leukocytosis. The mainstay of treatment is cessation of neuroleptic treatment and supportive care, including intravenous hydration, reversal of fever with antipyretics and cooling blankets, and careful monitoring of vital signs because of the risk of cardiac and respiratory disturbance.

All patients receiving traditional neuroleptic treatment should be monitored regularly for any signs of a movement disorder. If tardive dyskinesia is suspected, the benefits of antipsychotic treatment must be carefully weighed against the risk of tardive dyskinesia. This should be discussed with the patient, and the antipsychotic should be removed if clinically feasible or at least maintained at the lowest possible dose that provides antipsychotic effect. Unfortunately, there is no specific treatment of tardive dyskinesia, although some investigators have proposed the use of adrenergic agents such as clonidine, calcium channel blockers, vitamin E, benzodiazepines, valproic acid, or reserpine to reduce the spontaneous movements.

The introduction of the dibenzodiazepine clozapine marks a major breakthrough in the treatment of schizophrenia since chlorpromazine became available for clinical use. Double-blind, controlled studies have demonstrated the superior clinical efficacy of clozapine compared with standard neuroleptics, without the associated extrapyramidal symptoms. It is clearly superior to traditional neuroleptics for psychosis. Studies of chronic and treatment-resistant schizophrenia in the United States suggest that approximately 50% of patients derive a better response from clozapine than from traditional neuroleptics.

Unfortunately, clozapine is associated with agranulocytosis, and because of this risk, requires weekly white blood cell testing. Approximately 0.8% of patients taking clozapine and receiving weekly white blood cell monitoring develop agranulocytosis. Women and the elderly are at higher risk than other groups. The period of highest risk is the first 6 months of treatment.

The superior antipsychotic efficacy of clozapine has inspired an abundance of research in the field of modern psychopharmacology for the treatment of schizophrenia. Risperidone was approved by the U.S. Food and Drug Administration 4 years after clozapine gained its approval for use in treatment-resistant patients. Risperidone, unlike clozapine, is associated with extrapyramidal symptoms in a dose-dependent manner. However, it is an effective antipsychotic agent with minimal extrapyramidal symptoms. Risperidone may lead to side effects including insomnia or sedation, agitation, headache, constipation, and palpitations. Because it is relatively new, there are no data yet indicating associated risks of tardive dyskinesia, and investigation is required to address its efficacy for treatment-resistant patients. Unlike clozapine, risperidone does not have the risk of agranulocytosis and therefore does not require weekly blood drawing.

Nonpharmacological Treatment of Schizophrenia

Although psychopharmacological intervention has proved to be the foundation on which the treatment of schizophrenia depends, other approaches to the management of these patients serve a critical function. Studies have shown repeatedly that symptoms of schizophrenia have not only a genetic component but also an environmental aspect, and interactions with family and within the community can alter the course of the illness. It has become clear that psychopharmacological treatment strategies are most efficacious if combined with some type of psychosocial intervention and vice versa. Because of schizophrenia's chronic nature, one or more treatments may be required throughout the illness, and they are likely to need modifying as symptoms change over time.

INDIVIDUAL PSYCHOTHERAPY

The psychiatrist using individual psychotherapy should focus on forming and maintaining a therapeutic alliance (which is also a necessary part of psychopharmacological treatment) and providing a safe environment in which the patient is able to discuss symptoms openly. Sound therapy provides clear structure about the therapist-patient relationship and helps the patient to focus on personal goals.

Schizophrenia often strikes just as a person is leaving adolescence and entering young adulthood. The higher the premorbid level of social adjustment and functioning, the more devastating and confusing the onset of symptoms becomes. Young male patients with a high level of premorbid function are at increased risk of suicide, presumably in part because of the tremendous loss they face. These feelings can continue for years, with schizophrenic patients feeling isolated and robbed of a normal life. Therefore, a component of individual work (which can also be achieved to some degree in a group setting) with these patients is a focus on the impact schizophrenia has had on their lives. Helping patients to grieve for these losses is an important process that may ultimately help them achieve a better quality of life.

PSYCHOEDUCATIONAL TREATMENT

The literature suggests that schizophrenic patients can benefit from social skills training. This model is based on the idea that the course of schizophrenia is, in part, a product of the environment, which is inherently stressful because of the social deficits from which these patients suffer. The hypothesis is that if patients are able to monitor and reduce their stress, they could potentially decrease their risk of relapse.

For this intervention to be successful, patients must be aware of and set their own goals. Goals such as medication management, activities of daily living, and dealing with a roommate are achievable examples. Social skills and deficits can be assessed by patients' self-report, observation of behavioral patterns by trained professionals, or a measurement of physiological responses to specific situations (e.g., increased pulse when asking someone to dinner). Patients can then begin behavioral training in which appropriate social responses are shaped with the help of instructors.

FAMILY THERAPY

Based on these findings, it is clear that there is a significant interaction between the level of emotional involvement and criticism of relatives of schizophrenic probands and the outcome of their illness. Identifying the causative factors in familial stressors and educating involved family members about schizophrenia lead to long-term benefits for patients. Future work in this field must examine these interactions with an understanding of modern sociological and biological advances in genetics, looking at trait carriers, social skills assessments, positive and negative symptoms, and medication management with the novel antipsychotic agents.

SELF-DIRECTED TREATMENT

Structured self-help clubs have been effective means of bolstering patients' social, occupational, and living skills. Involved patients are called members of the club, giving them a sense of belonging to a group. They are always made to feel welcome, useful, and productive members of the club community.

The clubhouse model has expanded to provide services such as transitional employment programs, apartment programs, outreach programs, and medication management and consultation services, to name a few. A self-supportive rehabilitation program for mentally ill patients is an important option for many schizophrenic patients who might otherwise feel isolated and out of reach.

Bipolar Disorders

The diagnosis of bipolar disorder derives from the occurrence of individual episodes over time. Persons who experience a manic, hypomanic, or mixed episode, virtually all of whom also have a history of one or more major depressive episodes, are diagnosed with bipolar disorder. Those who experience major depressive and manic episodes are diagnosed with bipolar *type I* disorder, and those with major depressive and hypomanic (milder manic) episodes are diagnosed with bipolar *type II* disorder. It should not be construed that bipolar II disorder is in all respects milder than type I, although hypomania is by definition less severe than mania.

Persons who experience subsyndromal bipolar mood fluctuations over an extended period without major mood episodes are diagnosed with cyclothymic disorder. Much less is known about this milder disorder because afflicted persons present for medical attention less frequently than those with full-blown bipolar disorder. At various times cyclothymic disorder has been considered a temperament, apersonality disorder, and a disorder at the milder end of the bipolar spectrum. Available data clearly indicate that cyclothymic disorder is related to the more severe bipolar disorders.

DSM-IV Criteria

Manic Episode

A. A distinct period of abnormally and persistently elevated, expansive, or irritable mood, lasting at least 1 week (or any duration if hospitalization is necessary).

B. During the period of mood disturbance, three (or more) of the following symptoms have persisted (four if the mood is only irritable) and have been present to a significant degree:

(1) inflated self-esteem or grandiosity

(2) decreased need for sleep (e.g., feels rested after only 3 hours of sleep)

(3) more talkative than usual or pressure to keep talking

(4) flight of ideas or subjective experience that thoughts are racing

(5) distractibility (i.e., attention too easily drawn to unimportant or irrelevant external stimuli)

(6) increase in goal-directed activity (either socially, at work or school, or sexually) or psychomotor agitation

(7) excessive involvement in pleasurable activities that have a high potential for painful consequences (e.g., engaging in unrestrained buying sprees, sexual indiscretions, or foolish business investments)

C. The symptoms do not meet criteria for a mixed episode.

D. The mood disturbance is sufficiently severe to cause marked impairment in occupational functioning or in usual social activities or relationships with others, or to necessitate hospitalization to prevent harm to self or others, or there are psychotic features.

E. The symptoms are not due to the direct physiological effects of a substance (e.g., a drug of abuse, a medication, or other treatment) or a general medical condition (e.g., hyperthyroidism).

Note: Manic-like episodes that are clearly caused by somatic antidepressant treatment (e.g., medication, electroconvulsive therapy, light therapy) should not count toward a diagnosis of bipolar I disorder.

DSM-IV Criteria

Rapid-Cycling Specifier

Specify if:

With rapid cycling (can be applied to bipolar I disorder or bipolar II disorder). At least four episodes of a mood disturbance in the previous 12 months that meet criteria for a major depressive, manic, mixed, or hypomanic episode.

Note: Episodes are demarcated by either partial or full remission for at least 2 months or a switch to an episode of opposite polarity (e.g., major depressive episode to manic episode).

DSM-IV Criteria

Mixed Episode

A. The criteria are met both for a manic episode and for a major depressive episode (except for duration) nearly every day during at least a 1-week period.

B. The mood disturbance is sufficiently severe to cause marked impairment in occupational functioning or in usual social activities or relationships with others, or to necessitate hospitalization to prevent harm to self or others, or there are psychotic features.

C. The symptoms are not due to the direct physiological effects of a substance (e.g., a drug of abuse, a medication, or other treatment) or a general medical condition (e.g., hyperthyroidism).

Note: Mixed-like episodes that are clearly caused by somatic antidepressant treatment (e.g., medication, electroconvulsive therapy, light therapy) should not count toward a diagnosis of bipolar I disorder.

DSM-IV Criteria

Hypomanic Episode

A. A distinct period of persistently elevated, expansive, or irritable mood, lasting throughout at least 4 days, that is clearly different from the usual nondepressed mood.

B. During the period of mood disturbance, three (or more) of the following symptoms have persisted (four if the mood is only irritable) and have been present to a significant degree:

(1) inflated self-esteem or grandiosity

(2) decreased need for sleep (e.g., feels rested after only 3 hours of sleep)

(3) more talkative than usual or pressure to keep talking

(4) flight of ideas or subjective experience that thoughts are racing

(5) distractibility (i.e., attention too easily drawn to unimportant or irrelevant external stimuli)

(6) increase in goal-directed activity (either socially, at work or school, or sexually) or psychomotor agitation

(7) excessive involvement in pleasurable activities that have a high potential for painful consequences (e.g., the person engages in unrestrained buying sprees, sexual indiscretions, or foolish business investments)

C. The episode is associated with an unequivocal change in functioning that is uncharacteristic of the person when not symptomatic.

D. The disturbance in mood and the change in functioning are observable by others.

E. The episode is not severe enough to cause marked impairment in social or occupational functioning, or to necessitate hospitalization, and there are no psychotic features.

F. The symptoms are not due to the direct physiological effects of a substance (e.g., a drug of abuse, a medication, or other treatment) or a general medical condition (e.g., hyperthyroidism).

Note: Hypomanic-like episodes that are clearly caused by somatic antidepressant treatment (e.g., medication, electroconvulsive therapy, light therapy) should not count toward a diagnosis of bipolar II disorder.

DSM-IV Criteria 301.13

Cyclothymic Disorder

A. For at least 2 years, the presence of numerous periods with hypomanic symptoms and numerous periods with depressive symptoms that do not meet criteria for a major depressive episode.

Note: In children and adolescents, the duration must be at least 1 year.

B. During the above 2-year period (1 year in children and adolescents), the person has not been without the symptoms in criterion A for more than 2 months at a time.

C. No major depressive episode, manic episode, or mixed episode has been present during the first 2 years of the disturbance.

Box continued on following page

Cyclothymic Disorder *Continued*

D. The symptoms in Criterion A are not better accounted for by Schizoaffective Disorder and are not superimposed on Schizophrenia, Schizophreniform Disorder, Delusional Disorder, or Psychotic Disorder Not Otherwise Specified.

E. The symptoms are not due to the direct physiological effects of a substance (e.g., a drug of abuse, a medication) or a general medical condition (e.g., hyperthyroidism).

F. The symptoms cause clinically significant distress or impairment in social, occupational, or other important areas of functioning.

EPIDEMIOLOGY

Estimates of the lifetime risk for bipolar I disorder from epidemiological studies have ranged from 0.2% to 0.9%. The Epidemiological Catchment Area (ECA) study found a lifetime prevalence rate of 1.2% for combined type I or type II variants. These rates are approximately 10-fold greater than the prevalence rate for schizophrenia and about one fifth that for major depressive disorder. Little is known regarding the prevalence of cyclothymic disorder. Unlike major depressive disorder, bipolar disorder has an approximately equal sex distribution.

Of particular interest in regard to the epidemiology of bipolar disorder is that the incidence of bipolar disorder (and depressive disorders) appears to have increased since the 1940s. Reasons for this are not clear, although environmental factors, either physiological or psychosocial, may be responsible.

Occurrence of Bipolar Disorder with Other Psychiatric Disorders

Alcohol and drug abuse and dependence represent the most consistently described and most clinically important psychiatric comorbidities with bipolar disorder. Whereas rates of alcohol abuse combined with alcohol dependence are from 3% to 13% in the general population, lifetime rates for alcohol dependence from ECA data indicate that they are greater than 30% in persons with bipolar I disorder. The reasons for this co-occurrence are not clear. One hypothesis suggests that persons with bipolar disorder self-medicate with drugs or alcohol.

Other psychiatric comorbidities have been described in modest proportions of bipolar patients. Interestingly, data indicate that comorbidity may be higher in women with bipolar disorder than in men, which may contribute to the tendency for the female gender to be associated with more complex forms of bipolar disorder such as rapid cycling and dysphoric mania.

DIAGNOSIS

Mood episodes are discrete periods of altered feeling, thought, and behavior. Typically they have a distinct onset and offset, beginning over days or weeks and eventually ending gradually after several weeks or months. As noted earlier, bipolar disorder is defined by the occurrence of depressive plus manic, hypomanic, or mixed episodes.

Depressive episodes in bipolar disorder are indistinguishable from those in major depressive disorder. About half of persons with bipolar disorder experience depressive episodes characterized by decreased sleep and appetite, whereas about half experience more "atypical" symptoms of increased sleep and appetite. The diagnostic decision tree for bipolar disorder is given in Figure 26–1.

Manic episodes are defined by discrete periods of abnormally elevated, expansive, or irritable mood accompanied by marked impairment in judgment and social and occupational function. These symptoms are frequently accompanied by unrealistic grandiosity, excess energy, and increases in goal-directed activity that frequently have a high potential for damaging consequences.

Hypomanic and manic symptoms are identical, but hypomanic episodes are less severe. A person is "promoted" from hypomania to mania (type II to type I bipolar disorder) by the presence of one of three features: psychosis during the episode, sufficient severity to warrant hospitalization, or marked social role impairment.

Psychosis can occur in either pole of the disorder. If psychotic symptoms are limited to the major mood episode, persons are considered to have bipolar disorder with psychotic features. However, if psychotic symptoms endure significantly into periods of normal mood, the diagnosis of schizoaffective disorder is made.

Rapid cycling is defined by the occurrence of four or more mood episodes within 12 months. It should be noted that, despite the name, the episodes are not necessarily or even commonly truly cyclical; the diagnosis is based simply on episode counting. This subcategory is of significance because it predicts a relatively poorer outcome and worse response to lithium and other treatments.

History, Physical Examination, and Laboratory Studies

Although the diagnosis of bipolar disorder is made on the basis of phenomenology, there are several reasons for conducting a thorough medical history and physical examination. First, there are several general medical or substance-related causes of mania that, if treated, may lead to the resolution of mania (Table 26–1). Similarly, mania may be the first sign of a general medical illness that will be progressive and serious in its own right. Second, medical evaluation is necessary before starting medications used in the treatment of bipolar disorder.

Few general medical illnesses have been reliably associated with the development of bipolar disorder, and none can be considered specific risk factors. Administration of medications has been observed frequently in clinical practice to be associated with the onset of mania, particularly in patients with preexisting depression. Such medications are listed in Table 26–2.

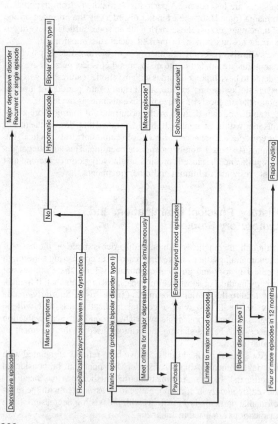

Figure 26–1 Decision tree for diagnosis of bipolar disorder. The building blocks for a diagnosis of bipolar disorder are individual episodes and their characteristics. This decision tree helps the psychiatrist through the steps that lead to diagnosis of bipolar disorder and identification of its subtypes.
*Does not apply to hypomanic episode, per DSM-IV.

Depressive episode → Manic symptoms → Hospitalization/psychosis/severe role dysfunction

Major depressive disorder Recurrent or single episode

Hypomanic episode

No

Bipolar disorder type II

Manic episode (probable bipolar disorder type I)

Meet criteria for major depressive episode simultaneously

Mixed episode*

Schizoaffective disorder

Psychosis

Endures beyond mood episodes

Limited to major mood episodes

Bipolar disorder type I

Four or more episodes in 12 months

Rapid cycling

268

TABLE 26–1 Medical Factors Associated with Mania

Neuroanatomical Lesions	Endocrine or Metabolic Disorders
Right frontotemporal lesions	Hyperthyroidism
Certain subcortical lesions	Addison's disease
Infections	Cushing's disease
	Vitamin B_{12} deficiency
Neurosyphilis	Postdialysis syndrome
Encephalitis	
Acquired immunodeficiency syndrome	

COURSE AND NATURAL HISTORY

Bipolar disorder has its onset in most persons in adolescence and young adulthood, between the ages of 15 and 30. However, prepubertal mania and first-onset disease in the ninth decade of life are not unheard of. Once developed, multiple episodes are the rule.

Episode length typically ranges from 4 to 13 months, with depressive episodes typically longer than manic or hypomanic episodes. Women appear to have more depressive relapses than manic ones, whereas men have a more even distribution.

TABLE 26–2 Treatments and Drugs Associated with Mania

Antidepressants	Dopaminergic Agents
Medications	Levodopa
Bright visible spectrum light treatment	Disulfiram
Electroconvulsive therapy	
Adrenergic Agents	**Drugs of Abuse**
Decongestants	Alcohol
Bronchodilators	Stimulants
Stimulants	Hallucinogens
Other Agents	
Isoniazid	
Corticosteroids	

When assessed 1.5 years after index hospitalization, between 7% and 32% of bipolar patients remain chronically ill, depending on polarity of index episode. The probability of remaining ill at 1, 2, 3, and 4 years after hospitalization for mania is, respectively, 51%, 44%, 33%, and 28%. Subsyndromal affective symptoms may remain in up to 13% to 34%, and substantial interepisode morbidity may remain despite adequate treatment.

GOALS OF TREATMENT

Traditionally, treatment for bipolar disorder has been categorized as acute versus maintenance; that is, treatment geared toward resolution of a specific episode versus continued treatment to prevent further symptoms. Treatment can also be considered along several other lines.

STANDARD TREATMENTS

Pharmacotherapy

Lithium is the mainstay of treatment for both phases of bipolar disorder. In mania, a large body of data indicates its superiority to placebo and effects equal to or surpassing those of neuroleptics. Certain factors predict relatively poorer response to lithium, including mixed mania and depression, rapid cycling, and substance abuse.

Controlled studies of the anticonvulsants carbamazepine and valproic acid indicated that these agents also have substantial antimanic efficacy. There is some evidence that certain predictors of nonresponse to lithium, such as mixed states or rapid cycling, may be predictors of response to carbamazepine. Other treatments for mania include electroconvulsive therapy (ECT) and a number of pharmacotherapeutic agents reported to be useful in case series or case reports. These are summarized in Chapter 54, which discusses mood stabilizers.

In contrast to evidence regarding acute mania, evidence is scarce concerning efficacy of specific agents for bipolar depression. Most treatment is undertaken primarily by extension from treatment experience in unipolar depression, which is summarized in Chapter 27 in its review of depression. However, several specific distinctions should be noted. First, lithium appears to be an effective antidepressant in bipolar depression, whereas the evidence is equivocal for its efficacy in unipolar depression. Second, it should be kept in mind that all somatic antidepressant treatments are promanic, with the probable exception of lithium. These two facts indicate that lithium should be the first-line treatment for unmedicated bipolar patients in the depressed phase.

Maintenance Treatment

Lithium and carbamazepine have thus far been shown to be effective prophylactic agents in prospective, randomized controlled trials. The antidepressant imipramine appears to be equally effective to lithium in preventing depressive but not manic relapse. There is little

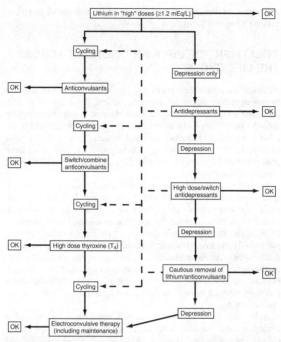

Figure 26-2 *Treatment algorithm for bipolar disorder. (Reprinted from Bauer M: Rapid cycling. In Joffe RT, Calabrese JR, (eds): Anticonvulsants in Mood Disorders. New York: Marcel Dekker, 1994:1-26, by courtesy of Marcel Dekker, Inc.)*

evidence that neuroleptics or benzodiazepines, used in the treatment of acute mania, have any prophylactic effect.

A treatment algorithm for refractory bipolar disorder, including strategies to deal with rapid cycling, is found in Figure 26-2. A summary of the most frequent or important side effects of anti-manic medications can be found in the discussion of mood stabilizers in Chapter 54.

Drug-drug interactions may lead to side effects. Such interactions are often associated with increases in serum levels of the drug of interest. For example, addition of thiazide, diuretics, or nonsteroidal antiinflammatory agents, the last mentioned now being available over the counter, is a common reason for an increase in lithium level and development of toxicity.

Psychotherapies

Data on specific psychotherapies in bipolar disorder are minimal, and we are therefore unfortunately left to rely on common sense clinical principles alone. These include psychoeducation regarding the disorder and the specific treatments, destigmatization, and enlistment of the patient and family in collaborative decision-making whenever possible.

TREATMENT OF BIPOLAR DISORDER ACROSS THE LIFE CYCLE

Although the somatotherapeutic and psychotherapeutic mainstays of treatment endure across the life cycle, several phases of life present particular challenges. There exist few data on treatment of bipolar disorder in childhood. Treatments are chosen by extension from the adult literature, with the one caveat that there have been rare cases of liver failure in conjunction with valproic acid use in children younger than 10 years of age who have been exposed to multiple anticonvulsants.

In pregnancy, there is some evidence that lithium may be teratogenic, associated with increased rates of cardiac abnormalities. Valproic acid and perhaps carbamazepine have been associated with neural tube defects, leaving the neuroleptics and antidepressants and ECT as the preferable management strategies during pregnancy, particularly the first trimester. It should be kept in mind, however, that treatment decisions are based on *risk,* not *certainty.* Risk of fetal malformation, parental attitude toward raising children with birth defects, severity of illness, and ease of management with alternative therapies all need to be considered in conjunction with the woman and her partner.

Aging also presents certain treatment concerns. Lithium, carbamazepine, and valproic acid are relatively well tolerated in the elderly once attention is given to the slower clearance of drugs generally in this population group. The risk of clinically significant renal toxicity with lithium is not great. Although glomerular filtration rate decreases with age in persons treated with lithium, the rate of decline does not appear to be accelerated by lithium treatment. Nonetheless, careful monitoring of renal function is needed in the elderly.

In addition, increasing age is clearly a risk factor for hypothyroidism, as is lithium use. Thus, elderly persons taking lithium should be followed up carefully for decrements in thyroid function, although hypothyroidism is not an indication for lithium discontinuation but rather simply for thyroid hormone supplementation.

Depressive Disorders

MAJOR DEPRESSIVE DISORDER

DEFINITION

The depressive disorders are characterized predominantly by lifelong vulnerability to episodes of disease, involving depressed mood or loss of interest and pleasure in activities, and continuing potential for cycling of mood from euthymia to depression to recovery and sometimes to hypomania. When the mood disorder is severe, the potential for psychosis leads to profound disruption of cognitive functioning.

The clinical syndrome of major depressive disorder (MDD) invariably involves alterations in mood experienced as a feeling of sadness, irritability, dejection, despair, or loss of interest or pleasure. Associated neurovegetative or biological signs of depression include impairment in sleep, appetite, energy level, libido, and psychomotor activity. These core symptoms of depression are evident in children or adolescents with MDD, although the depressed mood may be manifested by irritability or social withdrawal. Older adults may show a preponderance of somatic preoccupation and memory impairment in association with the signs of MDD.

Suicidal Phenomena

Suicidality is the essential feature of depressive disorder that currently poses substantial risk of mortality in the disease. Prevention of suicide, more than any other goal, demands immediate treatment or hospitalization. The risk of subsequent suicide for an individual hospitalized for an episode of severe MDD is estimated to be 15%.

EPIDEMIOLOGY

Prevalence and Incidence

Across epidemiological studies, MDD is found to be a common psychiatric disorder. Although the rates of MDD in prepubertal boys and girls are equal, women are two to three times more likely than men to have MDD after puberty. Estimates of lifetime risk for MDD in community samples vary from 20% to 25% for women and 7% to 12% for men.

Risk Factors

Primary risk factors for depression include 1) history of prior episodes of depression; 2) family history of depressive disorder, especially in first-degree relatives; 3) history of suicide attempts; 4) female sex; 5) age at onset before 40 years; 6) postpartum period; 7) comorbid medical illness; 8) absence of social support; 9) negative, stressful life events; and 10) active alcohol or substance abuse.

Comorbidity Patterns: General Medical Conditions

Symptoms of depression are found in 12% to 36% of patients with a general medical condition.

STROKE

After stroke, some patients manifest MDD that is causally related to cerebral infarction in left frontal and left subcortical brain regions. Other patients evidence MDD after stroke that can be understood as both a psychological and a physiological response to the insult.

The distinction between depressive disorders and dementing disorders is often complicated because co-occurring depression and dementia are the most common presentation. In addition, early stages of Alzheimer's disease and other dementia frequently involve depressive symptoms, sometimes with psychotic features.

PARKINSON'S DISEASE

Fifty percent of patients with Parkinson's disease experience MDD during the course of the illness.

DIABETES

It is estimated that depression in treated patients with diabetes is three times as prevalent as in the general population.

CORONARY ARTERY DISEASE

Depression is significantly associated with increased morbidity and mortality in myocardial infarction patients as well as in patients having coronary artery disease without myocardial infarction. Depressive disorders may promote poor adherence to cardiac rehabilitation and worse outcome. During the first year of recovery, more social problems have been observed in infarction patients with moderate to severe depression than in nondepressed infarction patients.

CANCER

MDD occurs in 25% of patients with cancer at some time during the illness and should be assessed and treated as an independent disorder.

DEPRESSION DUE TO MEDICATIONS

MDD caused by medications remains an important aspect of the differential diagnostic process. Medications reported to be associated with MDD include several drugs from the associated groups seen in Table 27–1.

TABLE 27–1 Medications Associated with Depression

Cardiovascular drugs	Hormones	Psychotropics
Methyldopa	Oral contraceptives	Benzodiazepines
Reserpine	Corticotropin and glucocorticoids	Neuroleptics
Propranolol	Anabolic steroids	
Guanethidine		
Clonidine		
Thiazide diuretics		
Digitalis		
	Antiinflammatory and Antiinfective Agents	**Others**
Anticancer Agents	Nonsteroidal antiinflammatory agents	Cocaine (withdrawal)
Cycloserine	Ethambutol	Amphetamines (withdrawal)
	Disulfiram	Levodopa
	Sulfonamides	Cimetidine
	Baclofen	Ranitidine
	Metoclopramide	

Other Clinical Psychiatric Disorders

More than 40% of patients with MDD meet criteria during their lifetime for one or more nonmood psychiatric disorders. Common comorbid illnesses include alcoholism, anxiety disorders, eating disorders, and personality disorders, especially borderline personality disorder.

GRIEF AND BEREAVEMENT

Depressive symptoms associated with normal grieving usually begin within 2 to 3 weeks of a loss by death and resolve spontaneously in 6 to 8 weeks. If signs of MDD persist for more than 2 months beyond the death of a loved one, an episode of MDD can be diagnosed.

RISK FACTORS

All attempts to develop integrated etiological models of depression have identified multiple psychosocial risk factors. In particular, the vulnerability to MDD appears to be influenced by female sex; limited social support; dependent, self-critical, and neurotic personality traits; and stressful life events.

Because genetic factors are operative in the etiology of MDD and prior depressive episodes place an individual at risk for future depression, indirect genetic factors operate in the vulnerability to lifetime risk. No specific biological etiology has yet been identified, although antidepressant drugs appear to exert their effect through modulation of catecholamine or serotonin systems in the brain. Psychological stress or loss is a known precipitant for depression.

DIAGNOSIS AND DIFFERENTIAL DIAGNOSIS

The detection of depression in both primary care settings and mental health settings is dependent on careful observation of mood disturbance or loss of interest and pleasure in activities for 2 weeks or more. Dysthymic disorder is characterized by at least 2 years of depressed mood accompanied by two or three depressive symptoms that does not meet threshold criteria for a major depressive episode. Depressive disorder not otherwise specified (NOS) includes a set of conditions that do not meet criteria for MDD, dysthymic disorder, or adjustment disorder with depressed mood. These syndromes include premenstrual dysphoric disorder, minor depressive disorder, recurrent brief depressive disorder, and postpsychotic depressive disorder occurring during the residual phase of schizophrenia.

DSM-IV Criteria

Major Depressive Disorder

A. Five (or more) of the following symptoms have been present during the same 2-week period and represent a change from previous functioning; at least one of the symptoms is either (1) depressed mood or (2) loss of interest or pleasure.

Note: Do not include symptoms that are clearly due to a general medical condition, or mood-incongruent delusions or hallucinations.

(1) depressed mood most of the day, nearly every day, as indicated by either subjective report (e.g., feels sad or empty) or observation made by others (e.g., appears tearful). **Note:** In children and adolescents, can be irritable mood.

(2) markedly diminished interest or pleasure in all, or almost all, activities most of the day, nearly every day (as indicated by either subjective account or observation made by others)

(3) significant weight loss when not dieting or weight gain (e.g., a change of more than 5% of body weight in a month), or decrease or increase in appetite nearly every day. **Note:** In children, consider failure to make expected weight gains.

(4) insomnia or hypersomnia nearly every day

(5) psychomotor agitation or retardation nearly every day (observable by others, not merely subjective feelings of restlessness or being slowed down)

(6) fatigue or loss of energy nearly every day

(7) feelings of worthlessness or excessive or inappropriate guilt (which may be delusional) nearly every day day (not merely self-reproach or guilt about being sick)

(8) diminished ability to think or concentrate, or indecisiveness, nearly every day (either by subjective account or as observed by others)

(9) recurrent thoughts of death (not just fear of dying), recurrent suicidal ideation without a specific plan, or a suicide attempt or a specific plan for committing suicide

B. The symptoms do not meet criteria for a mixed episode.

C. The symptoms cause clinically significant distress or impairment in social, occupational, or other important areas of functioning.

D. The symptoms are not due to the direct physiological effects of a substance (e.g., a drug of abuse, a medication) or a general medical condition (e.g., hypothyroidism).

E. The symptoms are not better accounted for by bereavement, i.e., after the loss of a loved one, the symptoms persist for longer than 2 months or are characterized by marked functional impairment, morbid preoccupation with worthlessness, suicidal ideation, psychotic symptoms, or psychomotor retardation.

DSM-IV Criteria 300.4

Dysthymic Disorder

A. Depressed mood for most of the day, for more days than not, as indicated either by subjective account or by observation by others, for at least 2 years. **Note:** In children and adolescents, mood can be irritable and duration must be at least 1 year.

B. Presence, while depressed, of two (or more) of the following:

    (1) poor appetite or overeating

    (2) insomnia or hypersomnia

    (3) low energy or fatigue

    (4) low self-esteem

    (5) poor concentration or difficulty making decisions

    (6) feelings of hopelessness

C. During the 2-year period (1 year for children or adolescents) of the disturbance, the person has never been without the symptoms in criteria A and B for more than 2 months at a time.

D. No major depressive episode has been present during the first 2 years of the disturbance (1 year for children and adolescents); i.e., the disturbance is not better accounted for by chronic major depressive disorder or major depressive disorder, in partial remission.

Note: There may have been a previous major depressive episode provided there was a full remission (no significant signs or symptoms for 2 months) before development of the dysthymic disorder. In addition, after the initial 2 years (1 year in children or adolescents) of dysthymic disorder, there may be superimposed episodes of major depressive disorder, in which case both diagnoses may be given when the criteria are met for a major depressive episode.

E. There has never been a manic episode, a mixed episode, or a hypomanic episode, and criteria have never been met for cyclothymic disorder.

F. The disturbance does not occur exclusively during the course of a chronic psychotic disorder, such as schizophrenia or delusional disorder.

G. The symptoms are not due to the direct physiological effects of a substance (e.g., a drug of abuse, a medication) or a general medical condition (e.g., hypothyroidism).

H. The symptoms cause clinically significant distress or impairment in social, occupational, or other important areas of functioning.

Specify if:

Early onset: if onset is before age 21 years

Late onset: if onset is age 21 years or older

Specify

(for most recent 2 years of dysthymic disorder):

With atypical features

The criteria for a major depressive episode are illustrated in the *Diagnostic and Statistical Manual of Mental Disorders,* Fourth Edition (DSM-IV).

The most common psychiatric syndrome associated with thoughts of death, suicidal ideation, or completed suicide is MDD. The preoccupation with suicide in MDD requires that the assessment always include careful monitoring of suicidality.

Assessment

To assess risk for suicide, one inquires about the presence of active suicidal ideation in relation to the current episode of depression and prior suicide attempts. The occurrence of significant life events such as separation, divorce, and death of significant others may precipitate the episode. When alcohol or other drug use co-occurs with such significant life events, the risk of suicidal behavior during an episode of depression increases. The history of a recent suicide attempt may suggest the need for immediate hospitalization and treatment.

The individual who presents for outpatient or hospital treatment for a primary depressive disorder will require a general medical examination, including a physical examination and laboratory testing to rule out an associated medical condition. When clinical signs suggest cognitive disruption or cognitive impairment, the clinician may also consider administering neuropsychological tests or conducting more focused neurological examination to explore cognitive, behavioral, and neurological correlates of brain function.

Certain inventories are commonly used in outpatient and inpatient settings to establish scores of clinical severity of depressive symptoms. Self-administered scales include the Beck Depression Inventory, the Zung Self-rating Depression Scale, and the Inventory for Depressive Symptomatology (self-report version). Psychiatrist-administered scales used for assessment of depressive symptoms include the Hamilton Depression Rating Scale, the Montgomery-Asberg Depression Rating Scale, and the Inventory for Depressive Symptomatology (psychiatrist rated).

COURSE AND NATURAL HISTORY

The mean age at onset of major depression is 27 years, although an individual can experience the onset of MDD at any age.

Symptoms of MDD develop in a period of days or weeks. Early manifestations of an MDD episode may include anxiety, sleeplessness, worry, and rumination before the experience of overt sadness. In a lifetime, the presence of one major depressive episode carries at least a 50% chance of leading to a subsequent episode. A history of two episodes carries at least a 70% chance of another episode, and three or more episodes yield at least a 90% chance of future episodes. Because the majority of MDD cases may recur, continuity of treatment and education about early warning signs of relapse or recurrence are essential in ongoing clinical care.

Untreated episodes of depression last 6 to 24 months. Symptom remission and a return to premorbid level of functioning characterize approximately 66% of depressed patients. By comparison, roughly 5% to 10% of patients continue to experience a full episode of depression for longer than 2 years, and approximately 20% to 25% of patients experience partial recovery between episodes.

Poor outcome and likelihood of recurrent episodes are associated with comorbid conditions such as personality disorder, active substance or alcohol abuse, organicity, or medical illness. Recurrence and outcome may be affected by the rapidity of clinical intervention. Inadequate treatment (e.g., insufficient dosing or duration of pharmacotherapy) contributes to poor outcome, including chronic MDD.

PROGNOSIS

Patients with MDD report health difficulties and actively use health services. Studies have indicated that as many as 23% of depressed patients report health difficulties severe enough to keep them bedridden. Furthermore, long-term diminished activity has been shown to characterize a community sample of depressed patients.

A significant relationship exists between MDD and mortality, characterized by suicide and accidents. Fifteen percent of patients with MDD that is severe enough to warrant hospitalization will die by suicide. Approximately 10% of patients with MDD who attempt suicide will eventually succeed in killing themselves. Roughly 50% of individuals who have successfully committed suicide carried a main diagnosis of depression.

GOALS OF TREATMENT

The goals of treatment in MDD are reduction and elimination of depression symptoms with restoration of full psychosocial functioning. Improved adaptive functioning after an episode is an associated goal. The establishment of a working relationship among patient, family, and psychiatrist promotes recovery and underlies psychiatric management and treatment.

Phases of Treatment

The phases of treatment include 1) an acute phase directed at reduction and elimination of depressive signs and symptoms and active restoration of psychosocial and work functioning, 2) a continuation phase directed at preventing relapse and reducing likelihood of recurrence through ongoing psychoeducation and continuation of pharmacotherapy and psychotherapy as indicated, and 3) a maintenance phase directed at preventing future episodes of depression based on a clinical understanding of the history of relapse or recurrence.

GENERAL APPROACHES TO TREATMENT

Pharmacotherapy and Other Somatic Treatment

Acute phase treatment with medication is highly effective for the reduction and resolution of all signs and symptoms of MDD. Medication appears to have a most direct effect on symptom reduction and is also associated with improved psychosocial functioning.

Antidepressant medications currently available for acute treatment of MDD are listed in Table 27–2. Choice of treatment with a specific medicine in a given clinical situation is based predominantly on determination of prior treatment response to a medication, consideration of potential side effects, history of response in first-degree relatives to medication, and presence of concurrent general medical illnesses or comorbid psychiatric disorders that might lead to a specific choice of antidepressant treatment. A typical algorithm for pharmacotherapy in MDD is seen in Table 27–3.

When antidepressant medicine is initiated, the medication treatment requires careful monitoring of initial dose and response, review of treatment with the patient soon after initiation, gradual increase of dose to therapeutic levels, and review of clinical response on a weekly basis in outpatient management. The ultimate goal of pharmacotherapy is complete remission of symptoms during the course of 6 to 12 weeks of treatment.

The most established therapeutic range for tricyclic antidepressants (TCAs) is for nortriptyline, which demonstrates a therapeutic window of 50 to 150 ng/p mL. The other TCAs appear to demonstrate a linear pattern of response as long as the blood level is above the established therapeutic level.

GENERAL PHARMACOTHERAPY RECOMMENDATIONS

If a trial of one medication within a class of antidepressants using adequate dose and duration has been completed, there is no clear evidence to recommend switching from one medication to another medication within the same class. Most authors recommend increasing the dose of the same medication, augmenting with lithium carbonate, or switching to another class of medication if there is incomplete response.

Electroconvulsive Therapy

Electroconvulsive therapy is an effective treatment in patients with severe MDD, including those with psychotic features. It is particularly useful in aborting acute suicidal drive for patients who require rapid resolution of symptoms. Electroconvulsive therapy requires active consultation of a psychiatrist familiar with the treatment and appropriately trained in modern procedures. The most common side

Text continued on page 286

TABLE 27-2 Typical Antidepressant Therapeutic Doses and Side Effects

Category and Trade Name	Compound	Usual Therapeutic Daily Dose	Sedation Effect	Hypotensive Effect (Decreased Blood Pressure)	Anticholinergic Effect (Dry Mouth, Constipation)	Cardiac Effect (Slowed Heart Rate)
Tricyclic Antidepressants						
Tertiary amines						
Anafranil	Clomipramine	150–300	High	High	High	Yes
Elavil	Amitriptyline	200–300	High	High	High	Yes
Sinequan, Adapin	Doxepin	200–300	High	Moderate	Moderate	Yes
Surmontil	Trimipramine	150–500	High	Moderate	Moderate	Yes
Tofranil	Imipramine	200–500	Moderate	High	Moderate	Yes
Secondary amines						
Norpramin	Desipramine	125–150	Low	Moderate	Low	Yes
Pamelor	Nortriptyline	50–150	Moderate	Low	Low	Yes
Vivactil	Protriptyline	30	Low	Low	High	Yes

Monoamine Oxidase Inhibitors

Marplan	Isocarboxazid	30	Low	Moderate	Low	Low
Nardil	Phenelzine	45–90	Low	Moderate	Low	Low
Parnate	Tranylcypromine	30–60	Low	Moderate	Low	Low
Atypical Agents						
Asendin	Amoxapine	200–300	Low	Moderate	Low	Yes
Desyrel	Trazodone	300–600	High	Low	Minimal	Low
Ludiomil	Maprotiline	150–200	Moderate	Low	Low	Yes
Wellbutrin	Bupropion	300	Minimal	Low	Minimal	Low
Selective Serotonin Reuptake Inhibitors						
Paxil	Paroxetine	2–50	Low	Minimal	Minimal	Low
Prozac	Fluoxetine	20–80	Minimal	Minimal	Minimal	Low
Zoloft	Sertraline	50–200	Minimal	Minimal	Minimal	Low
Luvox	Fluvoxamine	150–300	Low	Low	Low	Low

Table continued on following page

TABLE 27-2	Typical Antidepressant Therapeutic Doses and Side Effects *(Continued)*					
Category and Trade Name	Compound	Usual Therapeutic Daily Dose	Sedation Effect	Hypotensive Effect (Decreased Blood Pressure)	Anticholinergic Effect (Dry, Mouth, Constipation)	Cardiac Effect (Slowed Heart Rate)
	Serotonin-Norepinephrine Reuptake Inhibitor					
Effexor	Venlafaxine	75–300	Low	None (increased blood pressure)	None	Minimal
	Serotonin Transport Blocker and Antagonist					
Serzone	Nefazodone	200–600	Moderate	Low	Minimal	Low

TABLE 27–3	Pharmacotherapy Algorithm in Major Depressive Disorder

Major Depressive Disorder, Single or Recurrent Episode, Without Psychotic Features

Begin effective TCA, such as imipramine, nortriptyline, or desipramine (augment TCA with lithium carbonate, 600–900 mg).

or

Begin SSRI (augment with TCA, either nortriptyline or desipramine, recognizing important drug interactions).

or

Begin venlafaxine (Effexor), nefazodone (Serzone), bupropion (Wellbutrin).

If ineffective, consider tranylcypromine, augmented with lithium carbonate if necessary, for anergic features;

or

phenelzine, augmented with lithium carbonate if necessary, for anxious, dependent, and phobic features.

Major Depressive Disorder, Single or Recurrent Episode, with Psychotic Features

Begin antipsychotic medication to adequate doses to interrupt delusional features, augmented with standard TCA, either nortriptyline or desipramine, recognizing important drug interactions.

or

Begin electroconvulsive therapy as alternative in context of immediate suicide risk, physical deterioration, or prior response to electroconvulsive therapy.

or

Begin amoxapine as alternative.

Major Depressive Disorder with Atypical Features

Begin MAOI, either phenelzine or tranylcypromine, to therapeutic doses.

or

Begin SSRI beginning at low doses to minimize early side effects.

Major Depressive Disorder with Catatonic Features

Begin lorazepam, 1–3 mg daily, to interrupt catatonic symptoms; evaluate for presence of psychotic features and longitudinal history of bipolar disorder.

Add antipsychotic medication to therapeutic doses, augmented with lithium carbonate to therapeutic doses, if longitudinal history of bipolar or schizoaffective disorder emerges.

effect associated with electroconvulsive therapy is amnesia for the period of treatment and the several days that preceded the treatment.

There is no evidence to suggest chronic cognitive impairment as a result of electroconvulsive therapy. Acute treatment with electroconvulsive therapy is often followed by a continuation of medication treatment or a schedule of maintenance electroconvulsive therapy. Electroconvulsive therapy has been demonstrated as both safe and effective in depressive conditions that pose significant morbidity and mortality risk.

Light Therapy

Light therapy involves the exposure of individuals with MDD to 2500-lux light for 1 to 2 hours on awakening. It has been developed as a new therapy for patients who have MDD with a seasonal pattern. Most of these patients experience recurrent winter depression in the context of recurrent MDD or bipolar II disorder. The exposure to this bright light early in the morning has been associated with a favorable response within 4 to 7 days. At this time, light therapy is best administered by professionals who have experience in its use and who can appropriately evaluate the treatment indication and response. The side effects associated with light therapy involve ophthalmological complications and hypomania or mania with psychosis in those individuals vulnerable to bipolar I disorder.

Psychosocial Treatment

The past decade has led to the development of specific psychosocial treatments for MDD. These treatments include supportive psychiatric management, interpersonal psychotherapy, cognitive therapy, behavioral therapy, brief dynamic psychotherapy, and marital and family therapy.

Short-term focused psychotherapies for MDD have demonstrated efficacy in individuals with mild to moderate depressive symptoms. Psychotherapy alone is not indicated for individuals who demonstrate melancholic or psychotic features. The goals of the brief focused psychotherapy are similar to those of medication treatment and include 1) improved medication compliance, 2) reduction or elimination of active symptoms of depression, 3) prevention of relapse or recurrence, and 4) restoration of psychosocial functioning.

INTERPERSONAL PSYCHOTHERAPY

Interpersonal psychotherapy involves resolution of a set of current interpersonal difficulties including prolonged grief, role transitions, interpersonal disputes, and interpersonal deficits. The treatment requires initial education about the nature of depressive disorder and the relationship between symptoms and current interpersonal difficulties.

COGNITIVE THERAPY

Cognitive or cognitive-behavioral therapy for depression is a form of treatment aimed at symptom reduction through identification and correction of cognitive distortions and prevention of relapse by interrupting distorted schemas.

BEHAVIORAL THERAPY

Behavioral treatments of depression are based on a social learning theory, and the major goal involves increasing the positive reinforcement received by the depressed individual through specific social skills training.

BRIEF DYNAMIC PSYCHOTHERAPY

Brief dynamic psychotherapy focuses on current conflicts as manifestations of difficulties in early attachments and disruptions of early object relations. Dynamic psychotherapy that addresses demoralization, resolves conflicts, and promotes rehabilitation is effective in diminishing overall symptoms of depression and anxiety.

Factors Influencing Treatment Response

CLINICAL FEATURES

SUICIDE RISK. Patients with MDD are at increased risk for suicide. Clinical attention to suicide risk is indicated as patients begin to recover from depression with increased energy and sense of purpose. Persistent suicidal ideation, coupled with increased energy, can lead to impulsive suicidality.

MELANCHOLIC FEATURES. Melancholic features as defined in DSM-IV warrant trials of effective antidepressant pharmacotherapy or electroconvulsive therapy during the course of inpatient treatment.

PSYCHOTIC FEATURES. MDD with psychotic features requires active medical intervention with combined antipsychotic and antidepressant pharmacotherapy. Electroconvulsive therapy is effective in psychotic depression and should be considered a first-line treatment.

CATATONIC FEATURES. MDD with catatonic features may be life threatening owing to the patient's refusal to eat or drink. Treatment with benzodiazepines such as lorazepam at 1 to 3 mg often offers short-term response.

ATYPICAL FEATURES. Atypical features involve comorbid anxiety and reverse neurovegetative symptoms including increased sleep, appetite, and weight as well as fatigue and leaden paralysis. Although TCAs are not as effective, MAOIs yield response rates of 55% to 75%, which are comparable to responses in typical depression with TCAs. SSRIs are also likely to be helpful in MDD with atypical features.

SEVERITY. Individuals with mild to moderate depression can be effectively treated with psychotherapy or pharmacotherapy. Severe MDD requires treatment with antidepressant medication or electroconvulsive therapy as a first-line treatment.

RECURRENCE. Because MDD is often a recurrent disorder, treatment guidelines suggest maintenance antidepressant treatment at full therapeutic doses if there is a history of two episodes in 5 years or multiple (three or more) prior episodes.

HISTORY OF HYPOMANIA OR MANIA. Electroconvulsive therapy, light therapy, and antidepressant pharmacotherapy may induce hypomania or mania in individuals vulnerable to bipolar disorder. In such individuals, TCAs are also reported to induce rapid-cycling bipolar disorder. All individuals treated for depression should be evaluated for a history of hypomania or mania because they are at particular risk for antidepressant-induced mania. Up to 20% of individuals may experience induction of hypomania or mania with antidepressant treatment. Therefore, attention to antidepressant treatment response and longitudinal course is required.

ALCOHOL OR SUBSTANCE DEPENDENCE. Abstinence from alcohol or substance use is the first priority in treatment. Comorbid addiction complicates depressive disorders and promotes risk for suicide. If detoxification from alcohol or other substances is required, this should be accomplished before initiation of antidepressant therapy.

Refractory Major Depressive Disorder

Most authors consider a patient treatment refractory if a course of three or more treatments is offered without substantial clinical response. The standard approaches to the management of refractory depression include 1) increasing the antidepressant dose and monitoring for a full 8- to 12-week course, assuming that some patients will be late responders to treatment; 2) augmenting the treatment with one of several augmentation strategies; 3) using combinations of antidepressant drug treatment or combinations of pharmacotherapy and psychotherapy; and 4) switching to alternative somatic treatments including electroconvulsive therapy and specific forms of psychotherapy.

In general, the most common clinical predictors of lack of response are a history of prior nonresponse, poor interepisode recovery, and chaotic social history. Psychosocial factors in refractoriness include increased neuroticism, pathological dependency, and early developmental impairments involving low self-esteem.

DYSTHYMIC DISORDER

DEFINITION

Dysthymic disorder is characterized by chronic depressive symptoms that are present most of the day, more days than not, for at least 2 years. The longitudinal assessment of patients with dysthymic disorder reveals substantial risk for the development of MDD and comorbid personality disorder.

Early-onset dysthymic disorder is usually associated with subsequent episodes of MDD. Atypical dysthymic disorder may herald a bipolar I or bipolar II course.

EPIDEMIOLOGY

In the ECA study, a lifetime prevalence of 4.1% for women and 2.2% for men was found for dysthymic disorder. In adults, dysthymic disorder is more common in women than in men; in children, dysthymic disorder occurs equally in both sexes.

Comorbidity Patterns

Individuals with dysthymic disorder are at substantial risk for development of other psychiatric conditions, including alcohol or substance dependence, MDD, and personality disorders. Up to 15% of patients with dysthymic disorder also meet criteria for a comorbid alcohol or substance dependence. The most common personality disorders include those that are mixed, dependent, and borderline. Childhood- and adolescent-onset dysthymic disorder is associated with substantial risk for later onset of recurrent affective illness.

DIAGNOSIS AND DIFFERENTIAL DIAGNOSIS

The diagnosis of dysthymic disorder is not made if depressive symptoms occur during the course of nonaffective psychoses, including schizophrenia, schizoaffective disorder, and delusional disorder. A diagnosis of depressive disorder NOS is made if these symptoms meet criteria for MDD during the residual phase of a psychotic disorder. If dysthymic disorder is determined to be caused by a chronic medical condition, then one diagnoses mood disorder due to a general medical condition. If substance dependence is judged to be an etiological factor, a substance-induced mood disorder is diagnosed. Individuals with dysthymic disorder often manifest co-occurring personality disorders such that separate diagnoses on Axis I and Axis II are given.

COURSE AND NATURAL HISTORY

Often, dysthymic disorder begins in late childhood or adolescence and has a chronic course.

Results from the Medical Outcomes Study provide important information about the course of dysthymic disorder. Patients with dysthymic disorder, either with or without comorbid MDD, had more severe impairment in functional status (e.g., social, emotional, and physical functioning) than did patients with MDD alone. Those with dysthymic disorder and comorbid MDD evidenced a significantly lower probability of remission than patients who met criteria for MDD alone. Furthermore, patients with dysthymic disorder and comorbid MDD who had many severe symptoms at baseline evaluation demonstrated a particularly low probability of remission.

Overall, patients with MDD alone had intermediate outcomes, whereas patients with dysthymic disorder (with or without comorbid MDD) had a worse course of illness. Untreated dysthymic disorder results in significant occupational and financial burden. There are significant complaints of chronic restriction of activity, days spent in bed, complaints of poor health, and more disability days than in the general population.

GOALS OF AND APPROACHES TO TREATMENT

The goals of treatment in dysthymic disorder parallel those in MDD and include remission of symptoms and psychosocial recovery. MDD occurs commonly during the course of dysthymic disorder.

The presence of double depression (i.e., both MDD and dysthymic disorder) suggests maintenance antidepressant treatment with attention to recovery from chronic mood disturbance. Selective serotonin reuptake inhibitors (SSRIs) are also recommended in dysthymic disorder, and some claims of "personality change" may be due to medication-responsive chronic mood symptoms.

There are no randomized controlled studies of any depression-specific psychotherapy in dysthymic disorder, but clinical reports suggest response to interpersonal psychotherapy and cognitive therapy.

DEPRESSIVE DISORDER NOT OTHERWISE SPECIFIED

Depressive disorder NOS refers to a variety of diagnoses and includes several disorders listed in DSM-IV that may be distinguished from MDD, dysthymic disorder, or an adjustment disorder with depressed mood.

PREMENSTRUAL DYSPHORIC DISORDER

Premenstrual dysphoric disorder is characterized by depressed mood, anxiety, affective lability, and marked disability experienced during the last week of the luteal phase and remitting during the follicular phase of the menstrual cycle. This pattern occurs for most months during the year. The severity of the symptom pattern is comparable to that of MDD. The duration is usually briefer by definition because the symptoms completely disappear with the onset of menses.

Whereas up to 75% of women report minor premenstrual symptoms, 3% to 5% of women experience symptoms that may meet criteria for this disorder. Premenstrual dysphoric disorder worsens with increased age but diminishes at the time of menopause.

Premenstrual dysphoric disorder symptoms are likely to respond to fluoxetine or other SSRI treatment.

MINOR DEPRESSIVE DISORDER

Minor depressive disorder is characterized by one or more periods of depression lasting at least 2 weeks but with fewer symptoms (more than two but less than five) and less psychosocial impairment than in MDD. The point prevalence of minor depressive disorder in primary care settings ranges from 3.4% to 4.7%.

In differential diagnosis, one must consider an adjustment disorder with depressed mood and other experiences of sadness that may be part of living, including bereavement. Because minor depressive disorder frequently co-occurs with general medical conditions, one must rule out MDD and a mood disorder due to a general medical condition.

Minor depressive disorder tends to begin in late adolescence and affects men and women equally. In the elderly, minor depressive disorder is associated with greater impairment of routine activities in comparison with asymptomatic adults. There are limited data regarding treatment outcome with pharmacotherapy or psychotherapy.

RECURRENT BRIEF DEPRESSIVE DISORDER

Recurrent brief depressive disorder refers to episodes of depressive disorder that last 2 days to 2 weeks and meet full criteria (except duration) for MDD. These episodes occur once monthly for 12 months but are not associated with the menstrual cycle. These depressive episodes typically cause clinically significant distress and impairment in social and occupational functioning.

Associated clinical features may include comorbid substance dependence or anxiety disorders. The 1-year prevalence of recurrent brief depressive disorder is estimated to be 7%. The age at onset is typically during adolescence. There appears to be a higher than usual association of suicide attempts during the course of recurrent brief depressive disorder.

Recurrent brief depressive episodes are unrelated to menstrual cycles and are as common among men as among women.

Patients with recurrent brief depressive disorder have a higher rate of suicide attempts than a comparative MDD group.

Brief depressive disorder requires further distinction from comorbid personality disorder, especially borderline personality disorder.

POSTPSYCHOTIC DEPRESSIVE DISORDER OF SCHIZOPHRENIA

Postpsychotic depressive disorder of schizophrenia is an episode of MDD superimposed on schizophrenia that occurs during the residual phase of the illness. This mood disorder is not considered to be a result of substance abuse, neuroleptic-induced akinesia, other medication effects, or a general medical condition.

Associated clinical features include limited social support, several prior hospitalizations, and multiple relapses of psychosis. It is estimated that up to 25% of individuals with schizophrenia may experience postpsychotic depressive disorder.

Compared with individuals with psychotic disorders who are not depressed, individuals with postpsychotic depressive disorder of schizophrenia have an associated higher risk of suicide. Treatment studies demonstrate efficacy of antidepressant medication in postpsychotic depressive disorder of schizophrenia.

Panic Disorder with and Without Agoraphobia

DEFINITION AND HISTORICAL OVERVIEW

DSM-IV Criteria 300.01

Panic Disorder Without Agoraphobia

A. Both (1) and (2):

    (1) recurrent unexpected panic attacks

    (2) at least one of the attacks has been followed by 1 month (or more) of one (or more) of the following:

        (a) persistent concern about having additional attacks

        (b) worry about the implications of the attack or its consequences (e.g., losing control, having a heart attack, "going crazy")

B. Absence of agoraphobia.

C. The panic attacks are not due to the direct physiological effects of a substance (e.g., a drug of abuse, a medication) or a general medical condition (e.g., hyperthyroidism).

D. The panic attacks are not better accounted for by another mental disorder, such as social phobia (e.g., occurring on exposure to feared social situations), specific phobia (e.g., on exposure to a specific phobic situation), obsessive-compulsive disorder (e.g., on exposure to dirt in someone with an obsession about contamination), posttraumatic stress disorder (e.g., in response to stimuli associated with a severe stressor), or separation anxiety disorder (e.g., in response to being away from home or close relatives).

DSM-IV Criteria 300.21

Panic Disorder with Agoraphobia

A. Both (1) and (2):

    (1) recurrent unexpected panic attacks

    (2) at least one of the attacks has been followed by
        1 month (or more) of one (or more) of the
        following:

        (a) persistent concern about having additional
            attacks

        (b) worry about the implications of the attack or
            its consequences (e.g., losing control, having
            a heart attack, "going crazy")

B. The presence of agoraphobia.

C. The panic attacks are not due to the direct physiologi-
    cal effects of a substance (e.g., a drug of abuse, a
    medication) or a general medical condition (e.g.,
    hyperthyroidism).

D. The panic attacks are not better accounted for by
    another mental disorder, such as social phobia (e.g.,
    occurring on exposure to feared social situations),
    specific phobia (e.g., on exposure to a specific phobic
    situation), obsessive-compulsive disorder (e.g., on
    exposure to dirt in someone with an obsession about
    contamination), posttraumatic stress disorder (e.g.,
    in response to stimuli associated with a severe
    stressor), or separation anxiety disorder (e.g., in
    response to being away from home or close relatives).

Panic is defined as the unexpected onset and rapid escalation of a sense of fear or apprehension, accompanied by typical physical sensations such as heart palpitations, shortness of breath, dizziness, lightheadedness, trembling, shaking, and the like. Although panic episodes are identified in individuals with severe agoraphobia, it is clear that some patients with recurrent panic have few or no phobic complications. The experience of recurrent, unexpected panic attacks causes considerable distress and impairment, even without phobic complications. The prominent cardiovascular symptoms in panic episodes frequently bring patients to the cardiologist's office.

EPIDEMIOLOGY

Findings from epidemiological studies are summarized in Table 28–1.

There is evidence that a high percentage of individuals suffering from anxiety disorders are seen in general medical settings. Epide-

TABLE 28–1	Findings from Epidemiological Studies
Prevalence rates	
Panic disorder	3.5%
Unexpected panic attack	5%–10%
Any panic	20%
Typical age at onset	15–19 y
Sex distribution	Females affected twice as frequently as males
Associated behaviors	Frequent use of emergency services
	Impaired social functioning
	Financial dependency
	Substance use
	Suicide attempts

miological data indicate that 46% of the 6.4 million individuals treated for anxiety disorders in a 1-year period are seen in general medical settings.

The Epidemiological Catchment Area (ECA) data indicate a high degree of comorbidity among the anxiety disorders, between anxiety and affective disorders, and between anxiety disorders and substance abuse. There is also a high rate of comorbidity of panic disorder with personality disorders.

Epidemiological studies indicate that panic disorder occurs in 2% to 5% of the population and almost always in association with other psychiatric disorders. Sporadic or infrequent panic attacks are more prevalent than full panic disorder in community samples but are still found in only a small minority of the population. Panic is more prevalent in individuals with a family history of panic, is more prevalent in women than in men, and, in general, occurs at higher rates in individuals with fewer resources and less control over their lives. The occurrence of panic is associated with high levels of distress and impairment and a high frequency of help-seeking behaviors.

BIOLOGICAL THEORY

The first premise of the biological understanding is that panic is a psychophysiological phenomenon distinct from other forms of anxiety; panic is not just severe anxiety. A second premise is that failure of a biological regulatory mechanism results in misfiring of an inborn alarm response. The pathogenic role of panic in the development of associated symptoms is a third major premise of the neurobiological theory. It is the experience of recurrent panic that leads to anxious apprehension, phobic avoidance, demoralization, and comorbidity with other anxiety states and depression.

There are no childhood or adolescent antecedents of panic, with the exception of that seen in children who have an early onset manifested as panic attacks, school phobia, or separation anxiety. In particular, disturbances of self-concept, interpersonal relationships, maladaptive thoughts and behaviors, and even preexisting states of anxious apprehension are thought to play little or no role in predisposing to panic vulnerability.

COGNITIVE-BEHAVIORAL THEORY

Cognitive-behavioral therapists developed a model of panic episodes that was different from the neurobiological one. In this model, all anxiety or fear occurs as a reaction to stimulus. Pathological fear states occur via a mechanism of learned reactivity. Thus panic is a learned reaction to interoceptive cues and occurs because of cognitive misinterpretation of these cues or a conditioned fear response, or both. In the cognitive-behavioral model, physiological disturbance is seen as a concomitant of all fear reactions rather than as a pathogenic mechanism for the development of the symptom.

GENERAL NEUROSIS THEORY

This view includes considerations of the origin of panic incorporating both biological and psychological features. Described in its simplest form, the basic premises focus on 1) an inborn altered nervous system that displays heightened reactivity to everyday stimuli, such as novelty; 2) early experiences with caretakers experienced as cold, critical, controlling, and restrictive; 3) a chronic tendency to heightened fearfulness and anxiety (manifested in children as shyness, performance anxiety, and sometimes school phobia; in adolescents as social fearfulness; and in young adults as overall nervousness and safety seeking); and 4) the onset of panic occurring in a sensitized person or in a setting of life stress, often triggered by a situation that challenges self-confidence or raises uncomfortable feelings of potential abandonment or control by others. An extension of this model postulates that panic triggers are stimuli with psychological meaning.

DIAGNOSIS

The diagnosis of panic disorder is based on the report of discrete episodes that begin abruptly and escalate rapidly to peak intensity. There is an apprehensive affect, which is usually but not always fear, as well as typical somatic symptoms, including chest pain, heart palpitations, lightheadedness, breathing abnormalities, numbness or tingling of the extremities, dizziness, upset stomach, nausea, diarrhea, hot or cold sensations, sweating, or trembling. Depersonalization and derealization are sometimes seen. There is usually fear of some catastrophic event such as a stroke, heart attack, death, insanity, or loss of control. Often the first panic episode is misinterpreted as evidence of severe medical or psychiatric disturbance.

Differential Diagnosis

The differential diagnosis of panic disorder includes a variety of conditions in which panic attacks occur. Other anxiety disorders, depression, hypochondriasis, medical disorders, and substance abuse must be ruled out. In particular, panic disorder must be distinguished from each of the anxiety disorders, including social phobia, obsessive-compulsive disorder, generalized anxiety disorder, specific phobias, and even posttraumatic stress disorder (PTSD). The key differentiating feature required for the diagnosis of panic disorder is the unexplained, uncued, or spontaneous panic episode.

Key differential diagnosis issues are presented in Table 28–2.

Assessment

SPECIAL ISSUES IN PSYCHIATRIC EXAMINATION AND HISTORY

It is well known that patients with panic disorder suffer from agoraphobia, and determination of the degree of phobic avoidance

TABLE 28–2	Key Differential Diagnosis Issues	
Group	**Specific Disorder**	**Panic Disorder Feature**
Other anxiety disorders	Specific phobia Social phobia Obsessive-compulsive disorder	Unexpected, more widespread phobic symptoms
	Generalized anxiety disorder	Focus of worry is on panic attacks
	Posttraumatic stress disorder	Uncued panic, persistent fear of panic
Major depressive disorder		Relative prominence of panic compared with mood disturbance; mood disturbance attributed to panic
Substance abuse	Alcohol and other sedative-hypnotic use	Panic occurs in situations other than withdrawal
	Psychostimulant use	Panic occurs in situations other than intoxication
Medical conditions	Endocrinopathies (especially thyroid disease), seizure disorder, brain tumor, brain vascular event	Does not remit with treatment of the medical disorder

is an important component of psychiatric assessment. Less well known is the fact that other types of phobic symptoms are also common in patients with panic disorder. In particular, a patient with panic disorder often fears and avoids one or more situations that provoke uncomfortable physical sensations. Social phobia symptoms are also common in patients with panic disorder.

Psychiatrists treating patients with panic disorder need to be aware of the reported observation that panic disorder is associated with a heightened prevalence of suicidal behavior. They should pay attention to the issue of suicidal behavior even in patients who manifest panic disorder without concurrent depression.

RELEVANT PHYSICAL AND LABORATORY FINDINGS

A medical evaluation should always be performed in patients presenting with psychiatric symptoms. Although, in general, patients with panic disorder have few physical findings or laboratory abnormalities, they often have laboratory evidence of hyperventilation, as shown by low serum bicarbonate levels and the presence of functional respiratory abnormalities.

Patients with panic disorder are sensitive to a range of pharmacological agents that can provoke a panic episode, including sodium, lactate, caffeine, and carbon dioxide. Occasional patients are sensitive to antihistamines, and there are case reports in the literature suggesting that estrogen replacement may provoke panic attacks in some women, as may estrogen as well.

DIFFERENCES IN DEVELOPMENTAL, GENDER, AND CULTURAL PRESENTATIONS

Panic disorder, once thought to occur only in adults, is now recognized in children and adolescents as well.

There are few sex differences in symptom presentation in patients with panic disorder. However, agoraphobic complications are two to four times more prevalent in women than in men.

COURSE AND NATURAL HISTORY

Onset and Early Course

Panic disorder usually begins in late adolescence or early adulthood with a sudden unexpected panic episode in an ordinary, everyday life situation. The initial panic episode is likely to occur within 3 to 6 months after a significant life event—such as a death, a move, an engagement or marriage, or a change in job status—or after the onset of a physical illness. The onset of the disorder may occur as a sudden severe panic episode without prodromal symptoms.

Panic may also occur as a complication of substance use, especially with cocaine or amphetamine-like substances. This disorder has also been reported in reaction to a variety of prescription medications. Thus it is important to obtain a history of any prescription or over-the-counter medications the patient may have used immediately before the initial panic episode.

The usual course of a panic disorder is a relapsing-remitting pattern of panic attacks with persistent fear or apprehension about further episodes providing a more stable background. The anticipatory anxiety may be more or less prominent but is virtually always present and can be elicited on close questioning.

Phobic complications occur in most panic patients, but the degree and form of this problem are variable. The most serious phobic complication is severe agoraphobia, which can lead the patient to become housebound and debilitated.

Long-Term Outcome

The long-term outcome of panic disorder has not been well studied, but indications are that it is a chronic illness. Highly successful results have been achieved for short-term treatment using any of several different treatment approaches. However, studies suggest that residual symptoms and relapse are common with each. The natural history of the disorder appears to be variable, with many patients exhibiting a waxing and waning course, even without treatment. Many, however, progress to stable, debilitating illness if not adequately treated.

OVERALL TREATMENT GOALS

Treatment goals for panic disorder are summarized in Table 28–3.

Immediate Goals

The immediate goals of panic disorder treatment are to develop a rapport with the patient, to conduct a complete evaluation, to educate the patient about the disorder and treatment modalities available, and to begin a symptom-focused treatment intervention.

Effective treatment can be accomplished by using medication, cognitive-behavioral treatment, or a combination of the two. Medication works more rapidly than psychological strategies and requires less of the patient. Cognitive-behavioral treatment gives the patient a greater sense of control and avoids medication side effects. A combined treatment may offer the most advantages.

TABLE 28–3	Treatment Goals
Development of a therapeutic rapport	
Education of the patient	
Acute relief of panic and associated symptoms	
Continuation of treatment to solidify gains	
Maintenance treatment to prevent relapse	
Evaluation and treatment of comorbidity and of psychosocial dysfunction	
Maintenance of durability of treatment with long-term follow-up	

Short-Term Goals

The short-term treatment goal is optimal symptom relief. Relief of anticipatory anxiety and phobic avoidance are also short-term treatment goals. Symptom relief can be achieved by using medication, psychotherapy, or a combination of the two.

Long-Term Goals

Long-term goals are to decrease panic vulnerability and to maintain panic remission. Although prospective controlled studies of long-term treatment of patients with panic disorder are not yet available, current recommendations are for continued maintenance treatment. Other goals of long-term treatment include improvement of functional impairment and quality of life.

STANDARD TREATMENTS

The treating clinician needs to be aware of problems that may interfere with treatment acceptance. For the most part, these are related to fears concerning bodily sensation and loss of control. Either or both of these factors may interfere with medication acceptance. Fear of losing control may take the form of an inability to accept prescriptive treatment for behavioral exposure and other cognitive-behavioral interventions.

Pharmacotherapy

Pharmacological treatment is highly effective in blocking panic attacks. Tricyclic antidepressant medication is still considered by many clinicians to be the treatment of choice for patients with panic disorder, although selective serotonin reuptake inhibitors are first-line medications for growing numbers.

Patients with panic disorder are sensitive to medication side effects, and treatment should be started at low doses and increased gradually. If tricyclic antidepressants are used, medication dosages should be increased gradually until full panic-blocking effects occur.

When medication is prescribed appropriately and accepted by the patient, there is a high rate of response (70% to 90%). Treatment combining medication and psychotherapy may increase acceptance by the patient or decrease the required dose of medication, or both. Most psychiatrists continue treatment for 6 months to 1 year after symptom remission occurs.

Monoamine oxidase inhibitors and other non–tricyclic antidepressant medications have also been reported to be effective in alleviating panic and may have advantages over the tricyclic antidepressants.

Benzodiazepines have been extensively studied in the treatment of panic disorder. Benzodiazepines have the advantage of a rapid onset of action and relatively low side effect profile. Their major disadvantage is the possibility of withdrawal or rebound symptoms on discontinuation of treatment.

Some medications have been studied and proved no more effective than placebo. These include β-blockers such as propranolol and atenolol.

Psychosocial Treatments

The development of cognitive-behavioral treatment that is effective for the treatment of panic disorder has been called one of the major psychotherapy achievements of the century. This treatment centers on breaking the link between fear and somatic sensations, which is accomplished through 1) teaching slow abdominal breathing to correct any hyperventilation and lower the occurrence of the sensations, 2) teaching cognitive strategies to identify the origin of the sensations and to reduce the catastrophic meaning of the sensations, and 3) employing exposure to the feared sensations as a technique to decondition any automatic reaction and to allow practice of cognitive techniques. This treatment usually requires about 12 sessions and has been found to provide full panic relief in the majority of patients. A summary of strategies used in cognitive-behavioral treatment is presented in the discussion of cognitive and behavioral therapies in Chapter 46.

Although comorbidity with psychiatric and medical illness is common in patients with panic disorder, there is no evidence that patients with comorbidity respond differently to the standard treatments. Similarly, there appear to be no sex differences in response to treatment. Children may be less responsive to pharmacotherapy, although relatively few studies have been performed to date. Elderly patients require lower doses of medication but otherwise appear responsive to standard antipanic treatment. There appear to be no differences in response rates of different racial groups to panic disorder treatment, but this has not been well studied.

Social and Specific Phobias

Phobias are the most common of the anxiety disorders and among the most common of all mental disorders. However, despite the frequency with which phobias occur in the general population, they have tended to be relatively ignored by physicians and researchers. One of these, social phobia, is widespread and associated with significant functional impairment. Individuals with social phobia experience impairment in their work, home, and social relationships. Also, social phobia often presents comorbidly with other mental disorders.

With respect to specific phobias, the lack of attention is probably due to several factors. Few individuals with specific phobias present for treatment, and those who do seek help tend to differ from untreated individuals with phobias in respect to the number and types of specific phobias. As with social phobia, there has been an increase in attention paid to specific phobias, along with increased recognition that these phobias can interfere seriously with an individual's ability to function.

In the *Diagnostic and Statistical Manual of Mental Disorders, Fourth Edition* (DSM-IV), social phobia is defined as a "marked and persistent fear of one or more social or performance situations in which the person is exposed to unfamiliar people or to possible scrutiny of others." Typical situations feared by individuals with social phobia include meeting new people, interacting with others, attending parties or meetings, speaking formally, eating or writing in front of others, dealing with people in authority, and being assertive. Specific phobia is defined as a "marked and persistent fear that is excessive or unreasonable, cued by the presence or anticipation of a specific object or situation (e.g., flying, heights, animals, receiving an injection, seeing blood)."

EPIDEMIOLOGY

As discussed earlier, phobias are among the most common psychiatric disorders. Findings based on large community samples from five sites in the Epidemiological Catchment Area (ECA) Study yielded lifetime prevalence estimates of 11.25% for specific phobias and 2.73% for social phobia.

Most studies have found the mean age at onset of social phobia to be in the middle to late teens. Mean age at onset for specific phobias appears to differ depending on the type of phobia. Phobias of animals, blood, storms, and water tend to begin in early childhood, whereas phobias of heights tend to begin in the teens, and phobias of the situational type (e.g., claustrophobia) begin even later, with mean ages at onset in the late teens to middle 20s.

Having a phobia of one specific phobia type makes an individual more likely to have additional phobias of the same type than of other types. However, the clustering is not perfect; many studies show exceptions to this pattern. In addition, specific phobias often co-occur with other DSM-IV disorders. However, compared with individuals who have other anxiety disorders, an individual with a principal diagnosis of a specific phobia is less likely to have additional diagnoses.

Social anxiety is a feature of many disorders. Individuals with panic disorder, obsessive-compulsive disorder, or eating disorders often avoid social situations because of the possibility of being judged negatively if their symptoms are noticed by others. However, to meet diagnostic criteria for social phobia, one's concerns must not be exclusively related to the symptoms of another disorder.

As an additional diagnosis, social phobia is often assigned in patients with panic disorder along with agoraphobia, generalized anxiety disorder, obsessive-compulsive disorder, and major depressive disorder. Other studies have found social phobia to be common among patients with eating disorders and alcohol abuse as well. When social phobia coexists with a mood disorder, substance abuse disorder, or another anxiety disorder, the social phobia tends to predate the other disorder.

DIAGNOSIS

DSM-IV Criteria 300.295

Specific Phobia

A. Marked and persistent fear that is excessive or unreasonable, cued by the presence or anticipation of a specific object or situation (e.g., flying, heights, animals, receiving an injection, seeing blood).

B. Exposure to the phobic stimulus almost invariably provokes an immediate anxiety response, which may take the form of a situationally bound or situationally predisposed panic attack. **Note:** In children, the anxiety may be expressed by crying, tantrums, freezing, or clinging.

C. The person recognizes that the fear is excessive or unreasonable. **Note:** In children, this feature may be absent.

D. The phobic situation(s) is avoided or else is endured with intense anxiety or distress.

E. The avoidance, anxious anticipation, or distress in the feared situation(s) interferes significantly with the person's normal routine, occupational (or academic) functioning, or social activities or relationships, or there is marked distress about having the phobia.

F. In individuals under age 18 years, the duration is at least 6 months.

G. The anxiety, panic attacks, and phobic avoidance associated with the specific object or situation are not better accounted for by another mental disorder, such as obsessive-compulsive disorder (e.g., fear of dirt in someone with an obsession about contamination), posttraumatic stress disorder (e.g., avoidance of stimuli associated with a severe stressor), separation anxiety disorder (e.g., avoidance of school), social phobia (e.g., avoidance of social situations because of fear of embarrassment), panic disorder with agoraphobia, or agoraphobia without history of panic disorder.

Specify type:

Animal type

Natural environment type (e.g., heights, storms, water)

Blood-injection-injury type

Situational type (e.g., airplanes, elevators, enclosed places)

Other type (e.g., phobic avoidance of situations that may lead to choking, vomiting, or contracting an illness; in children, avoidance of loud sounds or costumed characters)

DSM-IV Criteria 300.235

Social Phobia

A. A marked and persistent fear of one or more social or performance situations in which the person is exposed to unfamiliar people or to possible scrutiny by others. The individual fears that he or she will act in a way (or show anxiety symptoms) that will be humiliating or embarrassing. **Note:** In children, there must be evidence of the capacity for age-appropriate social relationships with familiar people and the anxiety must occur in peer settings, not just in interactions with adults.

Box continued on following page

Social Phobia *Continued*

B. Exposure to the feared social situation almost invariably provokes anxiety, which may take the form of a situationally bound or situationally predisposed panic attack. **Note:** In children, the anxiety may be expressed by crying, tantrums, freezing, or shrinking away from social situations with unfamiliar people.

C. The person recognizes that the fear is excessive or unreasonable. **Note:** In children, this feature may be absent.

D. The feared social or performance situations are avoided or else are endured with intense anxiety or distress.

E. The avoidance, anxious anticipation, or distress in the feared social or performance situation(s) interferes significantly with the person's normal routine, occupational (or academic) functioning, or social activities or relationships, or there is marked distress about having the phobia.

F. In individuals under age 18 years, the duration is at least 6 months.

G. The fear or avoidance is not due to the direct physiological effects of a substance (e.g., a drug of abuse, a medication) or a general medical condition and is not better accounted for by another mental disorder (e.g., panic disorder with or without agoraphobia, separation anxiety disorder, body dysmorphic disorder, a pervasive developmental disorder, or schizoid personality disorder).

H. If a general medical condition or another mental disorder is present, the fear in criterion A is unrelated to it, e.g., the fear is not of stuttering, trembling in Parkinson's disease, exhibiting abnormal eating behavior in anorexia nervosa or bulimia nervosa.

Specify if:

Generalized: if the fears include most social situations (also consider the additional diagnosis of avoidant personality disorder)

Assessment

SPECIAL ISSUES IN PSYCHIATRIC EXAMINATION AND HISTORY

During all parts of the initial evaluation, the psychiatrist should be sensitive to several issues. First, for many patients with phobias, even discussing the phobic object can provoke anxiety. For example, some patients with spider phobias experience panic attacks when they discuss spiders. Certain patients with blood phobias faint when they discuss surgical procedures. Therefore, the psychiatrist should ask the patient whether discussing the phobic object or situation will provoke anxiety.

With respect to social phobia, the assessment itself may be considered a phobic stimulus. Because individuals with social phobia fear the evaluation of others, a psychiatric interview might be especially frightening. Even completing self-report questionnaires in the waiting room may be difficult for patients who fear writing in front of others. The psychiatrist should be sensitive to this possibility and provide reassurance when appropriate.

Behavioral testing is an important part of any comprehensive evaluation for a phobic disorder. Because most individuals with phobias avoid the objects and situations they fear, patients may find it difficult to describe the subtle cues that affect their fear in the situation. In addition, it is not unusual for patients to misjudge the amount of fear that they typically experience in the phobic situation. A behavioral approach test can be useful for identifying specific fear triggers as well as for assessing the intensity of the patient's fear in the actual situation.

To conduct a behavioral approach test, patients should be instructed to enter the phobic situation for several minutes and note the specific cues that affect the fear and the intensity of the fear. Patients should pay special attention to their physical sensations (e.g., palpitations, sweating, blushing), negative thoughts (e.g., I will fall from this balcony), and anxious coping strategies (e.g., escape, avoidance, distraction).

Before treatment, patients will often be reluctant to enter the feared situation. If this is the case, the information collected during the behavioral approach test may be elicited during the early part of behavioral treatment.

DEVELOPMENTAL ISSUES. Several studies have begun to look at the prevalence of phobias across the life span. Little is known about the prevalence of phobias among elderly persons, although there is some evidence that the prevalence of phobic disorders may decrease slightly after age 65 years.

Among children, specific and social fears are common. Because these fears may be transient, DSM-IV has included a provision that social and specific phobias not be assigned in children unless they are present for more than 6 months. Furthermore, children may be less likely than adults to recognize that their phobia is excessive or unrealistic. The specific objects feared by children are often similar to those feared by adults, although children may be more likely to fear objects and situations that are not easily classified by the four main specific phobia types in DSM-IV. In addition, children often report specific and social phobias having to do with school. Children with social phobia tend to avoid changing for gymnastics class in front of others, eating in the cafeteria, or speaking in front of the class. They may stay home sick on days when frightening situations arise or may make frequent trips to the school nurse. Whereas some investigators have found that boys and girls are equally likely to present for treatment of phobias, others have found social phobia to be more common among girls than boys.

Other diagnoses that should be considered before a diagnosis of specific phobia is assigned include posttraumatic stress disorder (if the fear follows a life-threatening trauma and is accompanied by the appropriate symptoms, such as reexperiencing the trauma), obsessive-compulsive disorder (if the fear is related to an obsession such as contamination), hypochondriasis (if the patient believes he or she has some serious illness), separation anxiety disorder (if the fear is of situations that might lead to separation from the family, such as traveling on an airplane without one's parents), eating disorders (if the fear is of eating certain foods but not related to a fear of choking), and psychotic disorders (if the fear is related to a delusion).

Social phobia should not be diagnosed if the fear is related to another disorder. For example, if an individual with obsessive-compulsive disorder avoids social situations only to avert the embarrassment of having others notice her or his excessive hand washing, a diagnosis of social phobia would not be given. Furthermore, individuals with depression, schizoid personality disorder, or a pervasive developmental disorder may avoid social situations because they lack interest in spending time with others. In the case of generalized social phobia, the diagnosis of avoidant personality disorder should be considered as well.

Finally, social and specific phobias should be distinguished from normal states of fear and anxiety.

Diagnostic decision trees for social and specific phobias are presented in Figures 29–1 and 29–2.

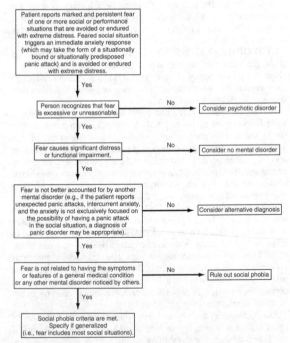

Figure 29–1 *Social phobia: diagnostic decision tree.*

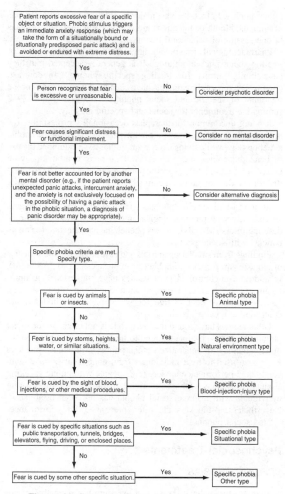

Figure 29–2 *Specific phobia: diagnostic decision tree.*

STANDARD APPROACHES TO TREATMENT

The main goal of treatment is to decrease fear and phobic avoidance to a level that no longer causes significant distress or functional impairment. In some cases, treatment includes strategies for improving specific skill deficits as well. For example, individuals with social phobia may lack adequate social skills and could benefit from social skills training.

Typically, effective treatment for social phobia lasts several months, although treatment of discrete social phobias (e.g., public speaking) may take less time. Specific phobias can usually be treated rather quickly. In fact, the vast majority of individuals with phobias of animals, blood, or injections are able to overcome their phobias in one session of behavioral treatment.

Pharmacological treatments have been used effectively for treating social phobia, although it is generally accepted that they have limited utility for treating specific phobias. In contrast, cognitive-behavioral treatments have been used with success for the treatment of specific and social phobias. Tables 29–1 and 29–2 summarize treatments for social and specific phobias.

It is not uncommon for therapists occasionally to prescribe low dosages of benzodiazepines for phobic patients to take in the phobic situation (e.g., while flying). Relevant studies have examined the use of benzodiazepines and β-blockers alone or in combination with behavioral treatments for specific phobias and in general have found that drugs do not contribute much to the treatment of specific phobias.

In contrast to specific phobias, social phobia has been treated successfully with pharmacological interventions. Monoamine oxidase inhibitors (MAOIs) such as phenelzine are effective for many patients with social phobia.

Findings from smaller open trials and case studies support the use of clonazepam for social phobia (mean dosages, 2.1 to 2.75 mg/d). In addition, uncontrolled pilot studies have suggested that alprazolam (mean dosage, 2.9 mg/d) and fluoxetine (mean dosage, 53.6 mg/d) may be effective for social phobia, although more controlled clinical trials are needed.

Other studies have found that buspirone is not effective for social phobia. Similarly, β-blockers tend to be no better than placebo for most patients with generalized social phobia. Although β-blockers have been used to treat individuals from nonpatient samples with heightened performance anxiety (e.g., people with public speaking anxiety, musicians with stage fright), their efficacy for treating individuals with discrete social phobia has not been established. Nevertheless, β-blockers are often prescribed for performance-related social phobia.

Psychosocial Treatments

SPECIFIC PHOBIAS

Numerous studies have shown that exposure-based treatments are effective for helping patients to overcome a variety of specific phobias including fears of blood, injections, dentists, animals, enclosed places, flying, heights, and choking. Furthermore, the way in which exposure is conducted may make a difference.

The following generalizations about exposure-based treatments should be considered: 1) Exposure seems to work best when sessions are spaced close together. 2) Prolonged exposure seems to be more effective than exposure of shorter duration. 3) During exposure sessions, patients should be discouraged from engaging in subtle avoidance strategies (e.g., distraction) and overreliance on safety signals (e.g., being accompanied during exposure). 4) Real-life exposure is more effective than exposure in imagination. 5) Some degree of therapist involvement seems to be more effective than exposure conducted exclusively without the therapist present. 6) In

TABLE 29–1 Treatments for Social Phobia

Treatment	Advantages	Disadvantages	Rating
Cognitive-behavioral therapy (e.g., exposure, cognitive restructuring, social skills training, education)	Good treatment response Brief course of treatment Treatment gains maintained at follow-up	May lead to temporary increases in discomfort or fear; therefore, patient must be highly motivated.	++++
MAOIs (e.g., phenelzine)	Good treatment response Early response	Side effects are common. Dietary restrictions must be followed. Potential exists for relapse after discontinuation.	+++
Moclobemide	Good treatment response (although slightly less than that for phenelzine) Fewer side effects than for phenelzine	Occasional side effects occur. More research is needed. Potential exists for relapse after discontinuation.	+++
Benzodiazepines (e.g., clonazepam, alprazolam)	Possibly beneficial	More controlled trials are needed. Side effects occur. Relapse after discontinuation is likely.	++
β-Blockers (e.g., atenolol)	Often used for performance anxiety	Drugs are not effective for generalized social phobia. Benefits for discrete social phobias are questionable. Side effects occur. Potential exists for relapse after discontinuation.	+

++++ First treatment of choice. Helpful for most patients, with few side effects. Good long-term benefits.
+++ Helpful for most patients. Potential for relapse after treatment is discontinued.
++ More controlled research needed, although preliminary studies suggest potential benefit.
+ Not especially effective for generalized social phobia.

TABLE 29-2	Treatments for Specific Phobias		
Treatment	Advantages	Disadvantages	Rating
In vivo exposure	Highly effective Early response Treatment gains maintained at follow-up	May lead to temporary increases in discomfort or fear; therefore, patient must be highly motivated.	++++
Applied tension	Highly effective for patients with blood-injection phobias who faint Early response Treatment gains maintained at follow-up	Treatment is relevant for a small percentage of patients with specific phobias.	+++
Applied relaxation	May be effective for some patients	Treatment has not been extensively researched for specific phobias. Treatment is probably not effective alone.	++
Cognitive therapy	May help to reduce anxiety about conducting exposure exercises	Treatment has not been extensively researched for specific phobias.	++
Benzodiazepines	May reduce anticipatory anxiety before patient enters phobic situation	Treatment has not been extensively researched for specific phobias. Treatment is probably not effective alone. Side effects (e.g., sedation) occur. Discontinuation of symptoms may undermine benefits of treatment.	++

++++ Treatment of choice. Effective for almost all patients.
+++ Very effective for a subset of patients.
++ May be helpful for some patients. More research needed.

the case of blood and injection phobias, the technique called applied muscle tension should be considered as an alternative or addition to exposure therapy. Applied muscle tension involves having patients repeatedly tense their muscles, which leads to a temporary increase in blood pressure and prevents fainting on exposure to blood or medical procedures.

Specific phobias are among the most treatable of the anxiety disorders. For example, in just one session of guided exposure, 90% of individuals with animal or injection phobias are judged much improved or completely recovered.

SOCIAL PHOBIA

Empirically validated psychosocial interventions for social phobia have come primarily from a cognitive-behavioral perspective and include four main types of treatment: 1) social skills training, 2) applied relaxation, 3) cognitive therapy, and 4) exposure-based strategies. Social skills training is designed to help patients become more socially competent when they interact with others. Treatment strategies may include modeling, behavioral rehearsal, corrective feedback, social reinforcement, and homework assignments. Applied relaxation involves learning to relax one's muscles during rest, during movement, and eventually in anxiety-provoking social situations. Cognitive therapy helps patients identify and change anxious thoughts (e.g., others will think I am stupid if I participate in a conversation at work) by teaching them to consider alternative ways of interpreting situations and to examine the evidence for their anxious beliefs. Finally, exposure-based treatments involve repeatedly approaching anxiety-provoking situations until they no longer elicit anxiety. Through repeated exposure, patients learn that their fearful predictions do not come true despite their having confronted the situation.

It seems clear that effective psychosocial treatments and medications for social phobia exist. Although both types of treatments appear to be equally effective, each has advantages and disadvantages. Medication treatments may work more quickly and are less time intensive for the patient and therapist. In contrast, improvement after cognitive-behavioral treatments appears to last longer. Furthermore, because of the side effects and dietary restrictions associated with phenelzine, cognitive-behavioral interventions may be more appropriate for some individuals. More studies are needed to examine the efficacy of combined medication and psychosocial treatments for social phobia.

Obsessive-Compulsive Disorder

Obsessive-compulsive disorder (OCD) is an intriguing and often debilitating syndrome characterized by the presence of two distinct phenomena: obsessions and compulsions. Obsessions are intrusive, recurrent, unwanted ideas, thoughts, or impulses that are difficult to dismiss despite their disturbing nature. Compulsions are repetitive behaviors, either observable or mental, intended to reduce the anxiety engendered by obsessions. Both obsessions and compulsions have been described in a wide variety of psychiatric and neurological disorders. However, obsessions and compulsions that clearly interfere with functioning and/or cause significant distress are the hallmark of OCD.

DSM-IV Criteria 300.3

Obsessive-Compulsive Disorder

A. Either obsessions or compulsions:

Obsessions as defined by (1), (2), (3), and (4):

  (1) recurrent and persistent thoughts, impulses, or images that are experienced, at some time during the disturbance, as intrusive and inappropriate and that cause marked anxiety or distress

  (2) the thoughts, impulses, or images are not simply excessive worries about real-life problems

  (3) the person attempts to ignore or suppress such thoughts, impulses, or images, or to neutralize them with some other thought or action

  (4) the person recognizes that the obsessional thoughts, impulses, or images are a product of his or her own mind (not imposed from without as in thought insertion)

Compulsions as defined by (1) and (2):

  (1) repetitive behaviors (e.g., hand washing, ordering, checking) or mental acts (e.g., praying, counting, repeating words silently) that the person feels driven to perform in response to an obsession, or according to rules that must be applied rigidly

    (2) the behaviors or mental acts are aimed at preventing or reducing distress or preventing some dreaded event or situation; however, these behaviors or mental acts either are not connected in a realistic way with what they are designed to neutralize or prevent or are clearly excessive

B. At some point during the course of the disorder, the person has recognized that the obsessions or compulsions are excessive or unreasonable. Note: This does not apply to children.

C. The obsessions or compulsions cause marked distress, are time consuming (take more than 1 hour a day), or significantly interfere with the person's normal routine, occupational (or academic) functioning, or usual social activities or relationships.

D. If another Axis I disorder is present, the content of the obsessions or compulsions is not restricted to it (e.g., preoccupation with food in the presence of an eating disorder; hair pulling in the presence of trichotillomania; concern with appearance in the presence of body dysmorphic disorder; preoccupation with drugs in the presence of a substance use disorder; preoccupation with having a serious illness in the presence of hypochondriasis; preoccupation with sexual urges or fantasies in the presence of a paraphilia; or guilty ruminations in the presence of major depressive disorder).

E. The disturbance is not due to the direct physiological effects of a substance (e.g., a drug of abuse, a medication) or a general medical condition.

Specify if:

With poor insight: if, for most of the time during the current episode, the person does not recognize that the obsessions and compulsions are excessive or unreasonable.

EPIDEMIOLOGY AND DEMOGRAPHIC FEATURES

In the National Epidemiological Catchment Area study, OCD was found to be the fourth most common psychiatric disorder (after the phobias, substance use disorders, and major depressive disorder), with a prevalence of 1.6% at 6 months and a lifetime prevalence of 2.5%.

Women appear to develop OCD slightly more frequently than do men. A predominance of males has been observed, however, in child and adolescent OCD populations. This finding may be due to the fact that males develop OCD at a younger age than do females. Genetic data show a significantly higher frequency of OCD in relatives of patients who manifest OCD before age 14 years, suggesting that in addition to gender distribution, there are differences between pediatric OCD and adult OCD.

COURSE AND NATURAL HISTORY

The mean age at onset of OCD is 19.8 ± 9.6 years. As noted previously, the age of male patients at onset of OCD is significantly earlier than that of female patients (17.5 ± 8.7 versus 21.2 ± 9.8 years). Eighty-three percent of patients with OCD experience the onset of significant symptoms between the ages of 10 and 24 years, whereas less than 15% experience onset of the disorder after the age of 35 years.

A further descriptive study shows that the course of OCD is usually waxing and waning—that is, once a patient acquires OCD, then obsessions or compulsions, or both, are present continuously, with varying degrees of intensity over time. Relatively few patients described either a progressively deteriorating course or a truly episodic course. Such a course has been found to occur even with adequate treatment.

PHENOMENOLOGY

The clinical presentation of OCD is characterized by phenomenological subtypes based on the content of the obsessions and corresponding compulsions. The list of subtypes in the Yale-Brown Obsessive-Compulsive Scale (YBOCS) was generated on the basis of clinical interviews with OCD subjects in the 1980s.

The most common obsession is fear of contamination, followed by pathological doubt, a need for symmetry, and aggressive obsessions. The most common compulsion is checking, which is followed by washing, symmetry, the need to ask or confess, and counting. Children with OCD present most commonly with washing compulsions, which are followed by repeating rituals.

Most patients have multiple obsessions and compulsions over time, with a particular fear or concern dominating the clinical picture at any one time. The presence of pure obsessions without compulsions is unusual. Patients who appear to have obsessions alone frequently have reassurance rituals or unrecognized mental compulsions, such as repetitive, ritualized praying, in addition to their obsessions. Pure compulsions are also unusual in adult patients but do occur in children with OCD, especially in the young (e.g., those 6 to 8 years of age).

INSIGHT

An awareness of the senselessness or unreasonableness of obsessions (often referred to as insight) and the accompanying struggle against the obsessions (referred to as resistance) have generally been accepted as fundamental to the diagnosis of OCD. However, numerous descriptions of OCD patients who are completely convinced of the reasonableness of their obsessions and need to perform compulsions have appeared in the psychiatric literature during the 20th century.

Patients with OCD do not always maintain good insight but rather have it in varying degrees. Although patients may be aware that their obsessions are senseless and unreasonable, in that they are excessively preoccupied, they may have little insight into the fact that the belief underlying their obsession (e.g., that they will get cancer from stepping on a chemically treated lawn) is senseless, unreasonable, and unrealistic. The *Diagnostic and Statistical Manual of Mental Disorders,* Fourth Edition (DSM-IV) acknowledges that the beliefs underlying OCD obsessions can be delusional and notes that in such cases an additional diagnosis of delusional disorder or psychotic disorder not otherwise specified may be appropriate.

COMORBIDITY

Obsessions and compulsions frequently occur in association with other Axis I disorders. In a study of 100 patients with primary OCD, 67% had a lifetime history of major depression, and 31% met criteria for current major depressive disorder.

The frequency of Tourette's disorder in patients with OCD is higher than in the general population, with a rate of approximately 7%. Conversely, patients with Tourette's disorder have a high rate of comorbid OCD and symptoms of OCD, with 30% to 40% reporting obsessive-compulsive symptoms. Other anxiety disorders frequently coexist with OCD, with relatively high lifetime rates of social phobia (18%), panic disorder (12%), and specific phobia (22%) reported in patients with OCD.

The coexistence of OCD and psychotic disorders has also been investigated. It appears important to differentiate OCD plus a comorbid psychotic disorder, which may have a relatively poor outcome, from delusional OCD, which may be more similar to OCD with insight and without comorbid psychosis.

DIFFERENTIAL DIAGNOSIS

OCD is sometimes difficult to distinguish from a number of other disorders. Obsessions and compulsions may appear in the context of other syndromes, which can lead to the question of whether the obsessions and compulsions are a symptom of another disorder or whether both OCD and another disorder are present. A general guideline is that if the content of the obsessions is not limited to the focused concern of another disorder (e.g., an appearance concern, as in body dysmorphic disorder, or food concerns, as in an eating disorder) and if the obsessions or compulsions are preoccupying as well as distressing or impairing, OCD should generally be diagnosed.

Obsessive-Compulsive Disorder Versus Obsessive-Compulsive Personality Disorder

Obsessive-compulsive personality disorder (OCPD) is defined as a lifelong maladaptive personality style characterized by perfectionism, overattention to detail, indecisiveness, rigidity, excessive devotion to work, restricted affect, lack of generosity, and hoarding. OCD and OCPD have historically been considered variants of the same disorder on a continuum of severity, with OCD being viewed as the more severe manifestation of illness. Contrary to this notion, studies using structured interviews to establish diagnosis have found that patients with OCD do not all have OCPD as well.

Unlike OCPD, OCD is characterized by distressing, time-consuming ego-dystonic obsessions and repetitive rituals aimed at diminishing the distress engendered by obsessional thinking. One hallmark that has traditionally been used to distinguish OCD from OCPD is that OCPD features are considered ego-syntonic. Age at onset may also be useful; OCD onset is typically in adolescence, although symptoms may begin earlier, whereas OCPD is lifelong. Although useful, these guidelines are not absolute, and some patients defy easy categorization.

Obsessive-Compulsive Disorder Spectrum Disorders

A number of disorders may be difficult to differentiate from OCD. Indeed, certain disorders other than OCD—such as body dysmorphic disorder, hypochondriasis, Tourette's disorder, and eating disorders—are characterized by obsessional thinking and/or ritualistic behaviors. On the basis of these apparent similarities, the concept of OCD spectrum disorders has been developed. OCD spectrum disorders have been defined as disorders that share features with OCD. These domains include not only symptoms but also treatment response, comorbidity, joint familial loading, sex ratio, age at onset, course, premorbid personality characteristics, and presumed cause.

TREATMENT

Both pharmacological and behavioral therapies have proved effective in the treatment of OCD. A flow chart that outlines treatment options for OCD is shown in Figure 30–1.

In general, the goals of treatment are to reduce both the frequency and intensity of symptoms as much as possible and to minimize the amount of interference the symptoms cause in the patient's life. It is of note that few patients experience a cure or complete remission of symptoms. Instead, OCD should be viewed as a chronic illness with a waxing and waning course. Symptoms are often worse during times of psychosocial stress. Individuals who suffer from OCD are often upset when they experience even a mild symptom exacerbation, expecting that their symptoms will revert to their worst, which is rarely if ever the case. Anticipating with the patient that stress will make the symptoms worse can often be helpful in the long-term treatment of these patients.

Pharmacological Treatments

The most extensively studied agents for the treatment of OCD are medications that affect the serotonin system. Many studies implicate the serotonin system in the pathophysiology of OCD, although

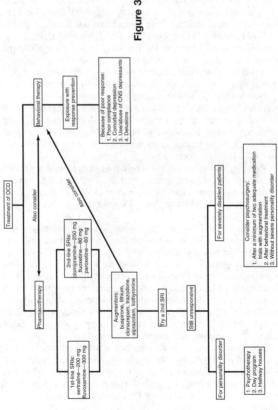

Figure 30–1 *Flow chart of treatment options for OCD.*

Treatment of OCD

Also consider

Pharmacotherapy

Behavioral therapy

Also consider

Exposure with response prevention

Because of poor response:
1. Poor compliance
2. Comorbid depression
3. Use/abuse of CNS depressants
4. Delusions

1st-line SRIs:
sertraline—200 mg
fluvoxamine—300 mg

2nd-line SRIs:
clomipramine—250 mg
fluoxetine—80 mg
paroxetine—60 mg

Augmentors:
buspirone, lithium,
clonazepam, trazodone,
alprazolam, liothyronine

Try a 2nd SRI

Still unresponsive

For personality disorder

1. Psychotherapy
2. Day program
3. Halfway houses

For severely disabled patients

Consider psychosurgery:
1. After a minimum of two adequate medication
   trials with augmentation
2. After behavioral treatment
3. Without severe personality disorder

317

comparative studies also seem to implicate other neurotransmitter systems, including the dopaminergic system, in treatment response. The principal pharmacological agents used to treat OCD are the selective serotonin reuptake inhibitors (SSRIs), which include clomipramine, fluoxetine, fluvoxamine, sertraline, and paroxetine.

The most extensively studied pharmacological agent in OCD is the tricyclic antidepressant clomipramine. This drug is unique among the antiobsessional agents in that in addition to its potency as an SSRI, it has significant affinity for dopaminergic, muscarinic, histaminic, and noradrenergic receptors.

Despite their different chemical structures, the SSRIs fluoxetine, fluvoxamine, sertraline, and paroxetine appear to be similar in their ability to treat OCD.

Behavioral Therapy

A growing body of data on the efficacy of behavioral therapy in OCD has emerged. This form of therapy is based on the principle of exposure and response prevention. The patient is asked to endure, in a graduated manner, the anxiety that a specific obsessional fear provokes while refraining from compulsions that allay that anxiety.

The principles behind the efficacy of behavioral treatment are explained to the patient in the following way. Although compulsions, either covert or overt, usually relieve anxiety immediately, this is only a short-term solution; the anxiety will ultimately return, requiring the performance of another compulsion. However, if the patient resists the anxiety and urge to ritualize, the anxiety will eventually decrease on its own (i.e., habituation will occur), and the need to perform the ritual will eventually disappear. Thus, rather than perpetuating a vicious circle of more obsessions and compulsions, behavioral therapy helps the patient habituate to the anxiety and extinguish the compulsions.

Compulsions, especially overt behaviors such as washing rituals, are more successfully treated by behavioral therapy than are obsessions or covert rituals such as mental checking. This is because covert rituals are harder to physically resist than are hand washing and checking a door.

For rituals that do not constitute overt behaviors, techniques other than exposure and response prevention have been used, although with less success. These approaches include imaginal flooding and thought stopping. In imaginal flooding, the anxiety provoked by the obsessions is evoked by continually repeating the thought, often with the help of a continuous-loop tape, until the thought no longer provokes anxiety. In thought stopping, an obsessional thought (e.g., continually repeating a short prayer in one's head) is stopped by simply shouting, making a loud noise, or snapping a rubber band on the wrist in an attempt to interrupt the thought.

Behavioral therapy can be used as the sole treatment of OCD, particularly in patients whose contamination fears or somatic obsessions make them resistant to taking medications. Behavioral treatment is also a powerful adjunct to pharmacotherapy. Some work appears to indicate that combined treatment may be more effective than pharmacotherapy or behavioral therapy alone, although these findings are still preliminary. From a clinical perspective, it may be useful to have patients begin treatment with medication to reduce the intensity of their symptoms; then they may be more amenable to experiencing the anxiety that will be evoked by the behavioral challenges they perform.

Psychoanalytic Psychotherapy

The use of psychotherapeutic techniques of either a psychoanalytic or a supportive nature have not proved successful in treating the specific obsessions and compulsions that are a hallmark of the Axis I disorder of OCD. However, the more characterological aspects that are part of the obsessive-compulsive personality may be helped by a more psychoanalytically oriented approach.

The initial phase of treatment is often the most difficult for the patient with OCD. This has to do with both risk aversion and a need to be in control. With pharmacological treatment, patients may occasionally experience a worsening of symptoms in addition to side effects. This can be terrifying to the patient and can lead to an abrupt discontinuation of the medication. Warning the patient before treatment that this might occur increases the patient's sense of control. Similarly, the antiobsessional effects of treatment often take 6 to 10 weeks to be seen and are often gradual in onset. This gradual response is usually delayed until after the patient experiences side effects. Thus, the early middle phase of treatment is frequently taken up with encouraging the patient to stay on medication despite side effects and no improvement. Side effects can often be framed as a good sign that the medication is being actively absorbed by the body. Again, preparing patients in advance allows them to feel in control and able to continue treatment. The gradual onset of improvement, although in some cases frustrating, is also reassuring to patients who might feel out of control if improvement occurred too rapidly.

Most patients with OCD do not have full recovery from their symptoms. Although the majority of patients, perhaps as many as 85%, experience some improvement in their symptoms, most tend to remain symptomatic to some degree. Nonetheless, improvement of symptoms of even 10% to 15% can have a dramatic effect on their lives.

Traumatic Stress Disorders

POSTTRAUMATIC STRESS DISORDER

DSM-IV Criteria 309.81

Posttraumatic Stress Disorder

A. The person has been exposed to a traumatic event in which both of the following were present:

  (1) the person experienced, witnessed, or was confronted with an event or events that involved actual or threatened death or serious injury, or a threat to the physical integrity of self or others

  (2) the person's response involved intense fear, helplessness, or horror. **Note:** In children, this may be expressed instead by disorganized or agitated behavior.

B. The traumatic event is persistently reexperienced in one (or more) of the following ways:

  (1) recurrent and intrusive distressing recollections of the event, including images, thoughts, or perceptions. **Note:** In young children, repetitive play may occur in which themes or aspects of the trauma are expressed.

  (2) recurrent distressing dreams of the event. **Note:** In children, there may be frightening dreams without recognizable content.

  (3) acting or feeling as if the traumatic event were recurring (includes a sense of reliving the experience, illusions, hallucinations, and dissociative flashback episodes, including those that occur on awakening or when intoxicated). **Note:** In young children, trauma-specific reenactment may occur.

  (4) intense psychological distress at exposure to internal or external cues that symbolize or resemble an aspect of the traumatic event

  (5) physiological reactivity on exposure to internal or external cues that symbolize or resemble an aspect of the traumatic event

C. Persistent avoidance of stimuli associated with the trauma and numbing of general responsiveness (not present before the trauma), as indicated by three (or more) of the following:

(1) efforts to avoid thoughts, feelings, or conversations associated with the trauma

(2) efforts to avoid activities, places, or people that arouse recollections of the trauma

(3) inability to recall an important aspect of the trauma

(4) markedly diminished interest or participation in significant activities

(5) feeling of detachment or estrangement from others

(6) restricted range of affect (e.g., unable to have loving feelings)

(7) sense of a foreshortened future (e.g., does not expect to have a career, marriage, children, or a normal life span)

D. Persistent symptoms of increased arousal (not present before the trauma), as indicated by two (or more) of the following:

(1) difficulty falling or staying asleep

(2) irritability or outbursts of anger

(3) difficulty concentrating

(4) hypervigilance

(5) exaggerated startle response

E. Duration of the disturbance (symptoms in criteria B, C, and D) is more than 1 month.

F. The disturbance causes clinically significant distress or impairment in social, occupational, or other important areas of functioning.

Specify:

Acute: if duration of symptoms is less than 3 months

Chronic: if duration of symptoms is 3 months or more

Specify if:

With delayed onset: if onset of symptoms is at least 6 months after the stressor

Community-based studies yield lifetime posttraumatic stress disorder (PTSD) prevalence rates ranging from 1% to 19%. Prevalence rates for at-risk populations (i.e., Vietnam veterans, rape victims, schoolchildren exposed to sniper attacks, and Armenian children after an earthquake) range from 14% to 75%. The wide range of prevalence rates reflects in part the variety of measurements that have been used to diagnose PTSD.

Epidemiological studies show that PTSD often remains chronic, with a significant number of people still symptomatic several years after the initial event. In support of this view are epidemiological data showing that recovery frequently does not occur. For example, the National Vietnam Veterans Readjustment study found lifetime and current prevalence rates of PTSD to be, respectively, 30.9% and 15.2% in men and 26.9% and 8.5% in women. In a population of rape victims, Kilpatrick and colleagues (1987) found a lifetime prevalence rate of 75.8% and a current prevalence rate of 39.4%.

DIAGNOSIS

The diagnosis of PTSD is based on a history of exposure to a traumatic stressor, the simultaneous appearance of three different symptom clusters, a minimal duration, and the existence of functional disturbance. To qualify for a traumatic stress, the event must have involved actual or threatened death or serious injury or a threat to the patient or others, and exposure to this event must arouse an intense affective response characterized by fear, helplessness, or horror. In children, disorganized or agitated behavior can be seen.

With regard to the symptoms as a whole, it is evident that they embody features of different psychiatric disorders, including obsessive-compulsive processes, generalized anxiety disorder, panic attacks, phobic avoidance, dissociation, and depression. An overlap with impulse control disorders could be conjectured in view of the anger and irritable outbursts that occur in PTSD, along with periodical recourse to violence. Symptoms must have lasted at least 1 month, and the disturbance must have caused clinically significant distress or impairment. Therefore, the psychiatrist must use judgment in deciding where to place the threshold when a person complains of PTSD-type symptoms.

DIFFERENTIAL DIAGNOSIS

PTSD symptoms may overlap with symptoms of other disorders, such as depression (e.g., affective constriction with anhedonia).

PTSD may be distinguished from adjustment disorder by assessing whether the traumatic stress meets the criteria described earlier. Also, if an insufficient number of symptoms qualify for the diagnosis, the case might merit a diagnosis of adjustment disorder. As another possibility, simple phobia may arise after traumatic exposure.

Generalized anxiety disorder consists of six symptoms, of which four are common to PTSD: being on edge, poor concentration, irritability, and sleep disturbance. PTSD requires the additional symptoms described in the *Diagnostic and Statistical Manual of Mental Disorders,* Fourth Edition (DSM-IV) and a source of worry different from the worry associated with generalized anxiety.

In obsessive-compulsive disorder, recurring and intrusive thoughts occur, but the patient recognizes these to be inappropriate and unrelated to any particular life experience. Obsessive-compulsive disorder is a common comorbid condition in PTSD and may develop with generalization (e.g., washing after rape to reduce contamination feelings).

Panic disorder is characterized by autonomic hyperarousal as a cardinal part of the panic attack. To distinguish between panic disorder and PTSD, the psychiatrist needs to assess whether panic attacks are related to the trauma or reminders of the same or whether they occur unexpectedly and spontaneously.

Depression and PTSD share a significant overlap, including four of the criterion C cluster symptoms and three of the criterion D cluster symptoms. Thus, an individual who presents with reduced interest, estrangement, numbing, impaired concentration, insomnia, irritability, and sense of a foreshortened future may manifest either disorder. PTSD may give rise to depression as well, and it is possible for the two conditions to coexist.

Dissociative disorders also overlap with PTSD. In the early aftermath of serious trauma, the clinical picture may be predominantly one of the dissociative state (see later section on Acute Stress Disorder [ASD]). ASD differs from PTSD in that the symptom pattern occurs within the first few days, lasts no longer than 4 weeks, and is accompanied by prominent dissociative symptoms.

More rarely, PTSD must be distinguished from other disorders producing perceptual alterations, such as schizophrenia and other psychotic disorders, delirium, substance abuse disorders, and general medical disorders producing psychosis.

Malingering may also be the cause of apparent PTSD. In this situation, it is important to make every effort to obtain corroborative evidence that the trauma did occur, and it may be noted that in PTSD the subject is usually distressed about, and reluctant to discuss, details of the trauma. This is not the case with factitious disorders.

The differential diagnosis is important but, notwithstanding, PTSD is unlikely to occur alone. Psychiatric comorbidity is the rule rather than the exception, and a number of studies have demonstrated that in both clinical and epidemiological populations a wide range of disorders is likely to occur at an increased probability. These include some depression, all of the anxiety disorders, alcohol and substance abuse disorders, somatization disorder, and schizophrenia and schizophreniform disorder.

COURSE AND NATURAL HISTORY

Immediately after severe trauma, a high percentage of individuals develop a mixed symptom picture, which includes disorganized behavior, dissociative symptoms, psychomotor change and, sometimes, paranoia. The newly introduced diagnosis of ASD (see later) accounts for many of these reactions. These reactions are generally short-lived, although by 1 month the symptom picture often settles into a more classic PTSD presentation, such that after rape, for example, as many as 90% of individuals may qualify for the diagnosis of PTSD. Approximately 50% of people with PTSD recover, and approximately 50% develop a persistent, chronic form of the illness still present 1 year later. The same holds true for subclinical states, which are below the diagnostic threshold of PTSD.

The longitudinal course of PTSD is variable. Permanent recovery occurs in some people, whereas others show a relatively unchanging course with only mild fluctuation. Still others show a more obvious fluctuation, with intermittent periods of well-being and recurrences of major symptoms. In a limited number of cases, the passage of time does not bring a resolution of symptoms, and the patient's condition tends to deteriorate with age. Particular symptoms that have been noted to increase with time in many people include startle response, nightmares, irritability, and depression.

OVERALL GOALS OF TREATMENT

General principles of treating PTSD involve explanation and destigmatization, which can be provided both to the patient and to family members. This often includes a description of PTSD symptoms and the way in which the disorder can affect behaviors and relationships. Regaining self-esteem and attaining greater control over impulses and affects are also desired.

PTSD is not always simple to treat. The initial history taking can evoke strong affects, to a greater degree than is customarily found in other disorders. In fact, it may take several interviews for the full details to emerge. This process can be draining to both patient and psychiatrist, and a sensitive yet persistent approach is needed on the part of the interviewer.

Mild and acute cases of PTSD may respond well to supportive psychotherapy and empathic listening, along with the passage of time. The availability of a support system is also crucial.

Pharmacotherapy

PTSD may be accompanied by enduring neurochemical and psychophysiological changes that lead to substantial impairment and distress. Sometimes the intensity of symptoms is severe enough to preclude the effective use of trauma-focused psychotherapy. For these reasons, the use of medication should be stressed and not delayed unnecessarily. At present, the tricyclic antidepressant and monoamine oxidase inhibitor drugs are the most extensively studied; however, the selective serotonin reuptake inhibitors are being used to an increasing extent, and it is only a matter of time before controlled trials are completed and published. Main drug groups relevant to PTSD, along with dose ranges and chief side effects, are listed in Table 31–1. A suggested sequencing of treatment is outlined in Table 31–2.

Often, patients need a combination of drugs, but polypharmacy should be carried out in a carefully planned fashion. Also, the time course of response may be slow, and it is advisable to persist with a particular course of action for at least 8 weeks before deciding that it has not been helpful.

Cognitive-Behavioral Therapy

Despite theoretical differences, most schools of psychotherapy recognize that cognitively oriented approaches to anxiety must

TABLE 31–1 Medications in Posttraumatic Stress Disorder: Dose Ranges and Side Effects

Drug Category	Dose Range (mg/d)	Common or Problematic Side Effects
Antidepressants		
Selective serotonin reuptake inhibitors		Gastrointestinal disturbance, sexual dysfunction, agitation
Fluoxetine	10–60	
Fluvoxamine	50–300	
Sertraline	50–200	Insomnia
Paroxetine	10–60	Tiredness
Tricyclic antidepressants		Anticholinergic effects, cardiovascular symptoms, weight gain, sexual dysfunction, sedation
Amitriptyline	50–300	
Imipramine	50–300	
Monoamine oxidase inhibitors		
Phenelzine	15–90	Weight gain, dizziness, sleep disturbance, sexual dysfunction, hypertensive reactions, hyperpyretic states
Anticonvulsants		
Carbamazepine	200–1500	Hematological effects
Valproic acid	15–60	Gastrointestinal disturbance, sedation
Mood Stabilizers		
Lithium carbonate	300–1200	Gastrointestinal disturbance, polyuria, headache

Table continued on following page

TABLE 31-1 Medications in Posttraumatic Stress Disorder: Dose Ranges and Side Effects *(Continued)*

Drug Category	Dose Range (mg/d)	Common or Problematic Side Effects
		Antiadrenergic drugs
Propranolol	20–160	Depression, hypertension, rebound hypertension
Clonidine	0.1–0.4	Memory problems, dizziness, tiredness
		Anxiolytics
Benzodiazepines		
Clonazepam	0.5–6	Sedation, memory problems, incoordination, dependence, withdrawal, rebound, disinhibition (for all benzodiazepines)
Alprazolam	0.25–4	
Diazepam	2–40	
Chlordiazepoxide	5–40	
Others		
		Azaspirone
Buspirone	5–60	Agitation, gastrointestinal disturbance, headaches
		Neuroleptics
Thioridazine	25–300	Extrapyramidal symptoms
Haloperidol	0.5–4	Sedation, anticholinergic effects
Others		

TABLE 31–2	Pharmacotherapy Steps for Posttraumatic Stress Disorder

Step 1

Selective serotonin reuptake inhibitor (SSRI)
Adjunctive medications:
  If prominent hyperarousal: benzodiazepine or buspirone
  If prominent mood liability or explosiveness: anticonvulsant
    or lithium
  If prominent dissociation: valproic acid
  If persistent insomnia: trazodone

Step 2

If no response or intolerance to SSRI:
  Tricyclic antidepressant
  Adjunctive medications as above

Step 3

If no response to steps 1 or 2:
  Monoamine oxidase inhibitor
  Adjunctive medications as above

Step 4

Other useful drugs:
  Bupropion—intrusive symptoms, numbing
  Propranolol—hyperarousal
  Clonidine—startle response
  Neuroleptics—poor impulse control

include an element of exposure. In dynamic psychotherapy of PTSD, successful abreaction results from "going over and over" the traumatic event, which is probably a form of exposure in fantasy.

In systematic desensitization, which emphasizes anxiety management training, people with PTSD listen to the psychiatrist present the traumatic event while deeply relaxed so that they come to associate traumatic cues with the relaxation response rather than with the symptoms of anxiety. Although some individuals respond to anxiety management strategies, relaxation per se often fails because of the overwhelming anxiety accompanying the presentation of traumatic reminders. Thus, exposure likely constitutes the active ingredient in systematic desensitization, with relaxation an inert component of the treatment picture or, at most, serving to facilitate exposure in vivo.

In contrast to systematic desensitization, prolonged exposure explicitly depends on the fact that anxiety will be extinguished in the absence of real threat, given a sufficient duration of exposure in vivo or in imagination to traumatic stimuli. In PTSD, the patient retells the traumatic experience as if it were happening again, until doing so becomes a pedestrian exercise and anxiety decreases. Between sessions, patients perform exposure homework, including listening to tapes of the flooding sessions and limited exposure in vivo.

Cognitive restructuring combined with exposure and response prevention probably contributes to recovery from both panic disorder and PTSD. Because PTSD involves aberrant and voluntary programs for the avoidance of danger that are conditioned by real experience, correction of these "fear structures" requires not only exposure to ensure habituation but also efforts to challenge and modify deviant beliefs stemming from the traumatic event.

There are several contraindications to exposure-based treatments in PTSD. Major depression attenuates the response to behavioral therapy and should be treated first with drug therapy. Ongoing substance abuse is a contraindication to behavioral psychotherapy in PTSD. Remitted substance abuse is a greater problem, as these persons are clearly at risk for relapse during prolonged exposure; substance abuse may pose a risk during gradual exposure as well. Finally, poor cooperation, especially when due to an intercurrent personality disorder, is a contraindication to intensive behavioral therapy because it reduces compliance and thus efficacy.

Anxiety Management Techniques and Stress Inoculation Training

Anxiety management techniques are designed to reduce anxiety by providing clients with better skills for controlling worry and fear. Among such techniques are muscle relaxation, thought stopping, control of breathing and diaphragmatic breathing, communication skills, guided self-dialogue, and stress inoculation training (SIT).

Psychodynamic Treatment

Psychodynamically based approaches emphasize the interpretation of the traumatic event as being a critical determinant of symptoms. Treatment is geared to alter attributions, usually by means of slow exposure through confrontation and awareness of the negative affects that have been generated by the trauma. Conflictual meanings begin to appear, and it is the task of treatment to reinterpret the experience in a more realistic and adaptive fashion. During such treatment, it is important to ensure that the affect intensity is not overwhelming or disorganizing. Obviously, support needs to be provided throughout, and sometimes other treatment approaches are used adjunctively. Excessive and maladaptive behaviors such as avoidance, use of alcohol or drugs, or risk taking may occur as means of coping with the experience, and these need to be identified and addressed.

SPECIAL FEATURES INFLUENCING TREATMENT

Psychiatric Features

Comorbid depression needs to be treated, as it is likely to interfere with the benefits of behavioral therapy or other psychotherapies.

In fact, in some instances guilt-bound issues may worsen with exposure. A suicidally depressive individual with PTSD needs to be adequately treated before dealing with issues of PTSD, which may in fact worsen suicidality in some instances.

Antisocial and severe borderline personality disorder may be contraindications to various forms of psychotherapy and are unlikely to respond well to pharmacotherapy.

General Medical Comorbidity

Many times patients with PTSD are likely to present with other general medical disorders. For instance, it has been demonstrated that these patients have an increased risk of hypertension, peptic ulcer disease, and bronchial asthma. There is also evidence that chronic pain and PTSD are commonly associated, and in situations in which PTSD has followed serious physical injury (e.g., burns, head injury, or multiple fractures), issues of physical disability not only need to be fully attended to but may affect and limit the impact of treatment for PTSD.

COMMON PROBLEMS IN MANAGEMENT

Much of the material offered by the traumatically stressed patient is charged with affect and, at times, may strain credibility and lead to high levels of doubt. The psychiatrist may fall into the error of not accepting such an emotionally charged experience, thus rejecting or denying its validity. Equally, the psychiatrist may fall into the error of overidentification with the patient such that impartiality is lost. It is important for psychiatrists not to become overinvolved with rescue nor to break down customary psychiatrist-patient boundaries.

Although not unique to PTSD, powerful violent urges may arise during treatment, which may challenge the psychiatrist's feeling of safety. Simple strategies, such as where the patient and psychiatrist sit with respect to proximity of escape, merit attention. Other simple yet important issues calling for attention are whether there is an available alarm if the psychiatrist is dealing regularly with violent or threatening patients.

With respect to the patient, there are times when decompensation occurs to such an extent that the psychiatrist will have to judge whether hospitalization is indicated. Denial of particularly painful issues can lead to avoidance of therapy and missed appointments. Similarly, the emergence of unpleasant or troubling side effects with medication may also lead to treatment discontinuation.

At times, it is helpful to engage the spouse or a significant family member in treatment because of the difficulties and stresses to which he or she may be subjected. Furthermore, he or she can provide information that might help the psychiatrist to acquire a better grasp of the severity of symptoms as well as their effects on the lives of others.

Given that many PTSD patients are receiving more than one treatment, coordination of effort is important.

ACUTE STRESS DISORDER

DSM-IV Criteria 308.3

Acute Stress Disorder

A. The person has been exposed to a traumatic event in which both of the following were present:

  (1) the person experienced, witnessed, or was confronted with an event or events that involved actual or threatened death or serious injury, or a threat to the physical integrity of self or others

  (2) the person's response involved intense fear, helplessness, or horror

B. Either while experiencing or after experiencing the distressing event, the individual has three (or more) of the following dissociative symptoms:

  (1) a subjective sense of numbing, detachment, or absence of emotional responsiveness

  (2) a reduction in awareness of his or her surroundings (e.g., "being in a daze")

  (3) derealization

  (4) depersonalization

  (5) dissociative amnesia (i.e., inability to recall an important aspect of the trauma)

C. The traumatic event is persistently reexperienced in at least one of the following ways: recurrent images, thoughts, dreams, illusions, flashback episodes, or a sense of reliving the experience; or distress on exposure to reminders of the traumatic event.

D. Marked avoidance of stimuli that arouse recollections of the trauma (e.g., thoughts, feelings, conversations, activities, places, people).

E. Marked symptoms of anxiety or increased arousal (e.g., difficulty sleeping, irritability, poor concentration, hypervigilance, exaggerated startle response, motor restlessness).

F. The disturbance causes clinically significant distress or impairment in social, occupational, or other important areas of functioning or impairs the individual's ability to pursue some necessary task, such as obtaining necessary assistance or mobilizing personal resources by telling family members about the traumatic experience.

G. The disturbance lasts for a minimum of 2 days and a maximum of 4 weeks and occurs within 4 weeks of the traumatic event.

H. The disturbance is not due to the direct physiological effects of a substance (e.g., a drug of abuse, a medication) or a general medical condition, is not better accounted for by brief psychotic disorder, and is not merely an exacerbation of a preexisting Axis I or Axis II disorder.

It has long been recognized that clinically significant dissociative states are seen in the immediate aftermath of overwhelming trauma. In addition, many individuals may experience less clinically severe dissociative symptoms or alterations of attention and time sense. Because such syndromes, even when short lasting, can produce major disruption of everyday activities, they may require clinical attention. During triage situations after a disaster, it can be important to recognize this clinical picture, which may require treatment intervention and which may also be predictive of later PTSD.

Acute stress disorder (ASD) represents the clinical features of PTSD along with conspicuous dissociative symptoms, of which at least three must be present. The possible dissociative symptoms in ASD are a subjective sense of numbing; detachment or absence of emotional response; reduced awareness of one's surroundings; derealization; depersonalization; and dissociative amnesia.

Little is known about the epidemiology of ASD as defined in DSM-IV, but after events such as rape and criminal assault, the clinical picture of acute PTSD is found in 70% to 90% of subjects, although frequency of the particular dissociative symptoms is unknown.

DIAGNOSIS AND DIFFERENTIAL DIAGNOSIS

ASD may need to be distinguished from several related disorders (Fig. 31–1). Brief psychotic disorder may be a more appropriate diagnosis if the predominant symptoms are psychotic. It is possible that major depressive disorder can develop posttraumatically and that there may be some overlap with ASD, in which case both disorders are appropriately diagnosed. When caused by direct physiological perturbation, ASD may be more appropriately diagnosed with reference to the etiological agent. Thus, an ASD-like picture that develops secondary to head injury is more appropriately diagnosed as mental disorder due to a general medical condition, whereas a clinical picture related to substance use (e.g., alcohol intoxication) is appropriately diagnosed as substance-induced disorder. Substance-related ASD is confined to the period of intoxication or withdrawal.

Because ASD by definition cannot last longer than 1 month, if the clinical picture persists, a diagnosis of PTSD is more appropriate.

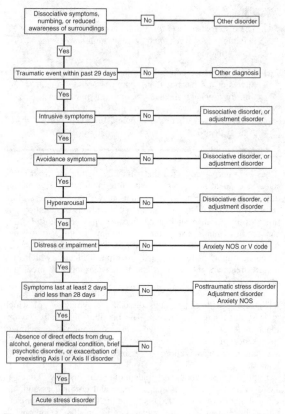

Figure 31–1 *Diagnostic decision tree for acute stress disorder.*

Some increased symptoms are expected in the great majority of subjects after exposure to major stress. These remit in most cases and only reach the level of clinical diagnosis if they are prolonged, exceed a tolerable quality, or interfere with everyday function. Resolution may be more difficult if there has been previous psychiatric morbidity, further subsequent stress, and lack of social support.

COURSE AND NATURAL HISTORY

Although data do not exist on the course and natural history of ASD as now defined, there is some indication that dissociative, cognitive, and psychotic symptoms, which are so common in the immediate wake of trauma, improve spontaneously with time. The likelihood of developing PTSD symptoms at 7 months' follow-up is more strongly related to the occurrence of dissociative symptoms than to anxiety symptoms immediately after disaster.

TREATMENT

Treatment of acute trauma is generally aimed at being brief, is provided immediately after the trauma whenever possible, is administered in a centralized and coordinated fashion with the expectation of the patient's return to normal function and as proximately as possible to the scene of the trauma, and is not directed at any uncovering or explorative procedures but rather at maintaining a superficial, reintegrating approach.

People most highly at risk, and therefore perhaps most in need of treatment, are survivors with psychiatric disorders; close relatives to traumatically bereaved people; children, especially when separated from their parents; individuals who are particularly dependent on psychosocial supports, such as the elderly, children, handicapped, and mentally retarded individuals; and traumatized survivors and body handlers.

Different components of treatment include information, psychological support, crisis intervention, and emotional first aid. Providing information about the trauma is important, as it can enable the survivor to fully recognize and accept all the details of what happened. Information needs to be given in a way that conveys hope and the possibility of coping with psychological pain and the threat of loss. Unrealistic hope needs to be balanced by the provision of realistic explanations as to what happened. Psychological support helps to strengthen coping mechanisms and promotes adaptive defenses. The survivor benefits if he or she ecognizes responsibility for successful outcome and is as actively involved with this as possible. Crisis intervention is often used after disasters, acts of violence, or other serious traumas. Emotional first aid is used to achieve any of the following: acceptance of feelings, symptoms, reality, and the need for help; recognition of psychologically distressing issues; identification of available resources and activities; acceptance of responsibility and absence of blame; cultivation of an optimistic attitude; and efforts to resume activities of daily life as much as possible.

It is not known whether early recognition and effective treatment of acute stress reactions prevent the development of PTSD, although it is safe to assume that they are likely to have beneficial effects in this regard.

Generalized Anxiety Disorder

DSM-IV Criteria 300.02

Generalized Anxiety Disorder

A. Excessive anxiety and worry (apprehensive expectation), occurring more days than not for at least 6 months, about a number of events or activities (such as work or school performance).

B. The person finds it difficult to control the worry.

C. The anxiety and worry are associated with three (or more) of the following six symptoms (with at least some symptoms present for more days than not for the past 6 months). **Note:** Only one item is required in children.

   (1) restlessness or feeling keyed up or on edge

   (2) being easily fatigued

   (3) difficulty concentrating or mind going blank

   (4) irritability

   (5) muscle tension

   (6) sleep disturbance (difficulty falling or staying asleep, or restless unsatisfying sleep)

D. The focus of anxiety and worry is not confined to features of an Axis I disorder, e.g., the anxiety or worry is not about having a panic attack (as in panic disorder), being embarrassed in public (as in social phobia), being contaminated (as in obsessive-compulsive disorder), being away from home or close relatives (as in separation anxiety disorder), gaining weight (as in anorexia nervosa), having multiple physical complaints (as in somatization disorder), or having a serious illness (as in hypochondriasis), and the anxiety and worry do not occur exclusively during posttraumatic stress disorder.

E. The anxiety, worry, or physical symptoms cause clinically significant distress or impairment in social, occupational, or other important areas of functioning.

F. The disturbance is not due to the direct physiological effects of a substance (e.g., a drug of abuse, a medication) or a general medical condition (e.g., hyperthyroidism) and does not occur exclusively during a mood disorder, a psychotic disorder, or a pervasive developmental disorder.

Generalized anxiety disorder (GAD) is currently defined as excessive anxiety and worry (apprehensive expectation) occurring more days than not for at least 6 months, about a number of events or activities (such as work or school performance). In individuals with GAD, the anxiety and worry are accompanied by at least three of six somatic symptoms (only one accompanying symptom is required in children), which include restlessness or feeling keyed up or on edge, being easily fatigued, difficulty concentrating or mind going blank, irritability, muscle tension, and sleep disturbance. In addition, the affected individual has difficulty controlling his or her worry, and the anxiety, worry, or somatic symptoms cause clinically significant distress or impairment in social, occupational, or other important areas of functioning. Furthermore, the GAD symptoms should not be due to the direct physiological effects of substances such as drugs or alcohol or a general medical condition and should not occur exclusively during a mood disorder, psychotic disorder, or pervasive developmental disorder.

Finally, it should be noted that worry and anxiety are part of normal human behavior, and it may be difficult to define a cutoff point distinguishing normal or trait anxiety (i.e., a relatively stable tendency to perceive various situations as threatening) from GAD. However, as described in the *Diagnostic and Statistical Manual of Mental Disorders,* Fourth Edition (DSM-IV) definition of GAD, individuals suffering from a "disorder" exhibit significant distress and impairment in functioning as a result of their anxiety symptoms.

EPIDEMIOLOGY

Current data indicate that GAD is probably one of the more common psychiatric disorders (Table 32–1). The Epidemiological Catchment Area study reported a lifetime prevalence rate for GAD of 4.1% to 6.6% in the three sites that assessed for GAD.

Overanxious anxiety disorder, the childhood equivalent of GAD, is also highly prevalent in the child and adolescent population. It is unclear whether overanxious anxiety disorder predisposes to or represents an early manifestation of adult GAD.

Comorbidity

Among the most prevalent current comorbid diagnoses are social phobia (16% to 59%), simple phobia (21% to 55%), panic disorder (3% to 27%), and depression (8% to 39%). Alcoholism also complicates the clinical course of GAD for some patients; however, the available literature suggests that alcohol abuse is not as prevalent in GAD as in other anxiety disorders, and the pattern of abuse is often a

TABLE 32–1	Lifetime Prevalence of Generalized Anxiety Disorder in the General Population	
Study		**Prevalence (%)**
Epidemiological Catchment Area study		
Durham, NC		6.6
St. Louis, MO		6.6
Los Angeles, CA		4.1
National Comorbidity survey		5.1

brief and nonpersistent one. Axis II disorders have been observed to co-occur in approximately 50% of patients with GAD. Cluster C personality disorders, specifically avoidant personality disorder and obsessive-compulsive personality disorder, have been the most prevalent personality disorders observed in patients with GAD.

DIAGNOSIS

GAD patients frequently report that they have been anxious all of their lives. Typically, they were moderately anxious during childhood, later developing full-blown GAD when their stress levels increased through activities such as attending college or starting to work. Patients with early onset of symptoms report experiencing significant anxiety and fears, social isolation, obsessionality, more academic difficulties, and disturbed home environment during their childhood.

Not all GAD patients have a lifelong history of abnormal anxiety. Some patients develop their disorder at a later age (i.e., in the third decade or later). These patients frequently report identifiable precipitating stressful events—specifically, unexpected, negative, important events in the year preceding development of GAD.

Patients commonly complain of feeling tense, jumpy, and irritable. They have difficulty falling or staying asleep and tire easily during the day. Particularly distressing to patients is the difficulty in concentrating and collecting their thoughts. Patients may complain of muscle tension, especially in their neck and shoulders. They may experience headaches, frequently described as frontal and occipital pressure or tension. They complain about sweaty palms, feel shaky and tremulous, complain of dryness of the mouth, and experience palpitations and difficulty breathing. Patients may also experience gastrointestinal symptoms such as heartburn and epigastric fullness. Approximately 30% of patients experience severe gastrointestinal symptoms of irritable bowel syndrome. The physical complaints frequently lead patients to seek medical attention, and most initially consult a primary care physician.

Special laboratory and diagnostic evaluation of patients with GAD may occasionally be required to exclude general medical disorders that mimic symptoms of generalized anxiety. An evaluation to identify these disorders includes a personal and family medical history, a review of systems, and a careful physical examination including neurological examination. The laboratory evaluation should include an electrocardiogram, screening for abusable substances, urinalysis, complete blood count, serum electrolyte levels, liver and thyroid function tests, and calcium, phosphorus, and blood urea nitrogen levels.

DIFFERENTIAL DIAGNOSIS

Anxiety can be a prominent feature of many psychiatric disorders. In addition, the substantial overlap of symptoms between GAD and other psychiatric disorders such as major depression often creates diagnostic and treatment dilemmas for the psychiatrist and may complicate the difficult task of differential diagnosis and treatment planning. The major disorders that should be considered in the differential diagnosis of GAD are found in Figure 32–1.

Many general medical conditions and medications may also present with prominent anxiety symptoms. If not identified and properly addressed, these conditions may adversely affect the treatment outcome of the anxious patient. Important medical conditions in the differential diagnosis of generalized anxiety are found in Table 32–2.

COURSE AND NATURAL HISTORY

Relatively little is known about the course of and long-term prognosis for GAD. For many years, GAD was conceptualized as a mild condition. However, an increasing amount of data indicates that GAD is a chronic, often intermittent (i.e., waxing and waning), distressing illness, frequently leading to moderate impairment. Thus, it appears that chronic, long-term treatment of this disorder may be required in many cases.

TREATMENT APPROACHES

Patients with milder forms of GAD may respond well to simple psychological interventions and require no medication treatment. In more severe forms of GAD, it may become necessary to see the patient regularly and to provide more specific psychological and pharmacological interventions (Table 32–3).

During the early (acute) phase of treatment, an attempt should be made to control the patient's symptoms. It may take 3 to 6 months to achieve an optimal response. However, there may be a considerable variation in the length of the initial treatment phase. For example, clinical response to benzodiazepines occurs early in treatment. Response to other anxiolytic medications, such as buspirone, or to cognitive-behavioral treatment generally requires longer periods. During the maintenance phase, treatment gains are consolidated. Unfortunately, studies suggesting how long treatment should be continued are limited. Routinely, pharmacological treatment is continued for a total of 6 to 12 months before an attempt is made to discontinue medications. Data indicate that maintenance psychotherapeutic treatments such as cognitive-behavioral therapy may be helpful in maintaining treatment gains in patients with anxiety dis-

Text continued on page 343

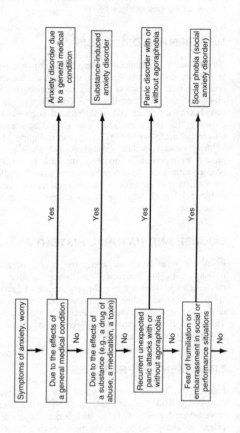

Symptoms of anxiety, worry

Due to the effects of a general medical condition → **Yes** → Anxiety disorder due to a general medical condition

No ↓

Due to the effects of a substance (e.g., a drug of abuse, a medication, a toxin) → **Yes** → Substance-induced anxiety disorder

No ↓

Recurrent unexpected panic attacks with or without agoraphobia → **Yes** → Panic disorder with or without agoraphobia

No ↓

Fear of humiliation or embarrassment in social or performance situations → **Yes** → Social phobia (social anxiety disorder)

No ↓

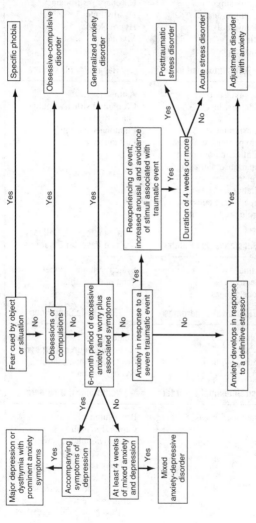

Figure 32-1 *Diagnostic decision tree for GAD.*

Specific phobia

Obsessive-compulsive disorder

Generalized anxiety disorder

Posttraumatic stress disorder

Acute stress disorder

Adjustment disorder with anxiety

Fear cued by object or situation — No →

Obsessions or compulsions — No →

6-month period of excessive anxiety and worry plus associated symptoms

Anxiety in response to a severe traumatic event

Reexperiencing of event, increased arousal, and avoidance of stimuli associated with traumatic event — Yes

Duration of 4 weeks or more — Yes / No

Anxiety develops in response to a definitive stressor — Yes

Yes ↑ (Specific phobia)

Yes ↑ (Obsessive-compulsive disorder)

Yes ↑ (Generalized anxiety disorder)

No →

Yes / No

Major depression or dysthymia with prominent anxiety symptoms

Accompanying symptoms of depression — Yes

At least 4 weeks of mixed anxiety and depression — Yes

Mixed anxiety-depressive disorder

TABLE 32–2 Medical Conditions and Drugs That May Cause Anxiety

Endocrine Disorders

Addison's disease
Cushing's syndrome
Hyperparathyroidism
Hyperthyroidism
Hypothyroidism
Carcinoid
Pheochromocytoma

Drug Intoxication

Anticonvulsants
Antidepressants

Antihistamines
Antihypertensive agents
Antiinflammatory agents
Antiparkinsonian agents
Caffeine
Digitalis
Sympathomimetics
Thyroid supplements

Substance Use Related

Cocaine
Hallucinogens
Amphetamines

Withdrawal Syndromes

Alcohol
Narcotics
Sedative-hypnotics

Gastrointestinal Disorders

Peptic ulcer disease

Infectious Diseases

Miscellaneous viral and bacterial infections

Cardiovascular and Circulatory Disorders

Anemia
Congestive heart failure
Coronary insufficiency
Dysrhythmia
Hypovolemia
Myocardial infarction

Respiratory Disorders

Asthma
Chronic obstructive pulmonary disease
Pulmonary embolism
Pulmonary edema

Immunological, Collagen, and Vascular Disorders

Systemic lupus erythematosus
Temporal arteritis

Metabolic Conditions

Acidosis
Acute intermittent porphyria
Electrolyte abnormalities
Hypoglycemia

Neurological Disorders

Brain tumors
Cerebral syphilis
Cerebrovascular disorders
Encephalopathies
Epilepsy (especially temporal lobe epilepsy)
Postconcussive syndrome
Vertigo
Akathisia

TABLE 32–3	Anxiolytic Agents*		
Drug	Daily Dosage Range (mg)	Advantages	Disadvantages
		Benzodiazepines†	
Alprazolam	2–6	Rapid onset of action	Sedation
Clonazepam	1–3	Favorable side effects profile	Multiple doses for shorter acting agents
Lorazepam	4–10		Physical dependence
Diazepam	15–20		Limited antidepressant effect
			Sexual side effects
		Tricyclic Antidepressants	
Imipramine	75–300	Once-daily dosage	Delayed onset
	50–250	Possibly better with concomitant depression	Activation
			Anticholinergic effects
			Orthostatic hypotension
			Weight gain
			Sexual side effects

Table continued on following page

TABLE 32–3   **Anxiolytic Agents*** (Continued)

Drug	Daily Dosage Range (mg)	Advantages	Disadvantages
		Atypical Antidepressants	
Trazodone	150–600	Once-daily dosage Possibley better with concomitant depression Low anticholinergic effects	Delayed onset Orthostatic hypotension Weight gain Sexual side effects Priapism (rare) Sedation
		Azapirones	
Buspirone	30–60	No withdrawal symptoms No physical dependence Favorable side effects profile	Multiple doses
		Selective Serotonin Reuptake Inhibitors	
Fluoxetine Sertraline Paroxetine Fluvoxamine	20–60 50–200 10–40 100–300	Unknown efficacy in generalized anxiety Possibly effective in mixed anxiety-depression Favorable side effects profile	Gastrointestinal side effects Activation Delayed onset Sexual side effects

*These recommendations are based on controlled studies, clinical reports, and the experiences of the authors.

†Higher doses may be necessary to ensure that other drugs/regimens may be effective.

orders after the discontinuation of pharmacotherapy. It is clear that many patients may experience chronic and continuous symptoms that require years of long-term treatment.

Pharmacotherapy

For many years, benzodiazepines have been the treatment of choice for GAD patients. The benzodiazepines have a broad spectrum of effects, including sedation, muscle relaxation, anxiety reduction, and decreased physiological arousal (e.g., palpitations, tremulousness). The main difference between individual benzodiazepines is potency and elimination half-life.

Interestingly, studies indicate that benzodiazepines have the most pronounced effect on hypervigilance and somatic symptoms of GAD but exhibit fewer effects on psychic symptoms such as dysphoria, interpersonal sensitivity, and obsessionality. Benzodiazepines exert their therapeutic effects quickly, often after a single dose, thus making their use particularly effective in the acutely anxious patient.

When treatment is initiated with benzodiazepines, it is helpful for patients to take an initial dose at home in the evening to see how it affects them. Gradual titration to an effective dose allows for limiting unwanted adverse effects. A final daily dosage of alprazolam at 2 to 4 mg/d, clonazepam at 1 to 2 mg/d, or diazepam at 15 to 20 mg/d is usually sufficient for the majority of patients.

The main side effect of benzodiazepines is daytime drowsiness, which usually subsides after several days of treatment. Mild cognitive and memory impairments have been demonstrated but are generally not serious except in the elderly patient. The reemergence of symptoms during tapering of benzodiazepines is common. Because GAD is often chronic, it should be expected that symptoms may reappear during tapering after successful benzodiazepine treatment. The distinction between withdrawal symptoms and reemergence of GAD can be difficult.

Possible factors that may contribute to the severity of withdrawal and the ultimate outcome of benzodiazepine taper include the dosage, the duration of treatment, the benzodiazepine elimination half-life and potency, and the rate of benzodiazepine taper (gradual versus abrupt). In addition, patient-related factors such as premorbid personality features have been implicated. It appears that the taper rate of 25% per week is probably too rapid for many patients.

The finding that the tricyclic antidepressants (TCAs), in particular imipramine, are effective anxiolytics provides additional treatment options for the psychiatrist, particularly if benzodiazepines are contraindicated. However, when treatment with TCAs is initiated, it is important to remember that the onset of the anxiolytic action of imipramine is gradual and that patients with GAD are typically sensitive to the side effects of TCAs.

The possible role of selective serotonin reuptake inhibitors (SSRIs) in the treatment of GAD remains largely unexplored. The SSRIs, such as sertraline and paroxetine, may have efficacy in some patients with GAD. However, controlled studies are required to define the potential of SSRIs in treating patients with GAD.

AZAPIRONES: BUSPIRONE

Comparative efficacy studies have shown that the anxiolytic response to buspirone is comparable to that of alprazolam, lorazepam, oxazepam, and clorazepate. However, in contrast to benzodiazepines, buspirone carries no apparent risk for abuse, physical dependence, or withdrawal and is not synergistic with alcohol or other sedative hypnotics. On the other hand, buspirone has the relative disadvantage of delayed onset of action. Whereas benzodiazepines can exert their effects quickly, often after a single dose, buspirone must be administered for nearly 2 weeks before a significant effect occurs. Perhaps the most significant problem with the use of buspirone has been that doses that are too low were advocated based on initial clinical trials. As a result, its efficacy in clinical practice may have been underestimated. To achieve optimal response, buspirone dosing may need to be in the range of at least 30 to 60 mg/d.

Nonpharmacological Treatments

SUPPORTIVE PSYCHOTHERAPY

Many patients with milder forms of GAD benefit from simple psychological interventions such as supportive psychotherapy. They may experience lessening of anxiety when given the opportunity to discuss their difficulties with a supportive psychiatrist and to become better informed about their illness. Thus, basic supportive techniques such as reassurance, clarification of patients' concerns, direct suggestions, and advice are often effective in reducing anxiety symptoms.

RELAXATION AND BIOFEEDBACK

Relaxation techniques such as progressive muscle relaxation and biofeedback have also been utilized in the treatment of patients with anxiety symptoms. Few controlled studies have examined their effectiveness.

It should be noted that relaxation may be associated with a paradoxical increase in anxiety and tension in patients with GAD. However, with repeated training, specifically in the context of cognitive-behavioral therapy, this phenomenon may be used to achieve habituation and anxiety extinction.

COGNITIVE-BEHAVIORAL THERAPY

There is evidence suggesting that cognitive-behavioral therapy may be more effective in the treatment of GAD than other psychotherapeutic interventions, such as behavioral therapy alone or nonspecific supportive therapy. A cognitive-behavioral treatment approach to GAD that concentrates on the behavioral procedure of directly exposing patients to the contents of their worry and apprehension (i.e., deconditioning strategy) in addition to relaxation techniques (i.e., progressive muscle relaxation) and cognitive restructuring has been found useful.

PSYCHODYNAMIC PSYCHOTHERAPY

The psychoanalytic literature offers a vast amount of clinical case report data supporting the efficacy of psychodynamic psychotherapies in the treatment of patients with anxiety disorders such as GAD.

The classical psychoanalytic theories view anxiety as an indicator of certain unconscious conflicts rather than as a primary target symptom to be alleviated. The psychiatrist should therefore use various techniques to help the patient uncover these unconscious conflicts. It is believed that the newly gained understanding of the underlying reasons for symptoms has a therapeutic effect, thereby reducing anxiety. Through interpretation of previously unconscious conflicts and unconscious origins of anxiety, patients are able to utilize new insights and find more adaptive outlets or solutions to their problems.

Another therapeutic approach to the treatment of anxiety symptoms was offered by object relations and self psychology theorists. In their view, anxiety results from the loss of or inadequate emotional relationships with significant others. Therefore, the primary focus of therapy shifts to emphasize the importance of the relationship to the psychiatrist, who functions as an emphatic object providing emotionally corrective experiences. For example, the patient may learn that an important person may be imperfect but still be trusted and nurturing.

The outcome of psychodynamic psychotherapy is determined in part by factors reflecting the patient's maturity and strength. Specifically, factors such as the patient's capacity for introspection and intelligence, as well as ability to relate to the psychiatrist and to bear painful feelings should be carefully evaluated.

Long-Term Management

Regardless of the actual drug prescribed, several general guidelines apply when long-term treatment of GAD is considered. We recommend use of the lowest dose of medication that can effectively control the patient's symptoms. Because some patients may experience periods of relative remission, it may be useful to attempt discontinuation of medications every 6 to 9 months. However, the clinician should be alert to the presence of any comorbid diagnoses that may prevent treatment discontinuation. Stress management and problem-solving techniques, along with specific psychotherapeutic approaches such as cognitive-behavioral therapy, should be attempted to further reduce the need for medication treatment.

Treatment in the Elderly

Evaluation of the available epidemiological data suggests that GAD is highly prevalent in the geriatric population (prevalence rates ranging from 0.7% to 7.1%), accounting for the majority of anxiety disorder cases in this group. In the elderly, anxiety symptoms are often associated with depression, medical conditions, and cognitive dysfunction. Thus, a careful differential diagnosis to eliminate exogenous causes of anxiety and to identify other coexisting conditions is necessary.

Benzodiazepines may be beneficial for treating GAD in the elderly. However, psychiatrists must be aware that these patients are more sensitive to the benzodiazepines than are younger patients. Buspirone may provide a reasonable alternative. Antidepressants may be beneficial, especially in anxious elderly patients with concurrent depression. As with benzodiazepines, the psychiatrist should pay special attention to the side effects of the antidepressants, mainly the TCAs, when treating the older patient with these agents.

Somatoform Disorders

The somatoform disorders class was created for clinical utility, not on the basis of an assumed common etiology or mechanism. In terms of the *Diagnostic and Statistical Manual of Mental Disorders, Fourth Edition* (DSM-IV), it was designed to facilitate the differential diagnosis of conditions in which the first diagnostic concern is the need to "exclude occult general medical conditions or substance-induced etiologies for the bodily symptoms." As shown in Figure 33–1, only after such explanations are reasonably excluded should somatoform disorders be considered.

The somatoform disorder concept should be distinguished from traditional concepts of "psychosomatic illness" and "somatization." The psychosomatic illnesses involved structural or physiological changes hypothesized as deriving from psychological factors. In DSM-IV somatoform disorders, such objective changes are generally not evident. The "classic" psychosomatic illnesses included bronchial asthma, ulcerative colitis, thyrotoxicosis, essential hypertension, rheumatoid arthritis, neurodermatitis, and peptic ulcer. In DSM-IV, most of these illnesses are diagnosed as a general medical condition on Axis III, in some cases with an additional designation of psychological factors affecting medical condition. By definition, the diagnosis "psychological factors affecting medical condition" does not denote a psychiatric disorder but is included under other conditions that may be a focus of clinical attention; it involves the presence of one or more specific psychological or behavioral factors that adversely affect a general medical condition.

The descriptive use of the term somatization in somatization disorder is not to be confused with theories that generally postulate a somatic expression of psychological distress. Empirical studies suggest that there is no single theory that can adequately explain somatization, which not only is multifactorially determined but is an exceedingly complex phenomenon.

DIAGNOSIS AND DIFFERENTIAL DIAGNOSIS

As shown in Figure 33–1, after it is determined that physical symptoms are not fully explained by a general medical condition or the direct effect of a substance, somatoform disorders must be differentiated from other mental conditions with physical symptoms.

In contrast to malingering and factitious disorder, symptoms in somatoform disorders are not under voluntary control; that is, they are not intentionally produced or feigned. Determination of intentionality may be difficult and must be inferred from the context in which symptoms present. Somatic symptoms may involve disorders in other diagnostic classes. However, in such instances, the overriding focus is on the primary symptom complex (i.e., anxiety, mood, or

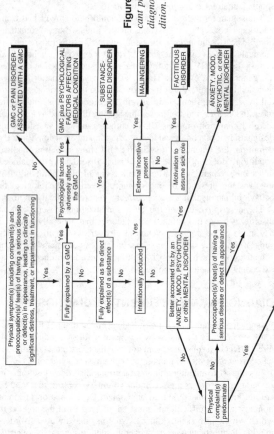

Figure 33–1 *Differential diagnosis of clinically significant physical symptoms. Shadowed boxes represent diagnostic categories. GMC, General medical condition.*

348

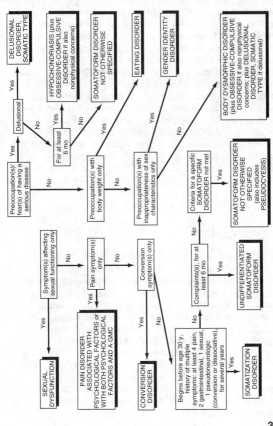

DELUSIONAL DISORDER, SOMATIC TYPE

Preoccupation(s)/fear(s) of having a serious disease — Yes → Delusional — Yes → DELUSIONAL DISORDER, SOMATIC TYPE

Delusional — No → For at least 6 mo — Yes → HYPOCHONDRIASIS (plus OBSESSIVE-COMPULSIVE DISORDER if also nonphysical concerns)

For at least 6 mo — No → SOMATOFORM DISORDER NOT OTHERWISE SPECIFIED

Preoccupation(s) with body weight only — Yes → EATING DISORDER

Preoccupation(s) with body weight only — No → Preoccupation(s) with inappropriateness of sex characteristics only — Yes → GENDER IDENTITY DISORDER

Preoccupation(s) with inappropriateness of sex characteristics only — No → BODY DYSMORPHIC DISORDER (plus OBSESSIVE-COMPULSIVE DISORDER if also nonphysical concerns; plus DELUSIONAL DISORDER, SOMATIC TYPE if delusional)

Symptom(s) affecting sexual functioning only — Yes → SEXUAL DYSFUNCTION

Symptom(s) affecting sexual functioning only — No → Pain symptom(s) only — Yes → PAIN DISORDER ASSOCIATED WITH PSYCHOLOGICAL FACTORS or WITH BOTH PSYCHOLOGICAL FACTORS AND A GMC

Pain symptom(s) only — No → Conversion symptom(s) only — Yes → CONVERSION DISORDER

Conversion symptom(s) only — No → Begins before age 30 y, history of multiple symptoms: at least 4 pain, 2 gastrointestinal, 1 sexual, 1 pseudoneurologic (conversion or dissociative), for several years — Yes → SOMATIZATION DISORDER

Begins before age 30 y... — No → Complaint(s), for at least 6 mo — Yes → UNDIFFERENTIATED SOMATOFORM DISORDER

Complaint(s), for at least 6 mo — No → Criteria for a specific SOMATOFORM DISORDER not met → SOMATOFORM DISORDER NOT OTHERWISE SPECIFIED (also includes PSEUDOCYESIS)

349

psychotic symptoms) rather than the physical symptoms. In both panic disorder and generalized anxiety disorder, physical symptoms such as chest pain, shortness of breath, palpitations, sweating, and tremulousness may occur. However, such somatic symptoms occur only in the context of fear or anxious foreboding. In general, there is a lack of a consistent physical focus. In mood disorders (particularly major depressive disorder) and in schizophrenia and other psychotic disorders, somatic preoccupations, fears, and even delusions and false perceptions may be evident. In the mood disorders, these are generally mood congruent (e.g., "I'm so worthless not even my organs work anymore"), whereas in the psychoses, bizarre and mood-incongruent beliefs are typical (e.g., "Half of my brain was removed by psychic neurosurgery").

DIFFERENTIATION AMONG THE VARIOUS SOMATOFORM DISORDERS

Whereas it is assumed that the specific disorders in the somatoform grouping are heterogeneous in terms of pathogenesis and pathophysiology, they are also phenomenologically diverse. In somatization disorder, undifferentiated somatoform disorder, conversion disorder, and pain disorder, the focus is on the physical complaints themselves, and thus on perceptions. In hypochondriasis and body dysmorphic disorder, however, emphasis is on physically related preoccupations or fears, and thus on cognitions. Somatization disorder and, to a lesser extent, undifferentiated somatoform disorder are characterized by multiple symptoms of different types; conversion disorder, pain disorder, hypochondriasis, and body dysmorphic disorder are defined on the basis of a single symptom or a few symptoms of a certain type (see Fig. 33–1). Whereas somatization disorder, undifferentiated somatoform disorder, and hypochondriasis are, by definition, at least 6 months in duration, conversion disorder, pain disorder, and somatoform disorder not otherwise specified (NOS) may be of short duration as long as they are associated with clinically significant distress or impairment.

EPIDEMIOLOGY

The vicissitudes of diagnostic approaches and the relative recency of the current somatoform disorder grouping has resulted, not surprisingly, in estimates of the frequency of this group of disorders in the general population and even in clinical settings that are inconsistent. Yet, existing data seem to indicate that such problems are indeed common and account for a major proportion of clinical services, especially in primary care settings. A World Health Organization study reported ICD-10 diagnoses of hypochondriasis in nearly 1% and of somatization disorder in nearly 3% of patients in primary care clinics in 14 countries. Another study using primary care sites found 14% of 1000 patients to be suffering from some somatoform disorder: 8% with "multisomatoform disorder," 4% with somatoform disorder NOS, 2% with hypochondriasis, and 1% with somatoform pain disorder.

TREATMENT

Whereas specific somatoform disorders indicate specific treatment approaches, some general guidelines apply to the somatoform disorders as a whole (Table 33–1). The therapeutic goals include 1) as a main goal, preventing adoption of the sick role and chronic invalidism; then 2) minimizing unnecessary costs and complications by avoiding unwarranted hospitalizations, diagnostic and treatment procedures, and medications (especially those of an addictive potential); and 3) effectively treating comorbid psychiatric disorders, such as depressive and anxiety syndromes. The three general treatment strategies include 1) consistent treatment, generally by the same physician, with careful coordination if multiple physicians are involved; 2) supportive office visits, scheduled at regular intervals rather than in response to symptoms; and 3) a gradual shift in focus from symptoms to an emphasis on personal and interpersonal problems.

SOMATIZATION DISORDER

As defined in DSM-IV, somatization disorder is a polysymptomatic somatoform disorder characterized by multiple recurring pains and gastrointestinal, sexual, and pseudoneurological symptoms occurring for a period of years with an age at onset younger than 30 years. The physical complaints are not intentionally produced and are not fully explained by a general medical condition or the direct effects of a substance. To warrant diagnosis, symptoms must result in medical attention or significant impairment in social, occupational, or other important areas of functioning.

DSM-IV Criteria 300.81

Somatization Disorder

A. A history of many physical complaints beginning before age 30 years that occur over a period of several years and result in treatment being sought or significant impairment in social, occupational, or other important areas of functioning.

B. Each of the following criteria must have been met, with individual symptoms occurring at any time during the course of the disturbance.

   (1) *four pain symptoms:* a history of pain related to at least four different sites or functions (e.g., head, abdomen, back, joints, extremities, chest, rectum, during menstruation, during sexual intercourse, or during urination)

   (2) *two gastrointestinal symptoms:* a history of at least two gastrointestinal symptoms other than pain (e.g., nausea, bloating, vomiting other than during pregnancy, diarrhea, or intolerance of several different foods)

Box continued on page 355

TABLE 33–1   Treatment of DSM-IV Somatoform Disorders

Somatoform Disorder	Treatment Goals	Psychotherapy and Psychosocial Strategies and Techniques	Pharmacological and Physical Strategies and Techniques*
Somatoform disorders, as a group	1. prevent adoption of the sick role and chronic invalidism 2. Minimize unnecessary costs and complications by avoiding unwarranted hospitalizations, diagnostic and treatment procedures, and medications 3. Pharmacological control of comorbid syndromes	1. Consistent treatment, generally by same physician, coordinated if multiple 2. Supportive office visits, schedules at regular intervals 3. Focus gradually shifted from symptoms to personal and social problems	1. Only as clearly indicated, or as time-limited empirical trial 2. Avoid drugs with abuse or addictive potential
Somatization disorder	1, 2, and 3; also • Instill, whenever possible, insight regarding temporal association between symptoms and personal, interpersonal, and situational problems	1, 2, and 3; also • Establish firm therapeutic alliance • Educate patient regarding manifestations of somatization disorder (psychoeducative approach) • Consistent reassurance	1 and 2, also • Antianxiety and antidepressant drugs for comorbid anxiety or depressive disorders; if diagnosis unclear, consider empirical trial
Undifferentiated somatoform disorder	1, 2, and 3	1, 2, and 3	1 and 2
Conversion disorder	1, 2, and 3; also • Prompt removal of symptoms	Acute: • Reassurance, suggestion to remove symptom	1 and 2; also • Consider macroanalysis as an interviewing or psychotherapy adjunct

Conversion disorder *Continued*		• Consider narcoanalysis (interview after drowsiness from amobarbital or other sedative-hypnotic, sometimes followed by methylphenidate or other stimulant), hypnotherapy, or behavioral therapy	
		Chronic: 1, 2, and 3	
		• Exploration of various conflict areas, particularly interpersonal relationships • Long-term, intensive, insight-oriented dynamic psychotherapy recommended by some	
Pain disorder	1, 2, and 3; also • Acute pain: relieve symptom • Chronic pain: maintain function and motility rather than focus on total pain relief	1, 2, and 3; also • Chronic pain: consider physical and occupational therapy, operant conditioning, cognitive-behavioral therapy	1 and 2; also • Acute: acetaminophen and NSAIDs alone or as adjuncts to opioids (if necessary) • Chronic: tricyclic antidepressants, acetaminophen, and NSAIDs; if necessary, milder opioids or pure opioid agonists, but these only if tied to nonpain objectives (such as increasing activity)

Table continued on following page

*NSAIDs, nonsteroidal antiinflammatory drugs; SSRIs, selective serotonin reuptake inhibitors.

353

TABLE 33–1   Treatment of DSM-IV Somatoform Disorders *(Continued)*

Somatoform Disorder	Treatment Goals	Psychotherapy and Psychosocial Strategies and Techniques	Pharmacological and Physical Strategies and Techniques*
			Consider acupuncture, transcutaneous electrical nerve stimulation
Hypochondriasis	1, 2, and 3; also • Pharmacological control of central syndrome itself	1, 2, and 3; also • Cognitive-behavioral therapy involving prevention of checking rituals and reassurance seeking	2; also • Attempt to decrease hypochondriacal symptoms with SSRIs at higher than antidepressant doses or clomipramine
Body dysmorphic disorder	1, 2, and 3, especially avoiding corrective surgery; also • Pharmacological control of central syndrome itself	1, 2, and 3; also • Cognitive behavioral therapy involving prevention of checking rituals and reassurance seeking	2; also • Attempt to decrease hypochondriacal symptoms with SSRIs at higher than antidepressant doses or clomipramine
Somatoform disorder NOS	1, 2, and 3; also • Evaluate carefully for alternative general medical or other psychiatric disorder to which the symptoms can be attributed	1, 2, and 3	1 and 2

DSM-IV Criteria 300.81

Somatization Disorder *Continued*

    (3) *one sexual symptom:* a history of at least one sexual or reproductive symptom other than pain (e.g., sexual indifference, erectile or ejaculatory dysfunction, irregular menses, excessive menstrual bleeding, vomiting throughout pregnancy)

    (4) *one pseudoneurological symptom:* a history of at least one symptom or deficit suggesting a neurological condition not limited to pain (conversion symptoms such as impaired coordination or balance, paralysis or localized weakness, difficulty swallowing or lump in throat, aphonia, urinary retention, hallucinations, loss of touch or pain sensation, double vision, blindness, deafness, seizures; dissociative symptoms such as amnesia; or loss of consciousness other than fainting)

C. Either (1) or (2):

    (1) after appropriate investigation, each of the symptoms in criterion B cannot be fully explained by a known general medical condition or the direct effects of a substance (e.g., a drug of abuse, a medication)

    (2) when there is a related general medical condition, the physical complaints or resulting social or occupational impairment is in excess of what would be expected from the history, physical examination, or laboratory findings

D. The symptoms are not intentionally produced or feigned (as in factitious disorder or malingering).

Three features generally characterize somatization disorder but rarely general medical disorders: 1) involvement of multiple organ systems, 2) early onset and chronic course without development of physical signs or structural abnormalities, and 3) absence of laboratory abnormalities characteristic of the suggested physical disorders (Table 33–2).

Somatization disorder is a chronic illness characterized by fluctuations in the frequency and diversity of symptoms. Full remissions occur rarely, if ever. Whereas the most active symptomatic phase is in early adulthood, aging does not appear to bring total remission.

TABLE 33–2	Discrimination of Somatization Disorder from General Medical Conditions

Features Suggesting Somatization Disorder	Features Suggesting a General Medical Condition
Involvement of multiple organ systems	Involvement of single or few organ systems
Early onset and chronic course without development of physical signs or structural abnormalities	If early onset and chronic course, development of physical signs and structural abnormalities
Absence of laboratory abnormalities characteristic of the suggested general medical condition	Laboratory abnormalities evident

Adapted from Martin RL, Yutzy SH: Somatoform disorders. In Hales RE, Yudofsky SC, Talbott JA (eds): The American Psychiatric Press Textbook of Psychiatry, 2nd ed. Washington, DC: American Psychiatric Press, 1994:600.

CONVERSION DISORDER

DSM-IV Criteria 300.11

Conversion Disorder

A. One or more symptoms or deficits affecting voluntary motor or sensory function that suggest a neurological or other general medical condition.

B. Psychological factors are judged to be associated with the symptom or deficit because the initiation or exacerbation of the symptom or deficit is preceded by conflicts or other stressors.

C. The symptom or deficit is not intentionally produced or feigned (as in factitious disorder or malingering).

D. The symptom or deficit cannot, after appropriate investigation, be fully explained by a general medical condition, or by the direct effects of a substance, or as a culturally sanctioned behavior or experience.

E. The symptom or deficit causes clinically significant distress or impairment in social, occupational, or other important areas of functioning or warrants medical evaluation.

F. The symptom or deficit is not limited to pain or sexual dysfunction, does not occur exclusively during the course of somatization disorder, and is not better accounted for by another mental disorder.

Specify type of symptom or deficit:

With motor symptom or deficit (e.g., impaired coordination or balance, paralysis or localized weakness, difficulty swallowing or lump in throat, aphonia, and urinary retention)

With sensory symptom or deficit (e.g., loss of touch or pain sensation, double vision, blindness, deafness, and hallucinations)

With seizures or convulsions (includes seizures or convulsions with voluntary sensory components)

With mixed presentation (if symptoms of more than one category are evident)

Because conversion symptoms by definition affect voluntary motor or sensory function (thus pseudoneurological), neurological conditions are usually suggested, but other general medical conditions may be implicated as well. Neurologists are generally first consulted by primary care physicians for conversion symptoms; psychiatrists become involved only after neurological or general medical conditions have been reasonably excluded. Nonetheless, psychiatrists should have a good appreciation of the process of making such exclusions. More than 13% of actual neurological cases are diagnosed as functional before the elucidation of a neurological illness.

Apparent conversion symptoms mandate a thorough evaluation for possible underlying physical explanation. This evaluation must include a thorough medical history; physical (especially neurological) examination; and radiographical, blood, urine, and other tests as clinically indicated. Reliance should not be placed on determination of whether psychological factors explain the symptom.

Although conversion symptoms may occur at any age, symptoms are most often first manifested in late adolescence or early adulthood. Conversion symptoms first occurring in middle age or later should increase suspicion of an occult physical illness.

Symptoms of many neurological illnesses may appear inconsistent with known neurophysiological or neuropathological processes, suggesting conversion and posing diagnostic problems. These illnesses include multiple sclerosis, in which blindness due to optic neuritis may initially present with normal fundi; myasthenia gravis, periodic paralysis, myoglobinuric myopathy, polymyositis, and other acquired myopathies, in which marked weakness in the presence of normal deep tendon reflexes may occur; and Guillain-Barré syndrome, in which early extremity weakness may be inconsistent.

Individual conversion symptoms are generally self-limited and do not lead to physical changes or disabilities. Rarely, physical sequelae such as atrophy may occur. Marital and occupational problems are not as frequent in patients with conversion disorder as they are in those with somatization disorder.

In acute cases, the most frequent initial aim is removal of the symptom. The pressure behind accomplishing this depends on the distress and disability associated with the symptom. If the patient is not in great distress and the need to regain function is not immediate, a conservative approach of reassurance, relaxation, and suggestion is recommended. With this technique, the patient is reassured that on the basis of evaluation, the symptom will disappear completely and, in fact, is already beginning to do so. The patient can then be encouraged to ventilate about recent events and feelings, without any causal relationships being suggested.

If symptoms do not resolve with such conservative approaches, a number of other techniques for symptom resolution may be instituted. It does appear that prompt resolution of conversion symptoms is important because the duration of conversion symptoms is associated with a greater risk of recurrence and chronic disability. The other techniques include narcoanalysis (e.g., amobarbital interview), hypnosis, and behavioral therapy.

HYPOCHONDRIASIS

DSM-IV Criteria 300.7

Hypochondriasis

A. Preoccupation with fears of having, or the idea that one has, a serious disease based on the person's misinterpretation of bodily symptoms.

B. The preoccupation persists despite appropriate medical evaluation and reassurance.

C. The belief in criterion A is not of delusional intensity (as in delusional disorder, somatic type) and is not restricted to a circumscribed concern about appearance (as in body dysmorphic disorder).

D. The preoccupation causes clinically significant distress or impairment in social, occupational, or other important areas of functioning.

E. The duration of the disturbance is at least 6 months.

F. The preoccupation is not better accounted for by generalized anxiety disorder, obsessive-compulsive disorder, panic disorder, a major depressive episode, separation anxiety, or another somatoform disorder.

Specify:

With poor insight: if, for most of the time during the current episode, the person does not recognize that the concern about having a serious illness is excessive or unreasonable.

As defined in DSM-IV, the essential feature in hypochondriasis is preoccupation with fears or the idea of *having* a serious disease based on the "misinterpretation of bodily symptoms." This is in contrast to somatization disorder, conversion disorder, and pain disorder, in which the symptoms themselves are the predominant focus.

As shown in Figure 33–1, the first step in approaching patients with distressing or impairing preoccupation with or fears of having a serious disease is to exclude the possibility of explanation on the basis of a general medical condition. Fears that seem excessive may also occur in patients with general medical conditions who have vague and subjective symptoms early in their disease course. These include neurological diseases, such as myasthenia gravis and multiple sclerosis; endocrine diseases; systemic diseases that affect several organ systems, such as systemic lupus erythematosus; and occult malignant neoplasms. The disease conviction of hypochondriasis may actually be less amenable to medical reassurance than the fears of patients with general medical illnesses, who may at least temporally accept such encouragement.

Initially, the generic treatment techniques outlined for the somatoform disorders in general should be followed. However, it has not been demonstrated that a specific psychotherapy for hypochondriasis is available.

Although controlled trials are lacking, anecdotal and open-label studies suggest that serotoninergic agents such as clomipramine and the SSRI fluoxetine may be effective in ameliorating hypochondriasis. Such pharmacotherapy is best combined with the generic psychotherapy recommendations for somatoform disorders, as well as with cognitive-behavioral techniques to disrupt the counterproductive checking and reassurance-seeking behaviors.

Dissociative Disorders

DISSOCIATIVE AMNESIA

DSM-IV Criteria 300.12

Dissociative Amnesia

A. The predominant disturbance is one or more episodes of inability to recall important personal information, usually of a traumatic or stressful nature, that is too extensive to be explained by ordinary forgetfulness.

B. The disturbance does not occur exclusively during the course of dissociative identity disorder, dissociative fugue, posttraumatic stress disorder, acute stress disorder, or somatization disorder and is not due to the direct physiological effects of a substance (e.g., a drug of abuse, a medication) or a neurological or other general medical condition (e.g., amnestic disorder due to head trauma).

C. The symptoms cause clinically significant distress or impairment in social, occupational, or other important areas of functioning.

This is the classical functional disorder of episodic memory. It does not involve procedural memory or problems in memory storage, as in Wernicke-Korsakoff syndrome. Dissociative amnesia is reversible, for example, by using hypnosis. It has three primary characteristics:

1. *Type of memory lost.* The memory loss is episodic. The first-person recollection of certain events, rather than knowledge of procedures, is lost.

2. *Temporal structure.* The memory loss is for one or more discrete time periods, ranging from minutes to years. It is not vagueness or inefficient retrieval of memories but rather a dense unavailability of memories that were encoded and stored. Unlike the situation in amnestic disorders, for example, resulting from damage to the medial temporal lobe in surgery, or that in Wernicke-Korsakoff syndrome, there is usually no difficulty in learning new episodic information. Thus, the amnesia is typically retrograde rather than anterograde. However, a dissociative syndrome of continuous difficulty in incorporating new information that mimics organic amnestic syndromes has been observed.

3. *Type of events forgotten.* The memory loss is usually for events of a traumatic or stressful nature. This fact has been noted in the language of the *Diagnostic and Statistical Manual of Mental Disorders,* Fourth Edition (DSM-IV) diagnostic criteria. In one study, the majority of cases involved child abuse (60%), but disavowed behavior such as marital problems, sexual activity, suicide attempts, criminal activity, and the death of a relative have also been reported as precipitants.

Dissociative amnesia most frequently occurs after an episode of trauma, and its onset may be gradual or sudden, most often in the third and fourth decades of life. It usually involves one episode, but multiple periods of lost memory are not uncommon. Comorbidity with conversion disorder, bulimia nervosa, alcohol abuse, and depression are common, and Axis II diagnoses of histrionic, dependent, or borderline personality disorders occur in a substantial minority of such patients.

Although information is kept out of consciousness in dissociative amnesia, it may well exert an influence on consciousness. For example, a rape victim with no conscious recollection of the assault nonetheless may behave like someone who has been sexually victimized.

Individuals with dissociative amnesia generally do not suffer disturbances of identity, except to the extent that their identity is influenced by the warded-off memory. It is not uncommon for such individuals to develop depressive symptoms as well, especially when the amnesia occurs in the wake of a traumatic stressor.

Some cases of dissociative amnesia revert spontaneously. In most cases, the amnesia can be breached by using techniques such as hypnosis. Most patients with dissociative disorder are highly hypnotizable on formal testing and are therefore easily able to make use of techniques such as age regression. Hypnosis can enable such patients to reorient temporally and therefore achieve access to otherwise dissociated and unavailable memories.

The psychotherapy of dissociative amnesia involves accessing the dissociated memories, working through affectively loaded aspects of these memories, and supporting the patient through the process of integrating these memories into consciousness.

DISSOCIATIVE FUGUE

DSM-IV Criteria 300.13

Dissociative Fugue

A. The predominant disturbance is sudden, unexpected travel away from home or one's customary place of work, with inability to recall one's past.

B. Confusion about personal identity or assumption of new identity (partial or complete).

Box continued on following page

DSM-IV Criteria 300.13

Dissociative Fugue *Continued*

C. The disturbance does not occur exclusively during the course of dissociative identity disorder and is not due to the direct physiological effects of a substance (e.g., a drug of abuse, a medication) or a general medical condition (e.g., temporal lobe epilepsy).

D. The symptoms cause clinically significant distress or impairment in social, occupational, or other important areas of functioning.

In dissociative fugue failure to integrate certain aspects of personal memory is combined with loss of customary identity and automatisms of motor behavior. It involves one or more episodes of sudden, unexpected, purposeful travel away from home, coupled with an inability to recall portions or all of one's past and a loss of identity or the assumption of a new identity. The onset is usually sudden, and it frequently occurs after a traumatic experience or bereavement. A single episode is not uncommon, and spontaneous remission of symptoms can occur without treatment.

Many cases of dissociative fugue remit spontaneously. Again, hypnosis can be useful in accessing dissociated material.

Patients with dissociative fugue may be helped with a psychotherapeutic approach that facilitates conscious integration of dissociated memories and motivations for behavior previously experienced as automatic and unwilled. It is often helpful to address current psychosocial stressors, such as marital conflict, with the involved individuals. To the extent that current psychosocial stress triggers fugue, resolution of that stress can help resolve it and reduce the likelihood of recurrence.

In the past, sodium amobarbital or other short-acting sedatives were used to reverse dissociative amnesia or fugue. However, such techniques offer no advantage over hypnosis and are not especially effective. Not infrequently, the ceremony of injecting the drug elicits spontaneous hypnotic phenomena before the pharmacological effect is felt, and sedation, respiratory depression, and other side effects can be troublesome.

DEPERSONALIZATION DISORDER

DSM-IV Criteria 300.6

Depersonalization Disorder

A. Persistent or recurrent experiences of feeling detached from, and as if one is an outside observer of, one's mental processes or body (e.g., feeling like one is in a dream).

B. During the depersonalization experience, reality testing remains intact.

C. The depersonalization causes clinically significant distress or impairment in social, occupational, or other important areas of functioning.

D. The depersonalization experience does not occur exclusively during the course of another mental disorder, such as schizophrenia, panic disorder, acute stress disorder, or another dissociative disorder, and is not due to the direct physiological effects of a substance (e.g., a drug of abuse, a medication) or a general medical condition (e.g., temporal lobe epilepsy).

This dissociative disorder involves lack of integration of one or more components of perception. The essential feature of depersonalization disorder is the occurrence of persistent feelings of unreality, detachment, or estrangement from oneself or one's body, usually with the feeling that one is an outside observer of one's own mental processes. Individuals suffering depersonalization are distressed by it. They are aware of some distortion in their perceptual experience and therefore are not hallucinating or delusional. Affected individuals often fear that they are "going crazy." The symptom is not infrequently transient.

Recurrent or persistent depersonalization should be thought of both as a symptom in itself and as a component of other syndromes requiring treatment, such as anxiety disorders and schizophrenia. The symptom itself may respond to training in self-hypnosis. Other relaxation techniques such as systematic desensitization, progressive muscle relaxation, and biofeedback may also be of help. Psychotherapy aimed at working through emotional responses to any traumatic or other stressors that tend to elicit the depersonalization is also helpful.

DISSOCIATIVE IDENTITY DISORDER (MULTIPLE PERSONALITY DISORDER)

DSM-IV Criteria 300.14

Dissociative Identity Disorder

A. The presence of two or more distinct identities or personality states (each with its own relatively enduring pattern of perceiving, relating to, and thinking about the environment and self).

B. At least two of these identities or personality states recurrently take control of the person's behavior.

Box continued on following page

DSM-IV Criteria 300.14

Dissociative Identity Disorder *Continued*

C. Inability to recall important personal information that is too extensive to be explained by ordinary forgetfulness.

D. The disturbance is not due to the direct physiological effects of a substance (e.g., blackouts or chaotic behavior during alcohol intoxication) or a general medical condition (e.g., complex partial seizures).
Note: In children, the symptoms are not attributable to imaginary playmates or other fantasy play.

Dissociative identity disorder (DID) is diagnosed in childhood with increasing frequency but typically emerges between adolescence and the third decade of life; it rarely presents as a new disorder after 40 years of age, but there is often considerable delay between initial symptom presentation and diagnosis.

Untreated, it is a chronic and recurrent disorder that rarely remits spontaneously, but the symptoms may not be evident for certain time periods. DID has been called "a disease of hiddenness." The dissociation itself hampers self-monitoring and accurate reporting of symptoms and history. Many patients with the disorder are not fully aware of the extent of their dissociative symptoms. They may be reluctant to bring up symptoms because of confusion or shame about the illness or because they encountered previous skepticism. Furthermore, because the majority of patients report histories of sexual and physical abuse, the shame associated with that and fear of retribution may inhibit reporting of symptoms as well.

The major comorbid psychiatric illnesses are the depressive disorders, substance use disorders, and borderline personality disorder. Sexual, eating, and sleep disorders co-occur less commonly. Such patients frequently display self-mutilative behavior, impulsiveness, and overvaluing and devaluing of relationships. Many such patients also meet criteria for posttraumatic stress disorder (PTSD), with intrusive flashbacks, recurrent dreams of physical and sexual abuse, avoidance of and loss of pleasure in usually pleasurable activities, and symptoms of hyperarousal, especially when exposed to reminders of childhood trauma.

Treatment

It is possible to help DID patients to gain control over the dissociative process underlying their symptoms in several ways. The fundamental psychotherapeutic stance should involve meeting patients halfway, a form of structured empathy in which their experience of themselves as fragmented is acknowledged while the reality that the fundamental problem is a failure of integration of disparate memories and aspects of the self is kept in view. In this sense, such individuals suffer from having less than one personality rather than more than one. Therefore, the goal in therapy is to facilitate integration of disparate elements.

TABLE 34–1	Stages of DID Therapy
Stage	**Technique**
Establishing treatment	Education, atmosphere of safety, instill confidence
Preliminary interventions	Confirm diagnosis, set limits, access dissociation with hypnosis
History gathering	Explore components of dissociative structure
Working through trauma	Grief work
Move toward integration	Enhance communication across dissociative states
Integration-resolution	Encourage development of integrated self
Learning coping skills	Help with life decisions and relationships
Solidification of gains	Transference examination
Follow-up	Maintenance

Adapted from Kluft RP: Multiple personality disorder. In Tasman A, Goldfinger SM (eds): American Psychiatric Press Review of Psychiatry. Volume 10. Washington, DC: American Psychiatric Press, 1991.

Because the loss of memory in DID is complex and chronic, its retrieval is likewise a more extended and integral part of the psychotherapeutic process. The therapy becomes an integrating experience of information sharing among disparate personality elements. Conceptualizing DID as a chronic PTSD, the psychotherapeutic strategy focuses on working through traumatic memories in addition to controlling the dissociation.

The therapeutic process can be thought of as a kind of grief work in which information retrieved from memory is reviewed, traumatic memories are put into perspective, and emotional expression is encouraged and worked through, thereby making it more possible to endure and disseminate the information as widely as possible among various parts of the patient's personality structure.

Given the intensity of the material that often emerges involving memories of sexual and physical abuse and sudden shifts in mental state accompanied by amnesia, the psychiatrist is called on to take a clear and structured role in managing the psychotherapy. Appropriate limits must be set concerning self-destructive or threatening behavior; agreements must be made regarding physical safety and treatment compliance; and other matters must be presented to the patient in such a way that dissociative ignorance is not an acceptable explanation for failure to live up to the agreements.

The stages of DID therapy are presented in Table 34–1. As with other dissociative disorders, there is little evidence that psychoactive drugs are of great help in reversing symptoms in DID.

Sexual Disorders

Sexual disorders are often clinically overlooked unless patients directly present with a sexual complaint. Both patients and psychiatrists, as citizens of a common general culture, initially experience discomfort about sexual matters. Patients are unaccustomed to verbalizing this aspect of their privacy and find it difficult to acknowledge sexual inadequacy. Psychiatrists fear not knowing how to help and are hesitant to risk feeling transient sexual excitement in a clinical setting.

Practicing psychiatrists cannot pretend that the problems of being a sexual person do not exist, however. The sexual disorders are a high-prevalence, high-incidence source of personal suffering. A sexual disorder is likely to affect almost every person at some time in the life cycle and often plays a role in the genesis of other psychiatric diagnoses. Patients assume that their psychiatrists know about sexual identity and function and frequently bring up their concerns during psychotherapy undertaken for other issues.

Human sexuality has seven psychological components: gender identity, orientation, intention, desire, arousal, orgasm, and emotional satisfaction. The first three components constitute sexual identity; sexual function comprises the second three; and emotional satisfaction derives from personal reflections on the first six (Table 35–1). The *Diagnostic and Statistical Manual of Mental Disorders,* Fourth Edition (DSM-IV) identifies impairments of five of these components as pathologic conditions. Variations in orientation and the failure to find ordinary sexual experience emotionally satisfying, although often the source of psychic pain for individuals and their families, are not designated as disorders.

SEXUAL DYSFUNCTIONS

Partner sexual behavior is an important means of establishing and reaffirming deep emotional attachments to others. The capacities to genuinely desire a partner and become aroused and attain orgasm when together are highly valued signs of personal sexual adequacy. They are also integral to placing the person in a position to experience the fullest physical expressions of love. Maintenance of desire, arousal, and orgasmic capacities tends to keep sexual behavior occurring regularly in an individual or a couple and often enables the couple to privately assume that they love and are loved. Dysfunctions are the most prevalent forms of sexual problems because the psychophysiology of sexual function is easily disrupted. However, they are also the most spontaneously changeable and the most treatable of the sexual problems.

TABLE 35–1	Components of Individual Sexual Life

Sexual Identity

Gender identity: the sense of the self as masculine or feminine

Orientation: the sex of others who are the object of the person's sexual and romantic predispositions

Intention: what a person wants to do to his or her partner during sexual behavior and what the person wants to have done to him or her by the partner

Sexual Function

Sexual desire: the fluctuating interest a person experiences about behaving sexually
Drive: biological aspects
Motive: psychological aspects
Wish: social aspects

Sexual arousal: the emotion of sexual excitement based on pelvic vasocongestion and autonomic arousal

Orgasm: the reflex sequence stimulated by high levels of arousal that creates a brief, intense physical pleasure and releases pelvic vasocongestion

Sexual Satisfaction

Private judgment that sexual behavior is pleasurable

DSM-IV DIAGNOSES

DSM-IV specifies three criteria for each sexual dysfunction. The first criterion describes the psychophysiological impairment (e.g., absence of sexual desire). The second and third criteria are the same for each impairment: the dysfunction causes marked distress or interpersonal difficulty, and the dysfunction is not better accounted for by another Axis I diagnosis. Table 35–2 lists the first criterion of each of the 12 sexual dysfunction diagnoses.

Diagnoses

DSM-IV Criteria 302.71

Hypoactive Sexual Desire Disorder

A. Persistently or recurrently deficient (or absent) sexual fantasies and desire for sexual activity. The judgment of deficiency or absence is made by the clinician, taking into account factors that affect sexual functioning, such as age and the context of the person's life.

B. The disturbance causes marked distress or interpersonal difficulty.

Box continued on following page

DSM-IV Criteria 302.71

Hypoactive Sexual Desire Disorder *Continued*

C. The sexual dysfunction is not better accounted for by another Axis I disorder (except another sexual dysfunction) and is not due exclusively to the direct physiological effects of a substance (e.g., a drug of abuse, a medication) or a general medical condition.

Specify type:

Lifelong type

Acquired type

Specify type:

Generalized type

Situational type

Specify:

Due to psychological factors

Due to combined factors

DSM-IV Criteria 302.79

Sexual Aversion Disorder

A. Persistent or recurrent extreme aversion to, and avoidance of, all (or almost all) genital sexual contact with a sexual partner.

B. The disturbance causes marked distress or interpersonal difficulty.

C. The sexual dysfunction is not better accounted for by another Axis I disorder (except another sexual dysfunction).

Specify type:

Lifelong type

Acquired type

Specify type:

Generalized type

Situational type

Specify:

Due to psychological factors

Due to combined factors

TABLE 35-2   Delineating Criteria of 12 Sexual Dysfunction Diagnoses

Sexual Desire Disorders	Sexual Arousal Disorders	Orgasmic Disorders	Sexual Pain Disorders
Hypoactive sexual desire disorder: persistently or recurrently deficient (or absent) sexual fantasies and desire for sexual activity Sexual aversion disorder: persistent or recurrent extreme aversion to, and avoidance of, all (or almost all) genital sexual contact with a sexual partner	Female sexual arousal disorder: persistent or recurrent inability to attain, or to maintain until completion of the sexual activity, an adequate lubrication-swelling response of sexual excitement Male erectile disorder: persistent or recurrent inability to attain, or to maintain until completion of the sexual activity, an adequate erection	Female orgasmic disorder: persistent or recurrent delay in, or absence of, orgasm after a normal sexual excitement phase Male orgasmic disorder: persistent or recurrent delay in, or absence of, orgasm after a normal sexual excitement phase during sexual activity Premature ejaculation: persistent or recurrent ejaculation with a minimal sexual stimulation before, on, or shortly after penetration and before the person wishes it	Dyspareunia: recurrent or persistent genital pain associated with sexual intercourse in either a male or a female Vaginismus: recurrent or persistent involuntary spasm of the musculature of the outer third of the vagina that interferes with sexual intercourse
Sexual Dysfunction due to a General Medical Condition:	**Substance-Induced Sexual Dysfunction:**	**Sexual Dysfunction Not Otherwise Specified:**	
any of the above-mentioned diagnoses must be judged to be exclusively due to the direct physiological effects of a medical condition	a sexual dysfunction that is fully explained by substance use in that it develops within a month of substance intoxication	for problems that do not meet the categories just described	

Two diagnoses are given to men and women whose desires for partner sexual behavior are deficient: hypoactive sexual desire disorder and sexual aversion disorder. The differences between the two revolve around the emotional intensity with which the patient avoids sexual behavior. When visceral anxiety, fear, or disgust is routinely felt as sexual behavior becomes a possibility, sexual aversion is diagnosed. Hypoactive sexual desire is far more frequently encountered than sexual aversion. These diagnoses, like all sexual dysfunctions, may be lifelong or may have been acquired after a period of ordinary fluctuations of sexual desire. Like all the sexual dysfunctions, acquired desire disorders may be partner specific (situational) or may occur with all subsequent partners (generalized).

Although sexual desire disorders have a broad range of etiological contributions, when the psychiatrist concludes that the patient's acquired generalized hypoactive sexual desire disorder is due to a medical condition, a medication, or a substance of abuse, the diagnosis is further elaborated to sexual dysfunction due to a general medical condition (e.g., hypoactive sexual desire disorder due to multiple sclerosis) or substance-induced sexual dysfunction.

DSM-IV Criteria

Sexual Dysfunction Due to . . . [Indicate the General Medical Condition]

A. Clinically significant sexual dysfunction that results in marked distress or interpersonal difficulty predominates in the clinical picture.

B. There is evidence from the history, physical examination, or laboratory findings that the sexual dysfunction is fully explained by the direct physiological effects of a general medical condition.

C. The disturbance is not better accounted for by another mental disorder (e.g., major depressive disorder).

Select code and term based on the predominant sexual dysfunction:

625.8 Female hypoactive sexual desire disorder due to . . . [indicate the general medical condition]: if deficient or absent, sexual desire is the predominant feature

608.89 Male hypoactive sexual desire disorder due to . . . [indicate the general medical condition]: if deficient or absent, sexual desire is the predominant feature

607.84 Male erectile disorder due to . . . [indicate the general medical condition]: if male erectile dysfunction is the predominant feature

625.0 Female dyspareunia due to . . . [indicate the general medical condition]: if pain associated with intercourse is the predominant feature

608.89 Male dyspareunia due to . . . [indicate the general medical condition]: if pain associated with intercourse is the predominant feature

625.8 Other female sexual dysfunction due to . . . [indicate the general medical condition]: if some other feature is predominant (e.g., orgasmic disorder) or no feature predominates

608.89 Other male sexual dysfunction due to . . . [indicate the general medical condition]: if some other feature is predominant (e.g., orgasmic disorder) or no feature predominates

Coding note: Include the name of the general medical condition on Axis I, e.g., 607.84 male erectile disorder due to diabetes mellitus; also code the general medical condition on Axis III.

DSM-IV Criteria

Substance-Induced Sexual Dysfunction

A. Clinically significant sexual dysfunction that results in marked distress or interpersonal difficulty predominates in the clinical picture.

B. There is evidence from the history, physical examination, or laboratory findings that the sexual dysfunction is fully explained by substance use as manifested by either (1) or (2):

   (1) the symptoms in criterion A developed during, or within a month of, substance intoxication

   (2) medication use is etiologically related to the disturbance

C. The disturbance is not better accounted for by a sexual dysfunction that is not substance induced. Evidence that the symptoms are better accounted for by a sexual dysfunction that is not substance induced might include the following: the symptoms precede the onset of the substance use or dependence (or medication use); the symptoms persist for a substantial period of time (e.g., about a month) after the cessation of intoxication, or are substantially in excess of what would be expected given the type or amount of the substance used or the duration of use; or there is other evidence that suggests the existence of an independent non-substance-induced sexual dysfunction (e.g., a history of recurrent non-substance-related episodes).

Box continued on following page

DSM-IV Criteria

Substance-Induced Sexual Dysfunction *Continued*

Note: This diagnosis should be made instead of a diagnosis of substance intoxication only when the sexual dysfunction is in excess of that usually associated with the intoxication syndrome and when the dysfunction is sufficiently severe to warrant independent clinical attention.

Code [specific substance]–induced sexual dysfunction:

(291.8 Alcohol; 292.89 Amphetamine [or Amphetamine-Like Substance]; 292.89 Cocaine; 292.89 Opioid; 292.89 Sedative, Hypnotic, or Anxiolytic; 292.89 Other [or Unknown] Substance)

Specify if:

With impaired desire

With impaired arousal

With impaired orgasm

With sexual pain

Specify if:

With onset during intoxication: if the criteria are met for intoxication with the substance and the symptoms develop during the intoxication syndrome.

The frequency of these last two diagnoses depends on the setting. In oncology settings, medical causes occur in high frequency. In drug rehabilitation programs, methodone maintenance is a common cause. In psychiatric settings, anger at a partner, loss of respect for the partner, hidden incompatibility of sexual identity between the self and the partner, an affair with a third partner, and negative parental transferences are the most common bases for hypoactive sexual desire disorder. When a major psychiatric illness, such as depression, is diagnosed, however, the desire disorder is often assumed to be related to what is inscribed in Axis I. This is often not correct; it is safer to assume that the two diagnoses are independently present. If the sexual problem improves as the depression does, it can then be reconsidered as merely another consequence of the depressed state.

Treatment

Sexual desire disorders have the reputation for being difficult to treat. This reputation is based on frequent failures of brief treatment approaches and, more important, on the realizations of psychiatrists about the serious psychosocial circumstances that often underlie these conditions.

Patients may be expected to do well when the psychiatrist correctly appraises the circumstances and has something meaningful to offer. For example, helping a couple resolve a marital dispute may return them to their usual normal sexual desire manifestations. However, for many individuals and couples, "doing well" may ultimately mean more calmly accepting the profound implications of continuing marital discord, infidelity, homosexuality, or other contributing factors.

PROBLEMS OF SEXUAL AROUSAL

The emotion synonymously referred to as sexual arousal or sexual excitement generates changes in respiration, pulse, and muscular tension as well as an increased blood flow to the genitals. This vasocongestion creates vaginal lubrication, clitoral tumescence, labial color changes, penile erection, testicular elevation, and penile color changes. How arousal is centrally coordinated in either sex remains unclarified. During lovemaking, men and women do not necessarily maintain or increase their arousal; rather, there is often a fluctuating intensity of arousal that is reflected in variations in vaginal wetness, penile turgidity, and other nongenital signs of arousal.

Female Sexual Arousal Disorder

DSM-IV Criteria 302.72

Female Sexual Arousal Disorder

A. Persistent or recurrent inability to attain, or to maintain until completion of the sexual activity, an adequate lubrication-swelling response of sexual excitement.

B. The disturbance causes marked distress or interpersonal difficulty.

C. The sexual dysfunction is not better accounted for by another Axis I disorder (except another sexual dysfunction) and is not due exclusively to the direct physiological effects of a substance (e.g., a drug of abuse, a medication) or a general medical condition.

Specify type:

Lifelong type

Acquired type

Specify type:

Generalized type

Situational type

Specify:

Due to psychological factors

Due to combined factors

Arousal problems usually present as diminished lubrication or painful intercourse. When these problems are not organic in origin, they often turn out to be understood as manifestations of a more basic sexual desire disorder.

Female sexual arousal disorder is usually an acquired diagnosis. Premenopausal women who are affected focus on the lack of moisture in the vagina or on their failure to be excited by the behaviors that previously and reliably brought pleasure. They have drive, motive, and wish but are enigmatically unable to sustain arousal. Something mental arises to distract them from their excitement during lovemaking. Therapy is focused, therefore, on the meaning of what preoccupies them. This often involves the dynamics of their current individual or partnered life or the influence of their past relationships on their present.

Male Erectile Disorder

DSM-IV Criteria 302.72

Male Erectile Disorder

A. Persistent or recurrent inability to attain, or to maintain until completion of the sexual activity, an adequate erection.

B. The disturbance causes marked distress or interpersonal difficulty.

C. The erectile dysfunction is not better accounted for by another Axis I disorder (other than a sexual dysfunction) and is not due exclusively to the direct physiological effects of a substance (e.g., a drug of abuse, a medication) or a general medical condition.

Specify type:

Lifelong type

Acquired type

Specify type:

Generalized type

Situational type

Specify:

Due to psychological factors

Due to combined factors

The prevalence of erectile dysfunction rises dramatically in the sixth decade of life, from less than 10% to 30%; it increases further during the seventh decade. The cardiovascular risk factors predict the most common pattern of organic erectile dysfunction in this age group.

Men in their 50s and older may have a (psychogenic) male erectile disorder, but this diagnosis is difficult to make unless the man has reliably present firm erections under some circumstances. At any age, selectivity of erectile failure is the single most important diagnostic feature of the diagnosis.

Lifelong male erectile disorder typically involves either a sexual identity dilemma—such as transvestism, transsexualism, homo-erotic orientation, or paraphilia—or another diagnosis that expresses the patient's fear of being sexually close to a partner. Sexual identity problems are often initially denied unless the psychiatrist is nonjudgmentally thorough during the inquiry.

With the exception of anxious beginners, men with lifelong male arousal disorder, when taken into individual therapy, are usually perceived as having a strong motive to avoid sexual behavior and, although dysfunctional with a partner, during much of their therapy might equally be diagnosed as having hypoactive sexual desire with normal drive but a motive to avoid partner sex. The prognosis with older men with lifelong erectile dysfunction is poor. Long-term therapy, even if it does not result in regular intercourse, may enable more emotional and sexual closeness to a partner.

In dramatic contrast, men with long-established good potency who recently lost their erectile capacities with their partner—acquired psychogenic male erectile disorder—have a far better prognosis. They may be treated in an individual or couples format, depending on the precipitants of the sexual problem and the status of their relationship with their partner.

Regardless of the precipitating factors, however, men with arousal disorders have performance anxiety. Performance anxiety has two faces: the anticipation of erectile failure before sex begins and the vigilant preoccupation with monitoring the state of tumescence during it. Performance anxiety is present in almost all impotent men, including those with organic and lifelong psychogenic impotence, but it plays a larger role in preventing recovery among the acquired types. Performance anxiety is efficiently addressed by identifying it for the patient and asking him to make love without trying intercourse on several occasions to demonstrate to himself how different lovemaking can feel for him when he is not risking failure. This enables many to relax, concentrate on sensation, and return to previous states of sensual abandon during lovemaking. This technique is known as sensate focus.

PROBLEMS WITH ORGASM

Female Orgasmic Disorder

DSM-IV Criteria 302.73

Female Orgasmic Disorder

A. Persistent or recurrent delay in, or absence of, orgasm following a normal sexual excitement phase. Women exhibit wide variability in the type or intensity of stimulation that triggers orgasm. The diagnosis of female orgasmic disorder should be based on the clinician's judgment that the woman's orgasmic capacity is less than would be reasonable for her age, sexual experience, and the adequacy of sexual stimulation she receives.

Box continued on following page

DSM-IV Criteria 302.73

Female Orgasmic Disorder *Continued*

B. The disturbance causes marked distress or interpersonal difficulty.

C. The orgasmic dysfunction is not better accounted for by another Axis I disorder (except another sexual dysfunction) and is not due exclusively to the direct physiological effects of a substance (e.g., a drug of abuse, a medication) or a general medical condition.

Specify type:

Lifelong type

Acquired type

Specify type:

Generalized type

Situational type

Specify:

Due to psychological factors

Due to combined factors

The lifelong generalized variety of female orgasmic disorder is recognized when a woman has never been able to attain orgasm alone or with a partner by any means, although she is regularly aroused. When a woman can readily attain orgasm only during masturbation, she is diagnosed as having the lifelong situational variety. Women with any form of lifelong female orgasmic disorder more clearly have conflicts about personal sexual expression due to fear, guilt, ignorance, or obedience to tradition than do those with the acquired variety. Women who can masturbate to orgasm often feel fear and embarrassment about sharing their private arousal with any other person.

The acquired varieties of this disorder are more common and are characterized by complete anorgasmia, too-infrequent orgasms, and too-difficult orgasmic attainment. Antidepressant medications, particularly serotoninergic antidepressants, are the most common new source of this dysfunction and are usually dealt with by lowering the dose or switching to another antidepressant of a different class. When medications are not the cause of an acquired female orgasmic disorder, the psychiatrist needs to assess carefully the meaning of the changes in the patient's life before the onset of the disorder. Both individual and couples psychotherapy are helpful in orgasmic disorders.

Premature Ejaculation

DSM-IV Criteria 302.75

Premature Ejaculation

A. Persistent or recurrent ejaculation with minimal sexual stimulation before, on, or shortly after penetration and before the person wishes it. The clinician must take into account factors that affect duration of the excitement phase, such as age, novelty of the sexual partner or situation, and recent frequency of sexual activity.

B. The disturbance causes marked distress or interpersonal difficulty.

C. The premature ejaculation is not due exclusively to the direct effects of a substance (e.g., withdrawal from opioids).

Specify type:

Lifelong type

Acquired type

Specify type:

Generalized type

Situational type

Specify:

Due to psychological factors

Due to combined factors

Premature ejaculation is a high-prevalence (25% to 40%) disorder seen primarily in heterosexuals, characterized by an untameably low threshold for the reflex sequence of orgasm. The problem, a physiological efficiency of sperm delivery, causes social and psychological distress.

The range of intravaginal containment times among self-diagnosed patients extends from immediately before or on vaginal entry (rare), to less than a minute (usual), to less than the man and his partner desire (not infrequent). Time alone is a misleading indicator, however. The essence of the self-diagnosis is an emotionally unsatisfying sexual equilibrium apparently due to the man's inability to temper his arousal.

There are three efficient approaches to this dysfunction: thoughtful discussion and refusal to confirm the rapid ejaculation as a dysfunction, serotoninergic medications, and focused psychotherapy.

Male Orgasmic Disorder

DSM-IV Criteria 302.74

Male Orgasmic Disorder

A. Persistent or recurrent delay in, or absence of, orgasm following a normal sexual excitement phase during sexual activity that the clinician, taking into account the person's age, judges to be adequate in focus, intensity, and duration.

B. The disturbance causes marked distress or interpersonal difficulty.

C. The orgasmic dysfunction is not better accounted for by another Axis I disorder (except another sexual dysfunction) and is not due exclusively to the direct physiological effects of a substance (e.g., a drug of abuse, a medication) or a general medical condition.

Specify type:

Lifelong type

Acquired type

Specify type:

Generalized type

Situational type

Specify:

Due to psychological factors

Due to combined factors

When a man can readily attain a lasting erection with a partner yet is consistently unable to attain orgasm in the vagina, he is diagnosed as having a male orgasmic disorder. The disorder has three levels of severity:

1. The most common form is characterized by the ability to attain orgasm with a partner outside of her body, either through oral, manual, or personal masturbation.

2. The more severe form is characterized by the man's inability to ejaculate in his partner's presence.

3. The rarest and most severe form is characterized by the inability to ejaculate when awake.

The disorder rarely is lifelong, but it is usually generalized—that is, it is not partner specific. Some of these men get better with therapy; others improve spontaneously with time; and for others, the dysfunction leads to the cessation of the aspiration for sex with a partner.

SEXUAL PAIN DISORDERS

The psychiatrist needs to consider a series of questions when dealing with a woman who reports painful intercourse. Does she have a known gynecological abnormality that is generally associated with pain? Is there anything about her complaint of pain that indicates a remarkably low pain threshold? Does she have an aversion to sexual intercourse now? At what level of physical discomfort did she develop the aversion? Does her private view of her current relationship affect her willingness to be sexual and her experience of pain? Does her partner's sexual style cause her physical or mental discomfort—for example, is he overly aggressive or does he stimulate memories of former abuse? What has been the partner's response to her pain? What role does her anticipation of pain play in her experience of pain?

The DSM-IV presents dyspareunia and vaginismus as distinct entities. These entities, however, have been viewed as inextricably connected in much of the modern sexuality literature—vaginismus is known to create dyspareunia, and dyspareunia has been known to create vaginismus.

Dyspareunia

DSM-IV Criteria 302.76

Dyspareunia

A. Recurrent or persistent genital pain associated with sexual intercourse in either a male or a female.

B. The disturbance causes marked distress or interpersonal difficulty.

C. The disturbance is not caused exclusively by vaginismus or lack of lubrication, is not better accounted for by another Axis I disorder (except another sexual dysfunction), and is not due exclusively to the direct physiological effects of a substance (e.g., a drug of abuse, a medication) or a general medical condition.

Specify type:

Lifelong type

Acquired type

Specify type:

Generalized type

Situational type

Specify:

Due to psychological factors

Due to combined factors

Recurrent uncomfortable or painful intercourse is known as dyspareunia. Although it rarely occurs in men, the term is used for both men and women. Women's dyspareunia varies from discomfort at intromission to severe, unsparing pain during penile thrusting, to vaginal irritation after intercourse. In both sexes, recurring coital pain leads to inhibited arousal and sexual avoidance.

The term dyspareunia is used as both a symptom and a diagnosis. When coital pain is caused solely by a clear-cut organic pathologic condition, vaginismus, or insufficient lubrication, dyspareunia is considered merely a symptom. The diagnosis is made when psychogenic etiologies are thought to be responsible for the pain. Because the symptom of dyspareunia is produced by numerous organic conditions, the psychiatrist should be certain that the patient has had a thorough pelvic examination by a physician equipped to assess a broad range of regional pathology.

Dyspareunia in men is usually organic in origin. Herpes, gonorrhea, prostatitis, and Peyronie's disease cause pain during intercourse. Remote trauma to the penis may cause penile chordee or bowing, which makes intercourse mechanically difficult and sometimes painful. Pain experienced on ejaculation can be a side effect of trazodone.

Vaginismus

DSM-IV Criteria 306.51

Vaginismus

A. Recurrent or persistent involuntary spasm of the musculature of the outer third of the vagina that interferes with sexual intercourse.

B. The disturbance causes marked distress or interpersonal difficulty.

C. The disturbance is not better accounted for by another Axis I disorder (e.g., somatization disorder) and is not due exclusively to the direct physiological effects of a general medical condition.

Specify type:

Lifelong type

Acquired type

Specify type:

Generalized type

Situational type

Specify:

Due to psychological factors

Due to combined factors

Vaginismus is an involuntary spasm of the musculature of the outer third of the vagina, which makes penile penetration difficult or impossible. The diagnosis is not made if an organic cause is known. Early episodic vaginismus may be common among women, but most of the cases brought to medical attention are chronic. Lifelong vaginismus is relatively rare. The psychiatrist needs to focus attention on what may have made the idea of intercourse so overwhelming to the patient: parental intrusiveness, sexual trauma, childhood genital injury, illnesses whose therapy involved orifice penetration, surgery?

In the course of assisting women with these problems, a variety of techniques may be utilized, including relaxation techniques, sensate focus, dilatation, marital therapy, and medication. Short-term therapies should not be expected to have lasting good results because once the symptom is relieved, other problematical aspects of the patient's sexual equilibrium and nonsexual relationships often come into focus.

GENDER IDENTITY DISORDERS

The organization of a stable gender identity is the first component of sexual identity to emerge during childhood. The processes that enable this accomplishment are so subtle that when a daughter consistently acts as though she realizes that "I am a girl and that is all right," or when a son's behavior announces that "I am a boy and that is all right," families rarely even remember their children's statements and behaviors to the contrary. Adolescent and adult gender problems are not rare, but they are commonly hidden from social view or evolve into other, less dramatic forms of sexual identity.

The clarity of distinctions between hetero-, bi-, and homosexual orientations rests on the assumption that the sex and gender of the person and the partner are known. The DSM-IV suggests that adults with gender identity disorders simply be subgrouped according to which sex the patient is currently sexually attracted: males, females, both, or neither. This makes sense for most patients with gender identity disorder because it is their gender identity that is most important to them.

The treatment of any gender identity disorder begins after evaluating parents, other family members, and spouses, by psychometric testing, and occasionally, by physical and laboratory examination. The details depend on the age of the patient. It is possible, of course, to have a gender identity disorder as well as mental retardation, a psychosis, dysthymic disorder, severe character pathology, or any other psychiatric diagnosis. Table 35–3 presents a flow chart showing the stages in treatment for the profoundly gender disordered.

PARAPHILIAS

A paraphilia is a disorder of intention, the final component of sexual identity to develop in children and adolescents. Intention refers to what individuals want to do with a sexual partner and what they want the partner to do with them during sexual behavior. Normally, the images and the behaviors of intention fall within ranges of peaceable

TABLE 35–3	Steps in Evaluation of the Profoundly Gender Disordered*

Formal evaluation and diagnosis—gender identity disorder or gender identity disorder NOS. Can the patient be referred to a gender program? Is another treatable psychiatric or physical disorder present?

Individual psychotherapy within the gender program or with an interested professional. Do the diagnoses remain the same? If yes, does the patient consistently want to

Discuss his (or her) situation but make no changes?

Increase cross-dressing toward cross-living?

Prepare the family for the real-life test?

Obtain permission to proceed with hormones?

Approval for hormones from a gender committee or on written recommendation from the psychiatrist to an endocrinologist. Individual or group psychotherapy should continue.

Real-life test of living and working full time in the aspired-to gender role for at least 1 year. Does the patient want to continue to surgery?

Gender committee approval for surgery. Many patients have cosmetic surgery other than that listed with only ordinary patient-surgeon consent. This most often involves breast augmentation but may include numerous other attempts to improve ability to pass as opposite sex and be attractive.

Men—genital reconstruction

Women—mastectomy, hysterectomy, genital reconstruction

*Most patients will not complete all of these steps.

mutuality. The disorders of intention are recognized by unusual eroticism (images) and often socially destructive behaviors, such as sex with children, rape, exhibitionism, voyeurism, masochism, obscene phone calling, or sexual touching of strangers. Although 5% of the diagnoses of paraphilia are given to women, most etiological speculations refer to male sexual identity development gone awry. The prevalence of paraphilic behaviors is likely to be far less than that of paraphilic imagery, but the actual frequency in the population is at best a guess.

The sine qua non in the diagnosis of paraphilia is unusual, often hostile, dehumanized eroticism that has occupied the patient for most of adolescent and adult life. To be paraphilic means that erotic imagery exerts a pressure to play out an often imagined scene. In its milder forms, the pressure results merely in a preoccupation with a behavior. In its more intense forms, it is described as a drivenness to act out the fantasy in sexual behavior, usually in masturbation. A severe sexual dysfunction involving desire, arousal, or orgasm with a partner, although not invariably present among paraphilics, often is.

TREATMENT

The treatment of paraphilia involves four general approaches: evaluation only, psychotherapy, medications, and external controls. The psychiatrist is often called on to prescribe the approach.

Evaluation only is often selected when the psychiatrist concludes that the paraphilia is benign in terms of society, the patient will be resistant to the other approaches, and the patient does not suffer greatly in terms of social and vocational functioning in ways that might be improved.

Psychiatrists need to be realistic about the limitations of various therapeutic ventures. Sexual acting out may readily continue during therapy beyond the awareness of the therapist: the more violent and destructive the paraphilic behavior to others, the less the psychiatrist should risk ambulatory treatment. Because paraphilia occurs in patients with other psychiatric conditions, the psychiatrist needs to remain vigilant in keeping the treatment program comprehensive and not lose sight of the paraphilia just because the depressive or compulsive symptoms are improved. Paraphilia may be improved by medications and psychotherapy, but the psychiatrist should expect that the intention disorder is the patient's lasting vulnerability.

Eating Disorders

ANOREXIA NERVOSA

Anorexia Nervosa

A. Refusal to maintain body weight at or above a minimally normal weight for age and height (e.g., weight loss leading to maintenance of body weight less than 85% of that expected; or failure to make expected weight gain during period of growth, leading to body weight less than 85% of that expected).

B. Intense fear of gaining weight or becoming fat, even though underweight.

C. Disturbance in the way in which one's body weight or shape is experienced, undue influence of body weight or shape on self-evaluation, or denial of the seriousness of the current low body weight.

D. In postmenarcheal females, amenorrhea, i.e., the absence of at least three consecutive menstrual cycles. (A woman is considered to have amenorrhea if her periods occur only following hormone, e.g., estrogen administration.)

Specify type:

Restricting type: during the current episode of anorexia nervosa, the person has not regularly engaged in binge-eating or purging behavior (i.e., self-induced vomiting or the misuse of laxatives, diuretics, or enemas)

Binge-eating/purging type: during the current episode of anorexia nervosa, the person has regularly engaged in binge-eating or purging behavior (i.e., self-induced vomiting or the misuse of laxatives, diuretics, or enemas)

The *Diagnostic and Statistical Manual of Mental Disorders,* Fourth Edition (DSM-IV) criteria require the individual to be significantly underweight for age and height. Although it is not possible to set a single weight loss standard that applies equally to all individuals, DSM-IV provides a benchmark of 85% of the weight considered normal for age and height as a guideline. Despite their abnormally low body weight, individuals with anorexia nervosa are intensely afraid of gaining weight and becoming fat, and remarkably, this fear typically intensifies as the weight falls.

Criterion C requires a disturbance in the person's judgment about his or her weight or shape. For example, despite being underweight, individuals with anorexia nervosa often view themselves or a part of their body as being too heavy.

DSM-IV suggests that individuals with anorexia nervosa be classed as having one of two variants, either the binge-eating/purging type or the restricting type. Individuals with the restricting type of anorexia nervosa do not engage regularly in either binge-eating or purging and, compared with individuals who have the binge-eating/purging form of the disorder, are not as likely to abuse alcohol and other drugs, exhibit less mood lability, and are less active sexually. There are also indications that the two subtypes may differ in their response to pharmacological intervention.

EPIDEMIOLOGY

Anorexia nervosa is a relatively rare illness. Even among high-risk groups, such as adolescent girls and young women, the prevalence of strictly defined anorexia nervosa is only about 0.5%. The prevalence rates of partial syndromes are substantially higher. Despite the infrequent occurrence of anorexia nervosa, most studies suggest that its incidence has increased significantly during the last 50 years, a phenomenon usually attributed to changes in cultural norms regarding desirable body shape and weight.

Anorexia nervosa usually affects women; the ratio of men to women is approximately 1:10 to 1:20. Anorexia nervosa occurs primarily in industrialized and affluent countries and, even within those countries, is more common among the higher socioeconomic classes. Anorexia nervosa appears more likely to develop in an environment with readily available food but in which, for women, being thin is somehow equated with higher or special achievement.

PATHOPHYSIOLOGY

An impressive array of physical disturbances has been documented in anorexia nervosa, and the physiological bases of many are understood (Table 36–1). Most of these physical disturbances appear to be secondary consequences of starvation, and it is not clear whether or how the physiological disturbances described here contribute to the development and maintenance of the psychological and behavioral abnormalities characteristic of anorexia nervosa.

DIAGNOSIS

In general, anorexia nervosa is not difficult to recognize. Uncertainty surrounding the diagnosis sometimes occurs in young adolescents, who may not clearly describe a drive for thinness and the fear of becoming fat. Rather, they may acknowledge only a vague concern about consuming certain foods and an intense desire to exercise. It can also be difficult to elicit the distorted view of shape and weight

TABLE 36–1	Medical Problems Commonly Associated with Anorexia Nervosa

Skin
  Lanugo
Cardiovascular system
  Hypotension
  Bradycardia
  Arrhythmias
Hematopoietic system
  Normochromic, normocystic anemia
  Leukopenia
    Diminished polymorphonuclear leukocytes
Fluid and electrolyte balance
  Elevated blood urea nitrogen and creatinine concentrations
  Hypokalemia
  Hyponatremia
  Hypochloremia
  Alkalosis
Gastrointestinal system
  Elevated serum concentration of liver enzymes
  Delayed gastric emptying
  Constipation
Endocrine system
  Diminished thyroxine level with normal thyroid-stimulating
    hormone level
  Elevated plasma cortisol level
  Diminished secretion of luteinizing hormone, follicle-
    stimulating hormone, estrogen, or testosterone
Bone
  Osteoporosis

(criterion C) in patients who have had anorexia nervosa for many years. Such individuals may state that they realize they are too thin and may make superficial efforts to gain weight, but they do not seem particularly concerned about the physical risks or deeply committed to increasing their calorie consumption.

Assessment

In assessing individuals who may have anorexia nervosa, it is important to obtain a weight history, including the individual's highest and lowest weights and the weight he or she would like to be now. For women, it is useful to know the weight at which menstruation last occurred, because it provides an indication of what weight is normal for that individual. The patient should be asked to describe a typical day's food intake and any food restrictions and dietary practices, such as vegetarianism. The psychiatrist should ask whether the patient ever loses control over eating and engages in binge-eating and, if so, the amounts and types of food eaten during such episodes. The use of self-induced vomiting, laxatives, diuretics, enemas, diet pills, and syrup of ipecac to induce vomiting should also be queried.

Probably the greatest problem in the assessment of patients with anorexia nervosa is their denial of the illness and their reluctance to participate in an evaluation. A straightforward but supportive and nonconfrontational style is probably the most useful approach, but it is likely that the patient will not acknowledge significant difficulties in eating or weight and will rationalize unusual eating or exercise habits. It is therefore helpful to obtain information from other sources, such as the patient's family.

PHYSICAL EXAMINATION AND LABORATORY FINDINGS

The patient should be weighed, or a current weight should be obtained from the patient's general physician. Blood pressure, pulse, and body temperature are often below the lower limit of normal. On physical examination, lanugo, a fine, downy hair normally seen in infants, may be present on the back or the face. The extremities are frequently cold and have a slight red-purple color (acrocyanosis). Edema is rarely observed at the initial presentation but may develop transiently during the initial stages of refeeding.

Common findings are a mild to moderate normochromic, normocytic anemia and leukopenia, with a deficit in polymorphonuclear leukocytes leading to a relative lymphocytosis. Elevations of blood urea nitrogen and serum creatinine concentrations may occur because of dehydration, which can also artificially elevate the hemoglobin and hematocrit. A variety of electrolyte abnormalities may be observed, reflecting the state of hydration and the history of vomiting as well as diuretic and laxative abuse. Serum levels of liver enzymes are usually normal but may transiently increase during refeeding. Cholesterol levels may be elevated.

The electrocardiogram typically shows sinus bradycardia and, occasionally, low QRS voltage and a prolonged QT interval; a variety of arrhythmias have also been described.

Differential Diagnosis

A wide variety of medical problems cause serious weight loss in young people and may at times be confused with anorexia nervosa. Examples of such problems include gastric outlet obstruction, Crohn's disease, and brain tumors. Individuals whose weight loss is due to a general medical illness usually do not show the drive for thinness, the fear of gaining weight, and the increased physical activity characteristic of anorexia nervosa.

COURSE AND NATURAL HISTORY

Most of the literature on course and outcome is based on individuals who have been hospitalized for anorexia nervosa. Whereas such individuals presumably have a relatively severe illness and adverse outcomes, a substantial fraction, probably between one third and one half, make full and complete psychological and physical recoveries.

On the other hand, anorexia nervosa is also associated with an impressive long-term mortality. The best data currently available suggest that 10% to 20% of patients who have been hospitalized for anorexia nervosa will, in the next 10 to 30 years, die as a result of their illness. Much of the mortality is due to severe and chronic starvation, which eventually terminates in sudden death. In addition, a significant fraction of patients commit suicide.

It is difficult to specify factors that account for the variability of outcome in anorexia nervosa. A significant body of experience suggests that the illness has a better prognosis when it begins in adolescence, but there are also suggestions that prepubertal onset may portend a difficult course. It is likely that the severity of the illness (e.g., the lowest weight reached, the number of hospitalizations) and the presence of associated symptoms, such as binge-eating and purging, also contribute to poor outcome. However, it is impossible to predict course and outcome in an individual with any certainty.

GOALS OF TREATMENT

The first goal of treatment is to engage the patient and her or his family. For most patients with anorexia nervosa, this is challenging. Patients usually minimize their symptoms and suggest that the concerns of family and friends, who have often been instrumental in arranging the consultation, are greatly exaggerated. It is helpful to identify a problem that the patient can acknowledge, such as weakness, irritability, difficulty concentrating, or trouble with binge-eating. The psychiatrist may then attempt to educate the patient regarding the pervasive physical and psychological effects of semistarvation and about the need for weight gain if the acknowledged problem is to be successfully addressed.

A second goal of treatment is to assess and address acute medical problems, such as fluid and electrolyte disturbances and cardiac arrhythmias. Depending on the severity of illness, this may require the involvement of a general medical physician.

The additional but most difficult and time-consuming goals are the restoration of normal body weight, the normalization of eating, and the resolution of the associated psychological disturbances. The final goal is the prevention of relapse.

A large percentage of patients with anorexia nervosa remain chronically ill: 30% to 50% of patients successfully treated in the hospital require rehospitalization within 1 year of discharge. Therefore, posthospitalization outpatient treatments are recommended by most psychiatrists to prevent relapse and improve overall short- and long-term functioning. Several studies have attempted to evaluate the efficacy of various outpatient treatments for anorexia nervosa, including behavioral, cognitive-behavioral, and supportive psychotherapy as well as a variety of nutritional counseling interventions. Whereas most of these treatments seem to be helpful, the clearest finding to date is that family therapy is effective for patients whose anorexia nervosa started before age 18 years and who have had the disorder for less than 3 years.

BULIMIA NERVOSA

DSM-IV Criteria 307.51

Bulimia Nervosa

A. Recurrent episodes of binge-eating. An episode of binge-eating is characterized by both of the following:

   (1) eating, in a discrete period of time (e.g., within any 2-hour period), an amount of food that is definitely larger than most people would eat during a similar period of time and under similar circumstances

   (2) a sense of lack of control over eating during the episode (e.g., a feeling that one cannot stop eating or control what or how much one is eating)

B. Recurrent inappropriate compensatory behavior in order to prevent weight gain, such as self-induced vomiting; misuse of laxatives, diuretics, enemas, or other medications; fasting; or excessive exercise.

C. The binge-eating and inappropriate compensatory behaviors both occur, on average, at least twice a week for 3 months.

D. Self-evaluation is unduly influenced by body shape and weight.

E. The disturbance does not occur exclusively during episodes of anorexia nervosa.

Specify type:

Purging type: during the current episode of bulimia nervosa, the person has regularly engaged in self-induced vomiting or the misuse of laxatives, diuretics, or enemas

Nonpurging type: during the current episode of bulimia nervosa, the person has used other inappropriate compensatory behaviors, such as fasting or excessive exercise, but has not regularly engaged in self-induced vomiting or the misuse of laxatives, diuretics, or enemas

The salient behavioral disturbance of bulimia nervosa is the occurrence of binge-eating episodes. During these episodes, the individual consumes an unusually large amount of food considering the circumstances under which it was eaten. Although this is a useful definition and conceptually reasonably clear, it can be operationally difficult to distinguish normal overeating from a small episode of binge-eating. Indeed, the available data do not suggest that there is a sharp dividing line between the size of binge-eating episodes and the size of other meals. On the other hand, whereas the border between normal and abnormal eating may not be a sharp one, both patients' reports and laboratory studies of eating behavior clearly indicate that, when binge-eating, patients with bulimia nervosa do indeed consume larger than normal amounts of food.

Episodes of binge-eating are associated, by definition, with a sense of loss of control. Once the eating has begun, the individual feels unable to stop until an excessive amount has been consumed. This loss of control is only subjective, in that most individuals with bulimia nervosa will abruptly stop eating in the midst of a binge episode if interrupted.

After overeating, individuals with bulimia nervosa engage in some form of inappropriate behavior in an attempt to avoid weight gain. Most patients who present to eating disorders clinics with this syndrome report self-induced vomiting or the abuse of laxatives. Other methods include misusing diuretics, fasting for long periods, and exercising extensively after eating binges.

In the DSM-IV nomenclature, the diagnosis of bulimia nervosa is not given to individuals with anorexia nervosa. Individuals with anorexia nervosa who recurrently engage in binge-eating or purging behavior should be given the diagnosis of anorexia nervosa, binge-eating/purging subtype, rather than an additional diagnosis of bulimia nervosa.

EPIDEMIOLOGY

Careful studies have found that whereas binge-eating is frequent, the full-blown disorder of bulimia nervosa is much less common, probably affecting 1% to 4% of young women in the United States. Although sufficient research data do not exist to pinpoint specific epidemiological trends in the occurrence of bulimia nervosa, research suggests that women born after 1960 have a higher risk for the illness than those born before 1960.

Among patients with bulimia nervosa who are seen at eating disorders clinics, there is an increased frequency of anxiety and mood disorders, especially major depressive disorder and dysthymic disorder; of drug and alcohol abuse; and of personality disorders. It is not certain whether this comorbidity is also observed in community samples or whether it is a characteristic of individuals who seek treatment. Bulimia nervosa primarily affects women; the ratio of men to women is approximately 1:10.

PATHOPHYSIOLOGY

Bulimia nervosa is associated with the development of fluid and electrolyte abnormalities that result from the self-induced vomiting or the misuse of laxatives or diuretics. The most common electrolyte disturbances are hypokalemia, hyponatremia, and hypochloremia. Patients who lose substantial amounts of stomach acid through vomiting may become slightly alkalotic; those who abuse laxatives may become slightly acidic.

There is an increased frequency of menstrual disturbances such as oligomenorrhea among women with bulimia nervosa.

Patients who induce vomiting for many years may develop dental erosion, especially of the upper front teeth. Some patients develop painless salivary gland enlargement, which is thought to represent hypertrophy resulting from the repeated episodes of binge-eating and vomiting. The serum level of amylase is sometimes mildly elevated in patients with bulimia nervosa because of increased amounts of salivary amylase.

Potentially life-threatening complications such as an esophageal tear or gastric rupture occur, but fortunately rarely.

The long-standing use of syrup of ipecac to induce vomiting can lead to absorption of some of the alkaloids and to permanent damage to nerve and muscle.

DIAGNOSIS

Bulimia nervosa typically begins after a young woman who sees herself as somewhat overweight starts a diet and, after some initial success, begins to overeat. Distressed by her lack of control and by her fear of gaining weight, she decides to compensate for the overeating by inducing vomiting or taking laxatives.

The binge-eating tends to occur in the late afternoon or evening and almost always while the patient is alone. The typical patient presenting to clinics for eating disorders has been binge-eating and inducing vomiting 5 to 10 times weekly for 3 to 10 years. Although there is substantial variation, binges tend to contain 1000 or more calories and to consist of sweet, high-fat foods that are normally consumed for dessert, such as ice cream, cookies, and cake.

Assessment

The assessment of individuals who may have bulimia nervosa is similar to that described for anorexia nervosa. The interviewer should explicitly inquire about self-induced vomiting and whether syrup of ipecac is ever used to promote vomiting. The interviewer should ask about the use of laxatives, diuretics, diet pills, and enemas. A weight history should be obtained, so the interviewer can determine whether the binge-eating was preceded by obesity or by anorexia nervosa, as is often the case. Because there is substantial comorbidity, the interviewer should ascertain whether there is a history of anxiety or mood disturbance or of substance abuse.

PHYSICAL EXAMINATION AND LABORATORY FINDINGS

The patient should be weighed and the presence of dental erosion noted. Routine laboratory testing reveals an abnormality of fluid and electrolyte balance such as those described in the section on pathophysiology in 25% to 50% of patients with bulimia nervosa.

Differential Diagnosis

Bulimia nervosa is not difficult to recognize if a full history is available. The binge-eating/purging type of anorexia nervosa has much in common with bulimia nervosa but is distinguished by the characteristic low body weight and, in women, amenorrhea.

Many individuals who believe they have bulimia nervosa fail to meet full diagnostic criteria because the frequency of their binge-eating is less than twice a week or because what they view as a binge does not contain an abnormally large amount of food. Individuals with these characteristics fall into the broad and heterogeneous category of atypical eating disorders. The term binge-eating disorder has been proposed for another atypical eating disorder characterized by recurrent binge-eating similar to that seen in bulimia nervosa but without the regular occurrence of inappropriate compensatory behavior.

COURSE AND NATURAL HISTORY

Perhaps because it was clearly recognized so recently, the natural history of bulimia nervosa is uncertain. In clinic samples, the eating disorder often appears to be chronic, with frequent fluctuations in symptom severity. On the other hand, some controlled clinical trials have reported that structured forms of psychotherapy have the potential to yield substantial and sustained recovery in a substantial fraction of patients who complete treatment. It is not clear what factors are most predictive of good outcome, but there are indications that those individuals who cease binge-eating and purging completely during treatment are least likely to relapse.

GOALS OF TREATMENT

The goals of the treatment of bulimia nervosa are straightforward. The binge-eating and inappropriate compensatory behaviors should cease, and self-esteem should become more appropriately based on factors other than shape and weight.

The treatment of bulimia nervosa has received considerable attention in recent years, and the efficacies of both psychotherapy and medication have been explored in numerous controlled studies. The form of psychotherapy that has been examined most intensively is cognitive-behavioral therapy, modeled on the therapy of the same type for depression. Although it was initially believed that cognitive-behavioral therapy was uniquely effective in the treatment of bulimia, it now appears that other forms of short-term structured psychotherapy, such as interpersonal therapy and supportive-expressive therapy, can also be effective.

The other commonly used mode of treatment that has been examined in bulimia nervosa is the use of antidepressant medication. This intervention was initially prompted by the high rates of depression among patients with bulimia nervosa. Most antidepressants appear to possess roughly similar antibulimic potency. Fluoxetine at a dose of up to 60 mg/d is favored by many investigators because it has been studied in several large trials and appears to be at least as effective as and better tolerated than most other alternatives. It is notable that it has not been possible to link the effectiveness of antidepressant treatment for bulimia nervosa to the pretreatment level of depression. Depressed and nondepressed patients with bulimia nervosa respond equally well in terms of their eating behavior to antidepressant medication.

SPECIAL FEATURES INFLUENCING TREATMENT

A major factor influencing the treatment of bulimia nervosa is the presence of other significant psychiatric or medical illness. For example, it can be difficult for individuals who are currently abusing drugs or alcohol to use the treatment methods described, and many psychiatrists suggest that the substance abuse needs to be addressed before the eating disorder can be effectively treated. Other examples include the treatment of individuals with bulimia nervosa and serious personality disturbance and those with insulin-dependent diabetes mellitus who "purge" by omitting insulin doses. In treating such individuals, the psychiatrist must decide which of the multiple problems must be addressed first and may elect to tolerate a significant level of eating disorder to confront more pressing disturbances. In nonresponsive patients, hospitalization should also be considered as a way to normalize eating behavior, at least temporarily, and perhaps to initiate a more effective outpatient treatment.

Sleep and Sleep-Wake Disorders

SLEEP DISORDERS

Sleep disorders usually take one of four forms: 1) insomnia, that is, subjectively insufficient, disturbed, or unrefreshing sleep; 2) excessive daytime sleepiness; 3) disturbances of the circadian sleep-wake cycle; and 4) abnormal behaviors or physiological events during sleep. By definition, the *Diagnostic and Statistical Manual of Mental Disorders,* Fourth Edition (DSM-IV) limits itself to chronic disorders (at least 1 month in duration). On the other hand, the *International Classification of Sleep Disorders* includes sleep disorders of short-term and intermediate duration, which in fact are more common than chronic disorders.

GENERAL APPROACH TO THE PATIENT WITH SLEEP DISORDER

Disorders of sleep and wakefulness are common. Insomnia complaints are reported by about one third of adult Americans during a 1-year period; clinically significant obstructive sleep apnea may be seen in as many as 10% of working, middle-aged men; and sleepiness is an underrecognized cause of dysphoria, automobile accidents, and mismanagement of patients by sleep-deprived physicians. Nearly all physicians will hear complaints of sleep problems. Psychiatrists may be even more likely than other medical specialists to receive these complaints. Of particular importance for mental disorders, prospective epidemiological studies suggest that persistent complaints of either insomnia or hypersomnia are risk factors for the later onset of depression, anxiety disorders, and substance abuse.

To assist the patient with a sleep complaint, the psychiatrist needs to have a diagnostic framework with which to obtain the information needed about the patient as a person and about his or her disorder. Two issues are particularly important:

1. How long has the patient had the sleep complaint? Transient insomnia and short-term insomnia, for example, usually occur in persons undergoing acute stress or other disruptions, such as admission to a hospital, jet lag, bereavement, or change in medications. Chronic sleep disorders, on the other hand, are often multidetermined and multifaceted.

2. Does the patient suffer from any preexisting or comorbid disorders? Does another condition cause the sleep complaint, modify a sleep complaint, or affect possible treatments? In general,

because common sleep disorders are frequently secondary to underlying causes, treatment should be directed at underlying medical, psychiatric, pharmacological, psychosocial, or other disorders.

A detailed history of the complaint and attendant symptoms must be obtained (Tables 37–1 and 37–2). Special attention should be given to the timing of sleep and wakefulness; qualitative and quantitative subjective measures of sleep and wakefulness; abnormal sleep-related behaviors; respiratory difficulties; medications or other substances affecting sleep, wakefulness, or arousal; expectations, concerns, attitudes about sleep, and efforts used by the patient to control symptoms; and the sleep-wake environment. The psychiatrist must be alert to the possibility that sleep complaints are somatic symptoms, which reflect individual ways of experiencing, expressing, and coping with psychosocial distress, stress, or psychiatric disorders.

TABLE 37–1	Office Evaluation of Chronic Sleep Complaints

Detailed history and review of the sleep complaint: predisposing, precipitating, and perpetuating factors

Review of difficulties falling asleep, maintaining sleep, and awakening early

Timing of sleep and wakefulness in the 24-h day

Evidence of excessive daytime sleepiness and fatigue

Bedtime routines, sleep setting, physical security, preoccupations, anxiety, beliefs about sleep and sleep loss, fears about consequences of sleep loss

Medical and neurological history and examination, routine laboratory examinations: look for obesity, short fat neck, enlarged tonsils, narrow upper oral airway, foreshortened jaw (retrognathia), and hypertension

Psychiatric history and examination

Use of prescription and nonprescription medications, alcohol, stimulants, toxins, insecticides, and other substances

Evidence of sleep-related breathing disorders: snoring, orthopnea, dyspnea, headaches, falling out of bed, nocturia

Abnormal movements or behaviors associated with sleep disorders: "jerky legs," leg movements, myoclonus, restless legs, leg cramps, cold feet, nightmares, enuresis, sleepwalking, epilepsy, bruxism, sleep paralysis, hypnagogic hallucinations, cataplexy, night sweats, and so on

Social and occupational history, marital status, living conditions, financial and security concerns, physical activity

Sleep-wake diary for 2 wk

Interview with bed partners or persons who observe patient during sleep

Tape recording of respiratory sounds during sleep to screen for sleep apnea

TABLE 37–2	Selected Disorders and Terms Used in Clinical Sleep Disorders Medicine
Term	**Definition**
Apnea index	Number of apneic events per hour of sleep; usually is considered pathological if ≥5.
Cataplexy	Sudden, brief loss of muscle tone in the waking stage, usually triggered by emotional arousal (laughing, anger, surprise), involving either a few muscle groups (i.e., facial) or most of major antigravity muscles of the body; may be related to muscle atonia normally occurring during REM sleep; is associated with narcolepsy.
Hypopnea	50% or more reduction in respiratory depth for 10 s or more during sleep.
Multiple Sleep Latency Test	An objective method for determining daytime sleepiness; sleep latency and REM latency are determined for four or five naps (i.e., a 20-min opportunity to sleep every 2 h between 10 AM and 6 PM; normal mean values are above 15 min.)
Periodic limb movements in sleep index	Number of leg kicks per hour of sleep; usually is considered pathological if ≥5.
Polysomnography	Describes detailed, sleep laboratory–based, clinical evaluation of patient with sleep disorder; may include electroencephalographical measures, eye movements, muscle tone at chin and limbs, respiratory movements of chest and abdomen, oxygen saturation, electrocardiogram, nocturnal penile tumescence, esophageal pH, as indicated.
Respiratory disturbance index	Number of apneas and hypopneas per hour of sleep.
Sleep apnea	Sleep-related breathing disorder characterized by at least five episodes of apnea per hour of sleep, each longer than 10 s in duration.

Sleep disorders vary with age and gender and, possibly, with culture and social class. The circadian timing of rest-activity, sleep duration at night, and daytime napping and sleepiness vary with age and gender. Sleep-wake patterns are also influenced by cultural or geographical factors, such as the siesta and late bedtime commonly associated with tropical climates, or the winter hypersomnia and summer hyposomnia said to occur near the Arctic Circle.

One approach to the differential diagnosis of persistent sleep disorders is suggested in the algorithm in Figure 37–1. First, determine whether the sleep complaint is due to another medical, psychiatric, or substance abuse disorder. Second, consider the role of circadian rhythm disturbances and sleep disorders associated with abnormal events predominantly during sleep. Finally, evaluate in greater detail complaints of insomnia (difficulty initiating or maintaining sleep) and excessive sleepiness.

The treatment approach is determined by the specific type of sleep disturbance. For example, patients with classic narcolepsy often

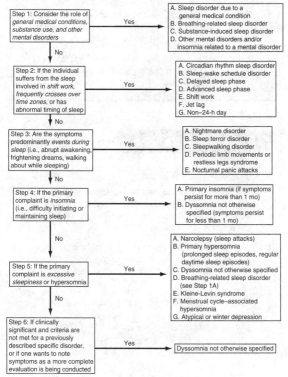

Figure 37–1 *An algorithm for the differential diagnosis of persistent sleep disorder complaints.*

respond partially to stimulants, such as pemoline, methylphenidate, or methamphetamine for the sleepiness, and to antidepressants for the cataplexy, which is part of the syndrome.

DSM-IV Criteria 307.42

Primary Insomnia

A. The predominant complaint is difficulty initiating or maintaining sleep, or nonrestorative sleep, for at least 1 month.

B. The sleep disturbance (or associated daytime fatigue) causes clinically significant distress or impairment in social, occupational, or other important areas of functioning.

C. The sleep disturbance does not occur exclusively during the course of narcolepsy, breathing-related sleep disorder, circadian rhythm sleep disorder, or a parasomnia.

D. The disturbance does not occur exclusively during the course of another mental disorder (e.g., major depressive disorder, generalized anxiety disorder, a delirium).

E. The disturbance is not due to the direct physiological effects of a substance (e.g., a drug of abuse, a medication) or a general medical condition.

DSM-IV Criteria 307.44

Primary Hypersomnia

A. The predominant complaint is excessive sleepiness for at least 1 month (or less if recurrent) as evidenced by either prolonged sleep episodes or daytime sleep episodes that occur almost daily.

B. The excessive sleepiness causes clinically significant distress or impairment in social, occupational, or other important areas of functioning.

C. The excessive sleepiness is not better accounted for by insomnia and does not occur exclusively during the course of another sleep disorder (e.g., narcolepsy, breathing-related sleep disorder, circadian rhythm sleep disorder, or a parasomnia) and cannot be accounted for by an inadequate amount of sleep.

D. The disturbance does not occur exclusively during the course of another mental disorder.

E. The disturbance is not due to the direct physiological effects of a substance (e.g., a drug of abuse, a medication) or a general medical condition.

Specify if:

Recurrent: if there are periods of excessive sleepiness that last at least 3 days occurring several times a year for at least 2 years

DSM-IV Criteria 347

Narcolepsy

A. Irresistible attacks of refreshing sleep that occur daily for at least 3 months.

B. The presence of one or both of the following:

(1) cataplexy (i.e., brief episodes of sudden bilateral loss of muscle tone, most often in association with intense emotion)

(2) recurrent intrusions of elements of REM sleep into the transition between sleep and wakefulness, as manifested by either hypnopompic or hypnagogic hallucinations or sleep paralysis at the beginning or end of sleep episodes

C. The disturbance is not due to the direct physiological effects of a substance (e.g., a drug of abuse, a medication) or another general medical condition.

DSM-IV Criteria 780.59

Breathing-Related Sleep Disorder

A. Sleep disruption, leading to excessive sleepiness or insomnia, that is judged to be due to a sleep-related breathing condition (e.g., obstructive or central sleep apnea syndrome or central alveolar hypoventilation syndrome).

B. The disturbance is not better accounted for by another mental disorder and is not due to the direct physiological effects of a substance (e.g., a drug of abuse, a medication) or another general medical condition (other than a breathing-related disorder).

Coding note: Also code sleep-related breathing disorder on Axis III.

Impulse Control
Disorders

Although dissimilar in behavioral expressions, impulse control disorders share the feature of impulse dyscontrol. Individuals who experience such dyscontrol are overwhelmed by the urge to commit certain acts that are often apparently illogical or harmful. The outcome of each of these behaviors is often harmful, either for the afflicted individual (e.g., trichotillomania, pathological gambling) or for others (e.g., intermittent explosive disorder, pyromania, kleptomania).

New research findings seem to associate various forms of impulsive behavior with biological markers of altered serotoninergic function. These include impulsive suicidal behavior, impulsive aggression, and impulsive fire setting. Impulsivity is also a focus of interest in the increasing attention paid to the behavioral phenomenology of borderline personality disorder. In all these circumstances, impulsivity is conceived of as the rapid expression of unplanned behavior, occurring in response to a sudden thought.

Although the sudden and unplanned aspect of the behavior may be present in the impulse disorders (e.g., intermittent explosive disorder and kleptomania), the primary connotation of the word impulsivity, as used to describe these conditions, is the irresistibility of the urge to act. In episodes of trichotillomania, pyromania, and pathological gambling, a sudden desire to commit the act of hair pulling, fire setting, or gambling may be followed by rapid expression of the behavior. But in these conditions, the individual may spend considerable amounts of time fighting off the urge, trying not to carry out the impulse. The inability to resist the impulse is the common core of these disorders, rather than the rapid transduction of thought to action. A decision tree for the differential diagnosis of impulsive behaviors may be seen in Figure 38–1.

High rates of comorbid mood disorder and anxiety disorder appear to be typical of these disorders. Although these conditions have historically been considered uncommon, later investigations suggest that some of them may be fairly prevalent. Trichotillomania, for example, was once considered rare. However, surveys indicate that the lifetime prevalence of the condition may exceed 1% of the population. Pathological gambling may be present in up to 3% of the population. Extrapolation from the known incidence of comorbid conditions suggests that kleptomania may have a 0.6% incidence. It seems reasonable to suspect that individuals with pyromania and kleptomania would seek to avoid detection and may therefore be underrepresented in research and clinical samples.

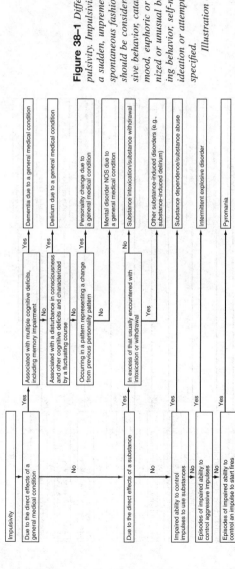

Figure 38-1 *Differential diagnosis of impulsivity. Impulsivity is a tendency to act in a sudden, unpremeditated, and excessively spontaneous fashion. Other decision trees that should be considered are those for aggressive behavior, catatonia, delusions, depressed mood, euphoric or irritable mood, disorganized or unusual behavior, distractibility, eating behavior, self-mutilation, and suicide ideation or attempt. NOS, Not otherwise specified.*

Illustration continued on following page

401

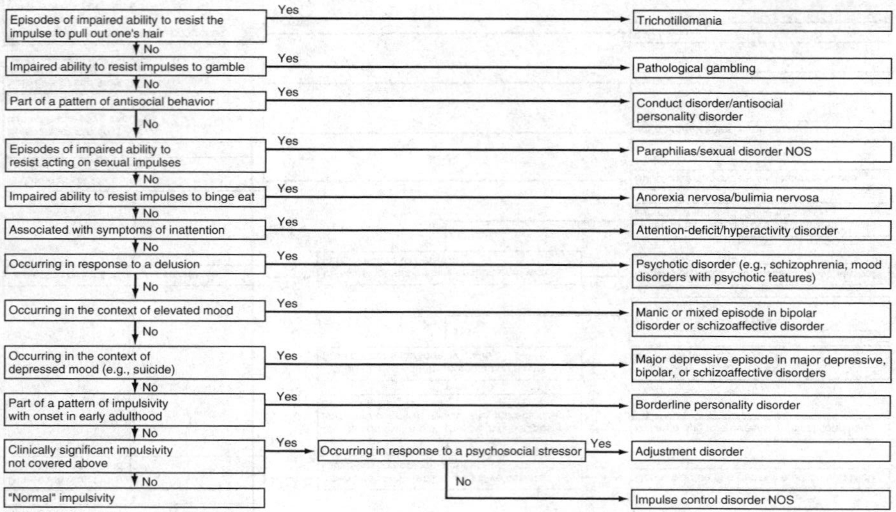

Figure 38-1 *Continued*

402

Treatment protocols for these conditions have not been well studied. Few treatment studies of these specific conditions have been performed. Attempts to treat these conditions are usually formulated by extrapolation from treatments that have been developed for other conditions, especially the frequently comorbid mood or anxiety disorders. For example, there has been some success in using serotonin reuptake inhibitor (SSRI) antidepressants in the treatment of trichotillomania.

The contemporary medical and psychological literature regarding treatment reflects prevailing general interests in current research and theory. As pharmacological treatments are applied to an increasing range of symptoms, the impulse disorders present new opportunities to widen the application of thymoleptic and anxiolytic medication. Some authors are now reconceptualizing the idea of mood and obsessional disorders, widening them into affective and obsessional spectrums and seeking to encompass various impulse disorders into these domains.

DSM-IV Criteria 312.34

Intermittent Explosive Disorder

A. Several discrete episodes of failure to resist aggressive impulses that result in serious assaultive acts or destruction of property.

B. The degree of aggressiveness expressed during the episodes is grossly out of proportion to any precipitating psychosocial stressors.

C. The aggressive episodes are not better accounted for by another mental disorder (e.g., antisocial personality disorder, borderline personality disorder, a psychotic disorder, a manic episode, conduct disorder, or attention-deficit/hyperactivity disorder) and are not due to the direct physiological effects of a substance (e.g., a drug of abuse, a medication) or a general medical condition (e.g., head trauma, Alzheimer's disease).

DSM-IV Criteria 312.32

Kleptomania

A. Recurrent failure to resist impulses to steal objects that are not needed for personal use or for their monetary value.

B. Increasing sense of tension immediately before committing the theft.

C. Pleasure, gratification, or relief at the time of committing the theft.

Box continued on following page

Kleptomania *Continued*

D. The stealing is not committed to express anger or vengeance and is not in response to a delusion or a hallucination.

E. The stealing is not better accounted for by conduct disorder, a manic episode, or antisocial personality disorder.

DSM-IV Criteria 312.33

Pyromania

A. Deliberate and purposeful fire setting on more than one occasion.

B. Tension or affective arousal before the act.

C. Fascination with, interest in, curiosity about, or attraction to fire and its situational contexts (e.g., paraphernalia, uses, consequences).

D. Pleasure, gratification, or relief when setting fires, or when witnessing or participating in their aftermath.

E. The fire setting is not done for monetary gain, as an expression of sociopathical ideology, to conceal criminal activity, to express anger or vengeance, to improve one's living circumstances, in response to a delusion or hallucination, or as a result of impaired judgment (e.g., in dementia, mental retardation, substance intoxication).

F. The fire setting is not better accounted for by conduct disorder, a manic episode, or antisocial personality disorder.

DSM-IV Criteria 312.31

Pathological Gambling

A. Persistent and recurrent maladaptive gambling behavior as indicated by five (or more) of the following:

    (1) is preoccupied with gambling (e.g., preoccupied with reliving past gambling experiences, handicapping or planning the next venture, or thinking of ways to get money with which to gamble)

    (2) needs to gamble with increasing amounts of money in order to achieve the desired excitement

(3) has repeated unsuccessful efforts to control, cut back, or stop gambling

(4) is restless or irritable when attempting to cut down or stop gambling

(5) gambles as a way of escaping from problems or of relieving a dysphoric mood (e.g., feelings of helplessness, guilt, anxiety, depression)

(6) after losing money gambling, often returns another day to get even ("chasing" one's losses)

(7) lies to family members, therapist, or others to conceal the extent of involvement with gambling

(8) has committed illegal acts such as forgery, fraud, theft, or embezzlement to finance gambling

(9) has jeopardized or lost a significant relationship, job, or educational or career opportunity because of gambling

(10) relies on others to provide money to relieve a desperate financial situation caused by gambling

B. The gambling behavior is not better accounted for by a manic episode.

DSM-IV Criteria 312.39

Trichotillomania

A. Recurrent pulling out of one's hair resulting in noticeable hair loss.

B. An increasing sense of tension immediately before pulling out the hair or when attempting to resist the behavior.

C. Pleasure, gratification, or relief when pulling out the hair.

D. The disturbance is not better accounted for by another mental disorder and is not due to a general medical condition (e.g., a dermatological condition).

E. The disturbance causes clinically significant distress or impairment in social, occupational, or other important areas of functioning.

Adjustment Disorder

By definition, the adjustment disorders are stress-related phenomena in which a designated psychosocial stressor results in the development of maladaptive states and psychiatric symptoms. The condition is presumed to be time limited (i.e., a transitory reaction), and symptoms recede when the stressor is removed or a new state of adaptation is defined. Other stress-related disorders are described in the *Diagnostic and Statistical Manual of Mental Disorders,* Fourth Edition (DSM-IV), such as posttraumatic stress disorder and acute stress disorder, those stress reactions that follow a disaster or cataclysmic personal event (i.e., *acute* distress disorder). The stress disorders are among the few conditions in DSM-IV, along with substance-induced disorders and mental disorders due to a general medical condition, with a *known cause* and for which the etiological agent is *essential* to establishing the diagnosis.

Diverse variables and modifiers are involved in determining who will experience an adjustment disorder after a stress. An objectively overwhelming stress could have little impact on one individual, whereas a minor one could be regarded as cataclysmic by another. A recent minor stress superimposed on a previous underlying (major) stress (which had no observable effect on its own) may have a significant impact, not operating independently but by its additive effect—the concatenation of events.

DIAGNOSIS

Each of the diagnostic constructs required for the diagnosis of adjustment disorder is difficult to assess and measure: 1) the stressor, 2) the maladaptive reaction to the stressor, and 3) the time and relationship between the stressor and the psychological response. None of these three components has been operationalized for a diagnostic decision tree, which consequently plagues the adjustment disorder diagnosis with limited reliability.

The psychiatrist needs to examine the patient's behavior to see whether it is beyond the normal range expected in a particular situation. The psychiatrist also needs to take into account the patient's cultural beliefs and practices, her or his developmental age, and the transient nature of the behavior. If the behavior lasts a few moments or is an impulsive outburst, it would not qualify for a maladaptive response to justify the diagnosis of adjustment disorder. The behavior in question should be maladaptive for that patient, in his or her culture, and sufficiently persistent to qualify for the maladaptation attribute of the adjustment disorder diagnosis.

TREATMENT

Treatment recommendations for the adjustment disorders remain based on consensus rather than evidence. At present, treatment is based on the understanding that this disorder emanates from an overwhelming psychological reaction to a stressor. The stressor needs to be identified, described, and shared with the patient; plans must be made to mitigate it, if possible. The abnormal response may be attenuated if the stressor can be eliminated or reduced. In the medically ill, the most common stressor may be the medical illness itself; the adjustment disorder may remit when the medical illness improves or the patient adapts to it.

REFRACTORY PATIENTS

Those patients who do not respond to counseling or the various modes of psychotherapy and to a trial of antidepressant or anxiolytic medications should be regarded as treatment nonresponders. Re-evaluation of the patient is essential to ensure that the diagnostic impression has not altered and, in particular, that the patient has not developed a major mental disorder, which would require a more aggressive treatment. The psychiatrist must also consider an Axis II disorder that might be interfering with the patient's resolution of the adjustment disorder. Finally, if the stressor continues and cannot be removed (e.g., the continuation of a seriously impairing chronic illness), additional support and management strategies must be employed to assist the patient in optimally adapting to the stressor that she or he is confronting (e.g., experiencing the progression of human immunodeficiency virus infection).

Personality Disorders

Each person has a personality, a characteristic manner of thinking, feeling, behaving, and relating to others. A personality disorder (PD) is a personality that results in clinically significant impairment in social or occupational functioning or in personal distress. PDs are defined in the *Diagnostic and Statistical Manual of Mental Disorders,* Fourth Edition (DSM-IV), as "an enduring pattern of inner experience and behavior that deviates markedly from the expectations of the individual's culture, is pervasive and inflexible, has an onset in adolescence or early adulthood, is stable over time, and leads to distress or impairment."

A number of points are worth emphasizing in this definition, as summarized in Table 40–1.

DSM-IV provides the diagnostic criteria for 10 PDs that are organized into three clusters: A, paranoid, schizoid, and schizotypal (placed within the odd-eccentric cluster); B, antisocial, borderline, histrionic, and narcissistic (dramatic-emotional-erratic cluster); and C, avoidant, dependent, and obsessive-compulsive (anxious-fearful cluster). There is some heuristic value in this cluster arrangement. For example, the paranoid PD (PPD), schizoid PD (SZPD), and schizotypal PD (STPD) do share the attribute of odd, eccentric behavior patterns, and they may have a common or at least similar etiology, pathology, and treatment.

Differentiation among the PDs is at times difficult. Few patients represent prototypical cases of a particular PD. That is, few patients have all of the features of one particular PD and none of the features of any of the other PDs. To facilitate the determination of which is most likely to be present, Table 40–2 presents a central feature and the most diagnostic symptom of each PD in DSM-IV.

TABLE 40–1	Central Features of a Personality Disorder

Onset in adolescence or young adulthood (i.e., evident since the age of approximately 18 y)

Stable in its appearance (i.e., no significant period in which it is not evident)

Pervasive in its effects (i.e., evident across a wide range of personal, social, and occupational situations)

Clinically significant maladaptivity (i.e., results in personal distress or in clear, explicit impairment in social and occupational functioning)

TABLE 40–2	**Central Features of Each Personality Disorder**

Paranoid: Distrust and suspiciousness (e.g., suspects, without sufficient basis, that others are exploiting, harming, or deceiving him or her)

Schizoid: Anhedonic detachment (e.g., neither desires nor enjoys close relationships)

Schizotypal: Interpersonal deficits and eccentricities (e.g., odd beliefs, magical thinking, and unusual perceptual experiences)

Antisocial: Disregard for and exploitation of others (e.g., repeatedly performs acts that are grounds for arrest)

Borderline: Instability in relationships, identity, behavior, and affect (e.g., unstable and intense interpersonal relationships)

Histrionic: Attention-seeking emotionality (e.g., uncomfortable when not the center of attention)

Narcissistic: Arrogance (e.g., grandiose sense of self-importance)

Avoidant: Social inhibition (e.g., avoids social and occupational activities that involve significant interpersonal contact)

Dependent: Emotional dependency (e.g., urgently and indiscriminantly seeks another relationship when close relationship ends)

Obsessive-compulsive: Preoccupation with orderliness, perfectionism, and control (e.g., preoccupied with details, rules, lists, order, organization, or schedules to the extent that the major point of the activity is lost)

Depressive: Depressive cognitions (e.g., pessimistic, gloomy, and cheerless)

Passive-aggressive: Negativistic attitudes (e.g., sullen, argumentative, and critical)

In DSM-IV, most of the PD diagnostic criteria are presented in a descending order of diagnostic value (i.e., the most diagnostic symptom is presented first). The list of features presented in Table 40–2, therefore, corresponds closely to the rank order of the criteria sets presented in DSM-IV.

PARANOID PERSONALITY DISORDER

DSM-IV Criteria 301.0

Paranoid Personality Disorder

A. A pervasive distrust and suspiciousness of others such that their motives are interpreted as malevolent, beginning by early adulthood and present in a variety of contexts, as indicated by four (or more) of the following:

Box continued on following page

DSM-IV Criteria 301.0

Paranoid Personality Disorder *Continued*

   (1) suspects, without sufficient basis, that others are exploiting, harming, or deceiving him or her

   (2) is preoccupied with unjustified doubts about the loyalty or trustworthiness of friends or associates

   (3) is reluctant to confide in others because of unwarranted fear that the information will be used maliciously against him or her

   (4) reads hidden demeaning or threatening meanings into benign remarks or events

   (5) persistently bears grudges, i.e., is unforgiving of insults, injuries, or slights

   (6) perceives attacks on his or her character or reputation that are not apparent to others and is quick to react angrily or to counterattack

   (7) has recurrent suspicions, without justification, regarding fidelity of spouse or sexual partner

B. Does not occur exclusively during the course of schizophrenia, a mood disorder with psychotic features, or another psychotic disorder and is not due to the direct physiological effects of a general medical condition.

Note: if criteria are met prior to the onset of schizophrenia, add "premorbid," e.g., paranoid personality disorder (premorbid).

PPD involves a pervasive and continuous distrust and suspiciousness of the motives of others. Persons with PPD believe that the intentions of most persons with whom they interact are malevolent. The presence of PPD is indicated by four or more of the seven DSM-IV diagnostic criteria.

There is some support for a genetic relationship of PPD with schizophrenia, but these findings have not always been replicated.

Differential Diagnosis

Paranoid symptoms are evident in a number of psychotic disorders. Paranoid ideation in PPD is inconsistent with reality and resistant to contrary evidence, but the beliefs are rarely absurd, inconceivable, or bizarre. PPD also lacks other features of a psychotic disorder (e.g., hallucinations) and is consistently evident since early adulthood, whereas a psychotic disorder can become evident at any time in a person's life. If PPD preceded the onset of schizophrenia, it should be noted that it was premorbid to the schizophrenia.

Course and Natural History

Premorbid traits of PPD may be evident before adolescence in the form of social isolation, hypersensitivity, hypervigilance, social anxiety, peculiar thoughts, and idiosyncratic fantasies. Adjustment in adulthood is particularly poor with respect to interpersonal relationships. Patients with PPD are prone to develop a variety of Axis I disorders, including substance-related, obsessive-compulsive, anxiety, agoraphobic, and depressive disorders.

Treatment

Persons with PPD rarely seek treatment for their paranoid personality traits (e.g., their suspiciousness and distrust). They typically experience these traits as simply the way they are, have been, and always will be (e.g., ego-syntonic).

The presence of paranoid personality traits complicates the treatment of an Axis I disorder or a relationship problem. Trust is central to the development of an adequate therapeutic alliance or rapport, and it is precisely the inability to develop such feelings that is central to this disorder. The goal of treatment is to develop a nonthreatening way of cultivating more self-reflection and self-questioning, as well as recognition of the way that paranoid traits and behaviors contribute to the difficulties the patients are experiencing in their lives. A useful approach can be to communicate a sincere and respectful willingness to explore the implications, logic, and reality of the suspicions. Whenever moving too quickly appears to be endangering rapport, the psychiatrist should retreat to a more neutral and accepting position.

SCHIZOID PERSONALITY DISORDER

DSM-IV Criteria 301.20

Schizoid Personality Disorder

A. A pervasive pattern of detachment from social relationships and a restricted range of expression of emotions in interpersonal settings, beginning by early adulthood and present in a variety of contexts, as indicated by four (or more) of the following:

   (1) neither desires nor enjoys close relationships, including being part of a family

   (2) almost always chooses solitary activities

   (3) has little, if any, interest in having sexual experiences with another person

   (4) takes pleasure in few, if any, activities

   (5) lacks close friends or confidants other than first-degree relatives

Box continued on following page

DSM-IV Criteria 301.20

Schizoid Personality Disorder *Continued*

(6) appears indifferent to the praise or criticism of others

(7) shows emotional coldness, detachment, or flattened affectivity

B. Does not occur exclusively during the course of schizophrenia, a mood disorder with psychotic features, another psychotic disorder, or a pervasive developmental disorder and is not due to the direct physiological effects of a general medical condition.

Note: if criteria are met prior to the onset of schizophrenia, add "premorbid," e.g., "schizoid personality disorder (premorbid)."

The SZPD is a pervasive pattern of social detachment and restricted emotional expression.

Differential Diagnosis

SZPD can be confused with schizotypal PD (STPD) and avoidant PD (AVPD), as both involve social isolation and withdrawal. STPD, however, also includes intense social anxiety and cognitive-perceptual aberrations. It is distinguished from AVPD by the absence of an intense desire for intimate social relationships. Avoidant persons also exhibit substantial insecurity and inhibition, whereas the schizoid person is largely indifferent to the reactions or opinions of others.

Course and Natural History

Persons with SZPD have been socially isolated and withdrawn as children. They may not have been accepted well by their peers and may even have experienced some ostracism. As adults, they have few friendships. They have had few sexual relationships and may never marry. Relationships fail to the extent that the other person desires or needs emotional support, warmth, and intimacy that the person with SZPD cannot provide. Persons with SZPD may do well and even excel in an occupation as long as substantial social interaction is not required. They would prefer to work in isolation. If they do eventually become parents, they have considerable difficulty providing warmth and emotional support and may appear neglectful, detached, and disinterested.

Treatment

Persons with SZPD rarely present for treatment, whether for their schizoid traits or a concomitant Axis I disorder. They feel little need for treatment because their isolation is often ego-syntonic.

If persons with SZPD are seen for treatment for a concomitant Axis I disorder (e.g., a sexual arousal disorder or a substance dependence), it is advisable to work within the confines and limitations of the schizoid personality traits. Charismatic, engaging, emotional, or intimate psychiatrists can be uncomfortable, foreign, and even threatening to persons with SZPD. A more business-like approach can be more successful.

SCHIZOTYPAL PERSONALITY DISORDER

DSM-IV Criteria 301.22

Schizotypal Personality Disorder

A. A pervasive pattern of social and interpersonal deficits marked by acute discomfort with, and reduced capacity for, close relationships as well as by cognitive or perceptual distortions and eccentricities of behavior, beginning by early adulthood and present in a variety of contexts, as indicated by five (or more) of the following:

   (1) ideas of reference (excluding delusions of reference)

   (2) odd beliefs or magical thinking that influences behavior and is inconsistent with subcultural norms (e.g., superstitiousness, belief in clairvoyance, telepathy, or "sixth sense"; in children and adolescents, bizarre fantasies or preoccupations)

   (3) unusual perceptual experiences, including bodily illusions

   (4) odd thinking and speech (e.g., vague, circumstantial, metaphorical, overelaborate, or stereotyped)

   (5) suspiciousness or paranoid ideation

   (6) inappropriate or constricted affect

   (7) behavior or appearance that is odd, eccentric, or peculiar

   (8) lack of close friends or confidants other than first-degree relatives

   (9) excessive social anxiety that does not diminish with familiarity and tends to be associated with paranoid fears rather than negative judgments about self

Box continued on following page

Schizotypal Personality Disorder *Continued*

B. Does not occur exclusively during the course of schizophrenia, a mood disorder with psychotic features, another psychotic disorder, or a pervasive developmental disorder.

Note: if criteria are met prior to the onset of schizophrenia, add "premorbid," e.g., "schizotypal personality disorder (premorbid)."

STPD is a pervasive pattern of interpersonal deficits, cognitive and perceptual aberrations, and eccentricities of behavior. The interpersonal deficits are characterized in large part by an acute discomfort with and reduced capacity for close relationships.

There is substantial empirical support for a genetic association of STPD with schizophrenia, which is not surprising because the diagnostic criteria were obtained from the observations of biological relatives of persons with schizophrenia.

Differential Diagnosis

AVPD and STPD share the features of social anxiety and introversion, but the social anxiety of STPD does not diminish with familiarity, whereas the anxiety of AVPD is concerned primarily with the initiation of a relationship. STPD is also a more severe disorder that includes a variety of cognitive and perceptual aberrations that are not seen in persons with AVPD.

The initial concern of many psychiatrists confronting a person with STPD is whether the more appropriate diagnosis is schizophrenia (or another psychotic disorder). Persons with STPD closely resemble persons within the prodromal or residual phases of schizophrenia. Premorbid schizotypal traits have prognostic significance for the course and treatment of schizophrenia, and such traits should be noted.

Course and Natural History

As children, persons with STPD are likely to have been rather isolated. They may have appeared odd to their peers and perhaps were teased or ostracized. As adults, they may drift toward esoteric, fringe groups that support their magical thinking and aberrant beliefs. These activities can provide structure for some persons with STPD, but they can also contribute to a further loosening and deterioration if they encourage psychosis-like or dissociative experiences. Only a small proportion of persons with STPD develop schizophrenia, but many may eventually develop a major depressive disorder. The symptoms of STPD do not appear to remit with age. The course appears to be relatively stable, with some proportion of schizotypal persons remaining marginally employed, withdrawn, and transient throughout their lives.

Treatment

Persons with STPD may seek treatment for their feelings of anxiousness, perceptual disturbances, or depression. Treatment of such persons should be cognitive, behavioral, supportive, and/or pharmacological because they often find the intimacy and emotionality of reflective, exploratory psychotherapy to be too stressful. They are also prone to regressive deterioration and decompensation.

Low doses of neuroleptic medications (e.g., thiothixene) have shown some effectiveness in the treatment of schizotypal symptoms, particularly the perceptual aberrations and social anxiousness. Group therapy has also been recommended for persons with STPD but only when the group is highly structured and supportive. The emotional intensity and intimacy of unstructured groups are usually too stressful. Schizotypal patients with predominant paranoid symptoms may even have difficulty in highly structured groups.

ANTISOCIAL PERSONALITY DISORDER

DSM-IV Criteria 301.7

Antisocial Personality Disorder

A. There is a pervasive pattern of disregard for and violation of the rights of others occurring since age 15 years, as indicated by three (or more) of the following:

   (1) failure to conform to social norms with respect to lawful behaviors as indicated by repeatedly performing acts that are grounds for arrest

   (2) deceitfulness, as indicated by repeated lying, use of aliases, or conning others for personal profit or pleasure

   (3) impulsivity or failure to plan ahead

   (4) irritability and aggressiveness, as indicated by repeated physical fights or assaults

   (5) reckless disregard for safety of self or others

   (6) consistent irresponsibility, as indicated by repeated failure to sustain consistent work behavior or honor financial obligations

   (7) lack of remorse, as indicated by being indifferent to or rationalizing having hurt, mistreated, or stolen from another

B. The individual is at least age 18 years.

C. There is evidence of conduct disorder with onset before age 15 years.

D. The occurrence of antisocial behavior is not exclusively during the course of schizophrenia or a manic episode.

ASPD is a pervasive pattern of disregard for and violation of the rights of others. This disorder has also been referred to as psychopathy, sociopathy, and dissocial PD.

Differential Diagnosis

It is at times difficult to differentiate ASPD from a substance dependence because many persons with ASPD develop a substance-related disorder and many persons with a substance dependence engage in antisocial acts. However, the requirement that the ASPD features be evident before the age of 15 years usually ensures the onset of ASPD before the onset of a substance-related disorder. If both are evident before the age of 15 years, it is likely that both disorders are in fact present and both diagnoses should then be provided. ASPD and substance dependence often interact, exacerbating and escalating each other's development.

Antisocial acts are also evident in histrionic PD (HPD) and borderline PD (BPD) because persons with these disorders display impulsivity, sensation seeking, self-centeredness, manipulativeness, and a low tolerance of frustration. Females with ASPD are often misdiagnosed with HPD. However, persons with HPD and BPD lack the childhood history of a conduct disorder and the cold, calculated exploitation, abuse, and aggression that are characteristic of ASPD.

Course and Natural History

In childhood ASPD is evident in the form of a conduct disorder. Evidence of a conduct disorder before the age of 15 years is in fact required for a DSM-IV ASPD diagnosis. The continuation into adulthood is particularly likely to occur if multiple delinquent behaviors are evident before the age of 10 years. As adults, persons with ASPD are unlikely to maintain steady employment, and they may even become impoverished or homeless or spend years in penal institutions.

There does tend to be a gradual remission of antisocial behaviors, particularly overt criminal acts, as persons with ASPD age. Such persons, however, are more likely than the general population to die prematurely by violent means (e.g., accidents or homicides) and to engage in quite dangerous, high-risk behavior. They are at a high risk for developing substance-related and impulse dyscontrol disorders.

Treatment

It is important to recognize the presence of ASPD in the treatment of any Axis I disorder because the tendency to be manipulative, dishonest, exploitive, aggressive, and irresponsible often disrupts and sabotages treatment.

ASPD is the most difficult PD to treat. Persons with ASPD usually lack motivation for or commitment to change. They see only the advantages of their antisocial traits and not the costs (e.g., risks of arrest and failure to sustain lasting or meaningful relationships). The immediate motivation for treatment is often provided by an external source, such as a court order or the demands of an employer or relative. The motivation may then last only as long as the external pressure remains. Outpatient therapy is rarely successful, and during inpatient therapy persons with ASPD are prone to manipulate, abuse, or exploit their fellow inpatients and the staff.

BORDERLINE PERSONALITY DISORDER

DSM-IV Criteria 301.83

Borderline Personality Disorder

A pervasive pattern of instability of interpersonal relationships, self-image, and affects, and marked impulsivity beginning by early adulthood and present in a variety of contexts, as indicated by five (or more) of the following:

(1) frantic efforts to avoid real or imagined abandonment. **Note:** do not include suicidal or self-mutilating behavior covered in criterion 5.

(2) a pattern of unstable and intense interpersonal relationships characterized by alternating between extremes of idealization and devaluation

(3) identity disturbance: markedly and persistently unstable self-image or sense of self

(4) impulsivity in at least two areas that are potentially self-damaging (e.g., spending, sex, substance abuse, reckless driving, binge eating). **Note:** do not include suicidal or self-mutilating behavior covered in criterion 5.

(5) recurrent suicidal behavior, gestures, or threats, or self-mutilating behavior

(6) affective instability due to a marked reactivity of mood (e.g., intense episodic dysphoria, irritability, or anxiety usually lasting a few hours and only rarely more than a few days)

(7) chronic feelings of emptiness

(8) inappropriate, intense anger or difficulty controlling anger (e.g., frequent displays of temper, constant anger, recurrent physical fights)

(9) transient, stress-related paranoid ideation or severe dissociative symptoms

---

BPD is a pervasive pattern of impulsivity and instability in interpersonal relationships and self-image. Many persons with BPD may also develop a variety of cognitive-perceptual aberrations and psychosis-like symptoms, including ideas of reference, hypnagogic experiences, transient hallucinations, and distortions of body image.

BPD is the most prevalent PD in most clinical settings. Approximately 15% of all inpatients (51% of inpatients with a PD)

and 8% of all outpatients (27% of outpatients with a PD) have BPD. Approximately 75% of those with BPD are female.

Research suggests an association with mood and impulse dyscontrol disorders, and there is consistent empirical support for a childhood history of physical or sexual abuse (as well as parental conflict, loss, and neglect).

Differential Diagnosis

Most persons with BPD develop mood disorders, and it is at times difficult to differentiate BPD from a mood disorder if the assessment is confined to the current symptoms. A diagnosis of BPD requires that the borderline symptoms be evident since adolescence, which should differentiate BPD from a mood disorder in all cases other than a chronic mood disorder.

Course and Natural History

As children, persons with BPD are likely to have been emotionally unstable, impulsive, and angry or hostile. Their chaotic impulsivity and intense affectivity may have contributed to a degree of popularity within rebellious groups during adolescence and may be confused with a normal adolescent rebellion or identity crisis. As adults, persons with BPD may require numerous hospitalizations because of their affect and impulse dyscontrol, psychosis-like and dissociative symptoms, and risk of suicide. They are at a high risk for developing depressive, substance-related, bulimic, and posttraumatic stress disorders. The potential for suicide is increased with a comorbid mood and substance-related disorder. Approximately 3% to 10% have committed suicide by the age of 30 years. Relationships tend to be unstable and explosive, and employment is poor. Affectivity and impulsivity, however, may begin to diminish as the person reaches the age of 30 years or with a supportive and patient sexual partner.

Treatment

Most persons with BPD have a comorbid Axis I disorder, such as an eating, mood, substance-related, dissociative, or anxiety disorder, and are in treatment for this disorder. It is important in such cases to recognize the presence and consider the effect of the borderline traits on the treatment for the respective Axis I disorder.

Persons with BPD tend to develop the same intense, dependent, hostile, unstable, and manipulative relationships with their psychiatrists as they do with others. At one time they might be compliant, responsive, and even idealizing but later angry, accusatory, and devaluing. Their tendency to be manipulatively self-destructive, as well as impulsively self-destructive, is often stressful and difficult to treat.

Persons with BPD are often highly motivated for treatment. Psychotherapeutic approaches tend to be both supportive and exploratory.

Pharmacological treatment of patients with BPD is varied because it depends primarily on the predominant Axis I symptoms. Persons with BPD can display a wide variety of Axis I symptoms, including anxiety, depression, hallucinations, delusions, and dissociations. It is important in their pharmacological treatment not to be influenced unduly by symptoms that are transient or readily addressed through exploratory or supportive techniques.

HISTRIONIC PERSONALITY DISORDER

DSM-IV Criteria 301.50

Histrionic Personality Disorder

A pervasive pattern of excessive emotionality and attention seeking, beginning by early adulthood and present in a variety of contexts, as indicated by five (or more) of the following:

(1) is uncomfortable in situations in which he or she is not the center of attention

(2) interaction with others is often characterized by inappropriate sexually seductive or provocative behavior

(3) displays rapidly shifting and shallow expression of emotions

(4) consistently uses physical appearance to draw attention to self

(5) has a style of speech that is excessively impressionistic and lacking in detail

(6) shows self-dramatization, theatricality, and exaggerated expression of emotion

(7) is suggestible, i.e., easily influenced by others or circumstances

(8) considers relationships to be more intimate than they actually are

HPD is a pervasive pattern of excessive emotionality and attention seeking. Histrionic persons tend to be emotionally manipulative and intolerant of delayed gratification.

Differential Diagnosis

To some extent HPD involves maladaptive variants of stereotypically feminine traits, such as emotionality. The DSM-IV diagnostic criteria for HPD are sufficiently severe that a normal woman would not meet these criteria, but a variety of studies have indicated that psychiatrists may at times diagnose HPD in women who in fact have antisocial traits. Both of these disorders can involve impulsivity, sensation seeking, low frustration tolerance, and manipulativeness, and the presence of the female gender may at times contribute to a false presumption of HPD. It is therefore important to adhere closely to the DSM-IV diagnostic criteria when confronted with histrionic and antisocial symptoms in female patients.

HPD overlaps BPD. However, BPD is the more severely dysfunctional disorder, involving self-destructiveness, identity disturbance, and chronic feelings of emptiness, as well as the affective instability and manipulativeness seen in HPD.

Course and Natural History

Little is known about the premorbid behavior pattern of persons with HPD. During adolescence they are likely to have been flamboyant, flirtatious, and attention seeking. As adults, persons with HPD readily form new relationships but have difficulty sustaining them. They have a tendency to make impulsive decisions that have a dramatic (or melodramatic) effect on their lives. They are prone to develop somatic, mood, dissociative, and perhaps substance-related disorders. However, the severity of the symptoms may diminish somewhat as the person ages.

Treatment

The presence of HPD can complicate the treatment of an Axis I mental disorder. Persons with HPD readily develop a rapport, but it is often superficial and unreliable.

A key task in treating patients with HPD is countering their global and diffuse cognitive style by insisting that they attend to structure and detail within sessions and to the practical, immediate problems of daily life. It is also important to explore within treatment the historical source of their needs for attention and involvement.

Many psychiatrists recommend the use of group therapy for persons with HPD. It is quite easy for them to become involved in a group, which may then be useful in helping them to recognize and explore their attention seeking, suggestibility, and manipulation, as well as to find alternative ways to develop more meaningful and sustained relationships. The intense affectivity of persons with HPD may also be responsive to antidepressant treatment, particularly in patients with substantial mood reactivity, hypersomnia, and rejection sensitivity.

NARCISSISTIC PERSONALITY DISORDER

DSM-IV Criteria 301.61

Narcissistic Personality Disorder

A pervasive pattern of grandiosity (in fantasy or behavior), need for admiration, and lack of empathy, beginning by early adulthood and present in a variety of contexts, as indicated by five (or more) of the following:

(1) has grandiose sense of self-importance (e.g., exaggerates achievements and talents, expects to be recognized as superior without commensurate achievements)

(2) is preoccupied with fantasies of unlimited success, power, brilliance, beauty, or ideal love

(3) believes that he or she is "special" and unique and can only be understood by, or should associate with, other special or high-status people (or institutions)

(4) requires excessive admiration

(5) has a sense of entitlement, i.e., unreasonable expectations of especially favorable treatment or automatic compliance with his or her expectations

(6) is interpersonally exploitative, i.e., takes advantage of others to achieve his or her own ends

(7) lacks empathy: is unwilling to recognize or identify with the feelings and needs of others

(8) is often envious of others or believes that others are envious of him or her

(9) shows arrogant, haughty behaviors or attitudes

NPD is a pervasive pattern of grandiosity, need for admiration, and lack of empathy. Persons with NPD may react defensively with rage, disdain, or indifference but are in fact struggling with feelings of shock, humiliation, and shame.

Differential Diagnosis

Individuals with NPD may often appear to function quite well. Exaggerated self-confidence may in fact contribute to success in a variety of professions, and narcissistic traits are at times seen in highly successful persons. A diagnosis of NPD, however, requires the presence of interpersonal exploitation, lack of empathy, a sense of entitlement, and other symptoms beyond simply arrogance and grandiosity.

Course and Natural History

Little is known about the premorbid behavior pattern of NPD, other than through retrospective reports of persons diagnosed with NPD as adults. As adolescents, those with NPD have probably been self-centered, assertive, gregarious, dominant, and perhaps arrogant. As adults, many people with NPD have experienced high levels of achievement. However, their relationships with colleagues, peers, and staff eventually become strained as their use of others and self-centered egotism become evident. Success may also be impaired by their difficulty in acknowledging or resolving criticism, deficits, and setbacks.

Treatment

Persons with narcissistic personality traits seek treatment for feelings of depression, substance-related disorders, and occupational or relational problems that are secondary to their narcissism. Their self-centeredness and lack of empathy are particularly problematical in marital, occupational, and other social relationships, and they usually lack an appreciation of the contribution of their conflicts regarding self-esteem, status, and recognition. It is difficult for them even to admit that they have a psychological problem or that they need help because this admission itself injures their self-esteem.

Group therapy can be useful for increasing awareness of the grandiosity, lack of empathy, and devaluation of others. However, these traits not only interfere with the narcissistic person's ability to sustain membership within groups (and within individual therapy) but also may become quite harmful and destructive to the rapport of the entire group. There is no accepted pharmacological approach to the treatment of narcissism.

AVOIDANT PERSONALITY DISORDER

DSM-IV Criteria 301.32

Avoidant Personality Disorder

A pervasive pattern of social inhibition, feelings of inadequacy, and hypersensitivity to negative evaluation, beginning by early adulthood and present in a variety of contexts, as indicated by four (or more) of the following:

(1) avoids occupational activities that involve significant interpersonal contact, because of fears of criticism, disapproval, or rejection

(2) is unwilling to get involved with people unless certain of being liked

(3) shows restraint within intimate relationships because of the fear of being shamed or ridiculed

(4) is preoccupied with being criticized or rejected in social situations

(5) is inhibited in new interpersonal situations because of feelings of inadequacy

(6) views self as socially inept, personally unappealing, or inferior to others

(7) is unusually reluctant to take personal risks or to engage in any new activities because they may prove embarrassing

AVPD is a pervasive pattern of timidity, inhibition, inadequacy, and social hypersensitivity. Persons with AVPD may have a strong desire to develop close, personal relationships but feel too insecure to approach others or to express their feelings.

Differential Diagnosis

The most difficult differential diagnosis for AVPD is with generalized social phobia. Both involve an avoidance of social situations, social anxiety, and timidity, and both may be evident since late childhood or adolescence. Many persons with AVPD in fact seek treatment for a social phobia. To the extent that the behavior pattern pervades the person's everyday functioning and has been evident since childhood, the diagnosis of a PD is more descriptive. However, both diagnoses can be given when the person meets the criteria for both disorders.

Course and Natural History

Persons with AVPD were shy, timid, and anxious as children. Many have been diagnosed with a social phobia. Adolescence was a particularly difficult developmental period, because of the importance at this time of attractiveness, dating, and popularity. Occupational success may not be significantly impaired for persons with AVPD, as long as there is little demand for public performance. Their avoidance of social situations impairs their ability to develop adequate social skills, and this then further handicaps any eventual efforts to develop intimate relationships. However, they may eventually develop an intimate relationship, to which they may cling dependently.

Persons with AVPD are prone to mood and anxiety disorders, particularly depression and social phobia. They may often seek treatment for a specific anxiety disorder (failing to recognize the pervasive nature of the disorder) and may develop a dependence on anxiolytics. The severity of the AVPD symptoms, however, tends to diminish as the person becomes older.

Treatment

Persons with AVPD seek treatment for their avoidant personality traits. However, many also seek treatment for symptoms of anxiety, particularly social phobia (generalized subtype). It is important in such cases to recognize that the shyness is not due simply to a dysregulation or dyscontrol of anxiousness. There is instead a more pervasive and fundamental mental disorder involving feelings of interpersonal insecurity, low self-esteem, and inadequacy.

Social skills training, systematic desensitization, and a graded hierarchy of in vivo exposure to feared social situations have been shown to be useful in the treatment of AVPD. However, it is also important to discuss the underlying fears and insecurities regarding attractiveness, desirability, rejection, or intimacy.

Persons with AVPD often find group therapies to be informative and helpful. Exploratory and supportive groups can provide them with an understanding environment in which to discuss their social insecurities, to explore and practice more assertive behaviors, and to develop an increased self-confidence in approaching others and to developing relationships outside the group.

Many persons with AVPD respond to anxiolytic medications and at times to antidepressants, particularly monoamine oxidase inhibitors such as phenelzine. General feelings of anxiousness (as well as more specific social phobias) can be suppressed or diminished through pharmacological interventions. This approach may in fact be necessary to overcome initial feelings of intense social anxiety that are markedly disruptive to current functioning (e.g., inability to give required presentations at work or to talk to new acquaintances). However, it is also important to closely monitor a reliance on medications. Persons with AVPD are prone to rely on substances to control their feelings of anxiousness, whereas their more general feelings of insecurity and inadequacy may require a more comprehensive treatment.

DEPENDENT PERSONALITY DISORDER

DSM-IV Criteria 301.6

Dependent Personality Disorder

A pervasive and excessive need to be taken care of that leads to submissive and clinging behavior and fears of separation, beginning by early adulthood and present in a variety of contexts, as indicated by five (or more) of the following:

(1) has difficulty making everyday decisions without an excessive amount of advice and reassurance from others

(2) needs others to assume responsibility for most major areas of his or her life

(3) has difficulty expressing disagreement with others because of fear of loss of support or approval. **Note:** Do not include realistic fears of retribution.

(4) has difficulty initiating projects or doing things on his or her own (because of a lack of self-confidence in judgment or abilities rather than a lack of motivation or energy)

(5) goes to excessive lengths to obtain nurturance and support from others, to the point of volunteering to do things that are unpleasant

(6) feels uncomfortable or helpless when alone because of exaggerated fears of being unable to care for himself or herself

(7) urgently seeks another relationship as a source of care and support when a close relationship ends

(8) is unrealistically preoccupied with fears of being left to take care of himself or herself

DPD involves a pervasive and excessive need to be taken care of that leads to submissiveness, clinging, and fears of separation. Persons with DPD also have low self-esteem and are often self-critical and self-denigrating.

Differential Diagnosis

Excessive dependency is often seen in persons who have developed debilitating mental and general medical disorders, such as agoraphobia, schizophrenia, mental retardation, severe injuries, and dementia. However, a diagnosis of DPD requires the presence of the dependent traits since late childhood or adolescence.

Deference, politeness, and passivity also vary substantially across cultural groups. It is important not to confuse differences in personality that are due to different cultural norms with the presence of a PD. The diagnosis of DPD requires that the dependent behavior be maladaptive, resulting in clinically significant functional impairment or distress.

Many persons with DPD also meet the criteria for HPD. Persons with DPD and those with HPD may both display strong needs for reassurance, attention, and approval. However, persons with DPD tend to be more self-effacing, docile, and altruistic, whereas persons with HPD tend to be more flamboyant, assertive, and self-centered.

Course and Natural History

Persons with DPD are likely to have been excessively submissive as children and adolescents, and some may have had a chronic physical illness or a separation anxiety disorder during childhood. Persons with DPD fear intensely a loss of concern, care, and support from others, particularly the person with whom they have an emotional attachment. They are unable to be by themselves, as their sense of self-worth, value, or meaning is obtained by or through the presence of a relationship. They have few other sources of self-esteem. They form new relationships quickly and often indiscriminately. Because of their intense fear of being alone, they may become quickly attached to persons who are unreliable, unempathic, and even exploitative or abusive. More desirable or reliable partners are at times driven away by their excessive clinging and continued demands for reassurance. Occupational functioning is impaired to the extent that independent responsibility and initiative are required.

Persons with DPD are prone to mood disorders, particularly major depressive and dysthymic disorders and to anxiety disorders, particularly agoraphobia, social phobia, and perhaps panic disorder. However, the severity of the symptoms tends to decrease with age, particularly if the person has obtained a reliable, dependable, and empathic partner.

Treatment

Persons with DPD are often in treatment for one or more Axis I disorders, particularly a mood (depressive) or an anxiety disorder. They tend to be agreeable, compliant, and grateful patients, often to excess. An important issue in the treatment of persons with DPD is not letting the relationship with the psychiatrist become an end in itself. Many persons with DPD find the therapeutic relationship to satisfy their need for support, concern, and involvement.

Exploring the breadth and source of the need for care and support is often an important component of treatment. Persons with DPD frequently have a history of exploitative, rejecting, and perhaps even abusive relationships that have contributed to their current feelings of insecurity and inadequacy. Cognitive-behavioral techniques are useful in addressing the feelings of inadequacy, incompetence, and helplessness. Social skills, problem solving, and assertiveness training also make important contributions.

Persons with DPD may also benefit from group therapy. A supportive group is useful in diffusing the feelings of dependency onto a variety of persons, in supplying feedback regarding their manner of relating to others, and in providing practice and role models for more assertive and autonomous interpersonal functioning. There is no known pharmacological treatment for DPD.

OBSESSIVE-COMPULSIVE PERSONALITY DISORDER

DSM-IV Criteria 301.4

Obsessive-Compulsive Personality Disorder

A pervasive pattern of preoccupation with orderliness, perfectionism, and mental and interpersonal control, at the expense of flexibility, openness, and efficiency, beginning by early adulthood and present in a variety of contexts, as indicated by four (or more) of the following:

(1) is preoccupied with details, rules, lists, order, organization, or schedules to the extent that the major point of the activity is lost

(2) shows perfectionism that interferes with task completion (e.g., is unable to complete a project because his or her own overly strict standards are not met)

(3) is excessively devoted to work and productivity to the exclusion of leisure activities and friendships (not accounted for by obvious economic necessity)

(4) is overconscientious, scrupulous, and inflexible about matters of morality, ethics, or values (not accounted for by cultural or religious identification)

(5) is unable to discard worn-out or worthless objects even when they have no sentimental value

(6) is reluctant to delegate tasks or to work with others unless they submit to exactly his or her way of doing things

(7) adopts a miserly spending style toward both self and
others; money is viewed as something to be hoarded
for future catastrophes

(8) shows rigidity and stubbornness

OCPD involves a preoccupation with orderliness, perfectionism,
and mental and interpersonal control.

Differential Diagnosis

Devotion to work and productivity varies substantially across
cultural groups. One should be careful not to confuse cultural
variation with the presence of a PD. A diagnosis of OCPD requires
that the devotion to work is maladaptive or to the exclusion of leisure
activities and friendships.

OCPD resembles to some extent obsessive-compulsive anxiety
disorder. However, many persons with OCPD fail to develop
obsessive-compulsive anxiety disorder and vice versa. Obsessive-
compulsive anxiety disorder involves intrusive obsessions and quite
specific and repetitively performed rituals whose purpose it is to
reduce or control feelings of anxiety. OCPD involves rigid behavior
patterns that are more ego-syntonic. However, if both behavior
patterns are present, both diagnoses should be given. These
disorders are sufficiently distinct that it is likely that in such cases
both disorders are in fact present.

Course and Natural History

As children, some persons with OCPD may have appeared to be
relatively well behaved, responsible, and conscientious. However,
they may also have been overly serious, rigid, and constrained. As
adults, many have good to excellent success in a job or career.
Relationships with a spouse and children are likely to be strained
because of their tendency to be detached and uninvolved, yet
authoritarian and domineering with respect to decisions.

Persons with OCPD may be prone to various anxiety and physical
disorders that are secondary to their worrying, indecision, and stress.
Those with concomitant traits of angry hostility and competitiveness
may be prone to cardiovascular disorders. Mood disorders may not
develop until the person recognizes the sacrifices that have been
made by their devotion to work and productivity, which may at
times not occur until middle age. However, most experience early
employment or career difficulties and even failures that may result
in depression.

Treatment

Persons with OCPD may fail to seek treatment for the OCPD
symptoms. They may seek treatment instead for disorders and problems that are secondary to their OCPD traits, including anxiety
disorders, health problems (e.g., cardiovascular disorders), and

problems in various relationships (e.g., marital, familial, and occupational). Treatment is complicated by their inability to appreciate the contribution of their personality to these problems and disorders.

Cognitive-behavioral techniques that address the irrationality of the excessive conscientiousness, moralism, perfectionism, devotion to work, and stubbornness, however, can be effective in the treatment of OCPD. Persons with OCPD may in fact appreciate the rational approach to treatment provided by cognitive-behavioral therapy.

Persons with OCPD can be problematical in groups. They tend to be domineering, constricted, and judgmental. However, many persons with OCPD find the effort to be more flexible, understanding, patient, and emotionally responsive to be rewarding and beneficial. There is no accepted pharmacological treatment for OCPD. Some persons with OCPD benefit from anxiolytic or antidepressant medications, but this typically reflects the presence of associated features or comorbid disorders. The core traits of OCPD may not be affected.

PERSONALITY DISORDER NOT OTHERWISE SPECIFIED

DSM-IV includes a diagnostic category, PD not otherwise specified, for persons with a PD who do not meet the diagnostic criteria for any of the 10 officially recognized PDs. PD not otherwise specified has in fact been the most commonly diagnosed PD category in almost every study in which it has been researched.

One usage of PD not otherwise specified is for the two PDs presented in an appendix to DSM-IV for criteria sets provided for further study, the passive-aggressive PD (PAPD) and the depressive PD (DPPD).

Passive-Aggressive (Negativistic) Personality Disorder

DSM-IV Criteria

Passive-Aggressive Personality Disorder

A. A pervasive pattern of negativistic attitudes and passive resistance to demands for adequate performance, beginning by early adulthood and present in a variety of contexts, as indicated by four (or more) of the following:

   (1) passively resists fulfilling routine social and occupational tasks

   (2) complains of being misunderstood and unappreciated by others

   (3) is sullen and argumentative

   (4) unreasonably criticizes and scorns authority

(5) expresses envy and resentment toward those apparently more fortunate

(6) voices exaggerated and persistent complaints of personal misfortune

(7) alternates between hostile defiance and contrition

B. Does not occur exclusively during major depressive episodes and is not better accounted for by dysthmic disorder

PAPD is a pervasive pattern of negativistic attitudes and passive resistance to authority, demands, responsibilities, or obligations. PAPD was an officially recognized PD diagnosis in DSM-III-R. It is in an appendix B to DSM-IV because there has been little research on its validity, and there was concern that the DSM-III-R diagnosis described a situational reaction rather than a pervasive and chronic PD.

DIFFERENTIAL DIAGNOSIS

Passive-aggressive behavior is often evident in settings in which persons have lost a freedom, responsibility, or decision-making authority that was previously available to them and overt expressions of assertiveness or opposition are discouraged. It is important in such settings to verify that the negativistic behavior was evident earlier and is currently evident in other situations.

PAPD overlaps substantially with DPPD. Both involve negativism and pessimism. However, persons with PAPD are much more critical of others than of themselves. Persons with DPPD feel excessively guilty and remorseful, whereas persons with PAPD are argumentative, scornful, defiant, and resentful.

COURSE AND NATURAL HISTORY

Many persons with PAPD may during childhood have met the criteria for an oppositional defiant disorder, which is also characterized by the tendency to be irritable, complaining, oppositional, argumentative, and negativistic. As adults, impairment is likely to be particularly evident with respect to employment. Persons with PAPD would be irresponsible, lax, and negligent employees, as well as resistant, oppositional, and even hostile. Resolution of interpersonal conflicts is difficult, because passive-aggressive persons tend to blame others. They are argumentative, sullen, and critical of their peers and friends, who may not tolerate their antagonism for too long.

TREATMENT

Persons with PAPD rarely enter treatment to make effective changes in their personality or behavior. They are more likely to seek treatment for Axis I disorders (e.g., depression, anxiety, or somatoform disorder) or for marital, family, or occupational problems. The initiation of treatment is often at the insistence of a spouse, relative, or employer. They can be difficult patients to treat because of their tendency to be blaming, argumentative, pessimistic, and passively resistant.

Cognitive treatment can be useful in directly addressing the false perceptions, assumptions, and attributions as long as the psychiatrist is not drawn into unproductive disagreements and arguments. It is common for psychiatrists to become frustrated, impatient, and defensive in response to the negativism, criticism, and complaints. Periodic consultations with colleagues are advisable. Group therapy is often helpful once the patient has developed a commitment to the group, as the various members can provide consistent and confirmatory feedback regarding the negativistic and passive-aggressive behavior. There is no known pharmacological treatment for PAPD.

Depressive Personality Disorder

DSM-IV Criteria

Depressive Personality Disorder

A. A pervasive pattern of depressive cognitions and behaviors beginning by early adulthood and present in a variety of contexts, as indicated by five (or more) of the following:

   (1) usual mood is dominated by dejection, gloominess, cheerlessness, joylessness, unhappiness

   (2) self-concept centers around beliefs of inadequacy, worthlessness, and low self-esteem

   (3) is critical, blaming, and derogatory toward self

   (4) is brooding and given to worry

   (5) is negativistic, critical, and judgmental toward others

   (6) is pessimistic

   (7) is prone to feeling guilty or remorseful

B. Does not occur exclusively during major depressive episodes and is not better accounted for by dysthymic disorder.

DPPD is a pervasive pattern of depressive cognitions and behaviors that have been evident since adolescence and characteristic of everyday functioning. Persons with DPPD characteristically display gloominess, cheerlessness, pessimism, brooding, rumination, and dejection.

DPPD was proposed for inclusion in DSM-III and DSM-III-R but there were concerns that it may not be adequately distinguished from the mood disorder of dysthymia. However, a field trial by the

DSM-IV Mood Disorders Work Group indicated that many persons do meet the diagnostic criteria for DPPD and not those for early-onset dysthymic disorder. In addition, many persons with early-onset dysthymia may not be adequately described as having a disorder confined to the regulation or control of their mood. However, the DSM-IV diagnostic criteria for DPPD lack sufficient empirical support to warrant full recognition at this time.

DIFFERENTIAL DIAGNOSIS

DPPD overlaps substantially early-onset dysthymia. Early-onset dysthymia was conceptualized as depressive personality or a characterological depression before DSM-III-R and the alternative criteria for dysthymia that were placed in an appendix to DSM-IV were based in part on research on DPPD. It is noted in DSM-IV that there may not be a meaningful distinction between these diagnoses. Some may prefer to use the diagnosis of early-onset dysthymia, but a dysregulation in mood may not adequately explain why some persons are characterized by chronic attitudes of pessimism, negativism, hopelessness, and dejection.

COURSE AND NATURAL HISTORY

As children, persons with DDPD have been pessimistic, gloomy, passive, and withdrawn. Performance in school was often inadequate to poor. This behavior pattern continues essentially unchanged into and through adulthood. Relationships with peers and sexual partners are invariably problematical. Persons with DDPD are gloomy and irritable company and have difficulty finding pleasure, joy, or satisfaction in leisure activities. They may also be quite withdrawn and lonely but lack an apparent motivation or energy to seek or maintain relationships.

TREATMENT

Many persons with DPPD seek or are referred for treatment of a depressive mood disorder. It is important for such persons to recognize the extent to which the depressed mood reflects their fundamental view of themselves and the world. Their pessimism involves more than simply a dysregulation of mood.

Cognitive-behavioral techniques have demonstrated efficacy in the treatment of depressive personality traits. Depressive individuals' pessimistic view of themselves and their future should be systematically challenged. Exploring the faulty reasoning, arbitrary inferences, selective perceptions, and misattributions can be influential in overcoming the pessimistic, gloomy, critical, and negativistic attitudes. Persons with DPPD are also responsive to antidepressant pharmacotherapy, particularly with tricyclic antidepressants.

Psychological Factors Affecting Medical Condition

This diagnostic category recognizes the variety of ways in which specific psychological or behavioral factors can adversely affect medical illnesses. Such factors may contribute to the initiation or the exacerbation of the illness, interfere with treatment and rehabilitation, or contribute to morbidity and mortality. Psychological factors may themselves constitute risks for medical diseases, or they may magnify the effects of nonpsychological risk factors. The effects may be mediated directly at a pathophysiological level (e.g., psychological stress inducing myocardial ischemia) or through the patient's behavior (e.g., noncompliance).

This diagnosis is structured in the *Diagnostic and Statistical Manual of Mental Disorders,* Fourth Edition (DSM-IV) so that both the psychological factor and the general medical condition are to be specified. The psychological factor can be an Axis I or Axis II mental disorder (e.g., major depressive disorder aggravating coronary artery disease), a psychological symptom (e.g., anxiety exacerbating asthma), a personality trait or coping style (e.g., type A behavior contributing to the development of coronary artery disease), maladaptive health behaviors (e.g., unsafe sex in a person with human immunodeficiency virus [HIV] infection), a stress-related physiological response (e.g., tension headache), or other or unspecified psychological factors. The medical condition is noted on Axis III.

The subject of psychological factors affecting medical condition (PFAMC) has become the focus of intense research because of the illumination it may provide of basic disease mechanisms (e.g., psychoneuroimmunology) and because of the intense interest in improving both the outcomes and the efficiency of health care delivery. In epidemiological studies, several psychiatric disorders increase the likelihood of mortality, especially depression, bipolar disorder, schizophrenia, and alcohol abuse or dependence. Psychiatric disorders or symptoms in patients with medical illness may increase their use of health care services, particularly the length of costly hospital stays.

It should be evident that this diagnosis is not really a discrete diagnostic category but rather a label for the interactive effects of psyche on soma. Mind-body interactions have long been a focus of interest, both in health and in disease. Psychiatric illness and medical disease frequently coexist. Psychiatrists and investigators of past eras were misled by this frequent comorbidity into premature conclusions that the psychological factors were preeminent in the causation of the medical disorders, and these were designated psychosomatic. A more modern approach has been to recognize that all medical illnesses are potentially affected by many different factors in the biological, psychological, and social realms.

In addition to promoting known risk factors for medical illness, psychological factors also have an impact on the course of illness by influencing how patients respond to their symptoms, including whether and how they seek care. For example, the defense mechanism of denial may lead an individual to ignore anginal chest pain, attribute it to indigestion, delay seeking medical attention, or minimize the pain when describing it to a physician.

Psychological factors can also reduce the patient's compliance with treatment and lifestyle change and can interfere with rehabilitation through impairment of motivation, understanding, optimism, or tolerance.

There is an increasing body of scientific evidence that psychological factors, in addition to their impact on classic (nonpsychological) risk factors and the physician-patient interaction, have direct effects on pathophysiological processes. For example, stress has been experimentally shown to cause myocardial ischemia in patients with coronary disease.

TREATMENT

Management of psychological factors affecting the patient's medical condition should be tailored both to the particular psychological factor of relevance and to the medical outcome of concern. Some general guidelines, however, can be helpful. The physician, whether in primary care or a specialty, should not ignore apparent psychiatric illness, although this occurs too often because of discomfort, stigma, lack of training, or disinterest. Referring the patient to a mental health specialist for evaluation is certainly better than ignoring the psychological problem but should not be regarded as "disposing" of it, because the physician must still attend to its potential impact on the patient's medical illness. Similarly, psychiatrists and other mental health practitioners should not ignore coincident medical disease and should not assume that referral to a nonpsychiatric physician absolves them of all responsibility for the patient's medical problem.

Relational Problems

A relational problem is a situation in which two or more emotionally attached individuals (i.e., family members, romantic partners) engage in communication or behavior patterns that are destructive, unsatisfying, or both, to one or more of the individuals. Relational problems deserve clinical attention because, once initiated, they tend to be perpetuating, chronic, and frequently contemporaneous with or followed by other serious problems, such as individual symptoms (e.g., depression) or social unit dissolution (e.g., divorce). These difficulties cause malfunction in the family or social unit beyond the area of specific difficulty, may create stress such that symptoms begin to appear in the most vulnerable members of the family, and may threaten the viability of the social unit. Relational problems may be diagnosed either in the presence or absence of an individual disorder.

Relational problems are placed in the *Diagnostic and Statistical Manual of Mental Disorders* (DSM-IV) section "Other Conditions That May Be a Focus of Clinical Attention." Five specific relational problems are described:

1. **Relational problem related to a mental disorder or general medical condition.** This is a category in which the focus of clinical attention is a pattern of impaired family interaction in the presence of a mental disorder or medical condition in a family member.
2. **Parent-child relational problem.** This category describes a pattern of family interaction between parent and child that shows signs of impairment, such as faulty communication, overprotection, and inadequate discipline. The family interaction is associated with clinically significant impairment or symptoms with clinically significant impairment or symptoms in an individual or in family functioning, or both.
3. **Partner relational problems.** This category focuses on a pattern of interaction between spouses or partners characterized by negative and distorted communication or noncommunication associated with clinically significant impairment in one or both partners.
4. **Sibling relational problem.** This category refers to a pattern of interaction between siblings that is associated with clinically significant impairment in individual or family members.

5. **Relational problem not otherwise specified.** This category refers to relational problems not listed here. It includes extrafamily relational problems and difficulties with others, such as coworkers.

Four major constructs (Table 42–1) have been investigated that describe nodal areas of relational difficulty in the family and marital environment: structure, communication, expression of affect, and problem solving. Relational difficulties in other environments (e.g., work) have not been described in the clinical literature.

TREATMENT

The primary goal of treatment is to bring the relational unit, such as the couple or the family, to a point of harmonious, conflict-minimized, organized, and satisfying level of functioning. The mediating goals of treatment are focused on improvement in the specific areas of functioning of the relational unit (i.e., structure, communication, affect expression, problem solving).

Relational problems are best observed and treated directly in a family format that has the conflicted family members together with the therapist. However, in certain situations relational problems may be more conducive to change within an individual treatment format.

TABLE 42–1	Empirically Derived Family Relational Constructs
Structure	Leadership and distribution of functions
Overinvolvement	Unclear boundaries; overdependence
Communication	Amount and clarity of information exchange
Communication deviance	Unclear, amorphous, fragmented, and/or unintelligible communication
Coercion	Behavior control by use of aversive communication
Expression of affect	Implicit or explicit verbalization of affective tone
Problem solving	Definition of problems, consideration of alternative lines of action, agreement to use optimal line of action
Conflict and its resolution	Process of resolving differences of opinion

For example, relational problems of an individual with a mental disorder (e.g., a schizophrenic son 25 years of age in conflict with his mother and father) in some cases may best be approached by individual sessions with the affected person. Furthermore, when one adult in a family unit is depressed, interpersonal or cognitive psychotherapies may be used individually and focused on interpersonal conflict resolution.

The specific techniques available to family therapists can be divided into five categories: psychoeducational, cognitive-behavioral, structural, strategic-systemic, and insight-oriented techniques. Psychoeducational approaches are most helpful when there is a family member with a specific medical or psychiatric disorder, and the family can utilize information on how to manage the disorder with the least tension and stress on the patient. Cognitive-behavioral techniques are useful in improving communication and problem-solving skills and the positive interactive behaviors in marital-family units. Structural and strategic-systemic approaches are most useful in rearranging the repetitive interactions in a family that constitute the boundaries and alliances in the social system.

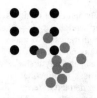

Therapeutics

Individual Psychoanalytic Psychotherapy

Psychoanalytic theory provides the modern clinician with a comprehensive system for the understanding of personality development, the meaningfulness of human conflict and emotional pain, and the mutative factors within the doctor-patient relationship. Psychoanalysis is a general psychology, a developmental theory, and a specific treatment. With respect to psychoanalysis as a treatment approach, since its inception psychoanalytic theory has undergone numerous and substantial revisions. Its history has been punctuated by persistent attempts both to simplify psychoanalytic technique and to shorten its duration of treatment. The synonymous terms psychoanalytic psychotherapy, psychoanalytically oriented psychotherapy, psychodynamic psychotherapy, and expressive psychotherapy have come to represent the most coherent of these attempts.

WHAT IS PSYCHOTHERAPY?

Strupp (1986) specified that psychotherapy is the systematic use of a human relationship for therapeutic purposes of alleviating emotional distress by effecting enduring changes in a patient's thinking, feelings, and behavior. The mutual engagement of the patient and the psychotherapist both cognitively and emotionally is the foundation for effective psychotherapeutic work.

The core task of the psychoanalytic psychotherapist is to make contact with and comprehend, as thoroughly as possible, the patient's subjective inner world in order to engage in an analytical (i.e., interpretive) conversation about it. This core task implies that all psychoanalytic psychotherapies may be further defined in terms of three operations: accepting, understanding, and explaining. More specifically, the therapist must engage with the patient by accepting the subjective experience of the patient's emotional pain and conflict. This is achieved through the establishment of a therapeutic dialogue based on an empathic, nonjudgmental rapport.

Second, within the process of listening to and feeling with the patient, the therapist will begin to develop an understanding of the intricacies of the patient's plight. Much of what the therapist observes may at first remain outside of the patient's conscious awareness, manifested in the form of reenactments and reliving of earlier experiences within the therapy rather than in deliberate, conscious, descriptive communication.

Finally, as the therapist shares this beginning understanding with the patient through a simultaneously empathic and interpretive mode, both arrive at a deeper appreciation for the genesis of and the reasons for the patient's symptoms. The shared relationship in which understanding is gained is no less instrumental in achieving change than are the insights and modified perceptions that may result from the psychotherapeutic experience.

EXPRESSIVE-SUPPORTIVE CONTINUUM

Traditionally, to the degree that psychoanalytic psychotherapy has focused on the recovery of repressed psychological material, it has been called expressive and has been distinguished from the supportive psychotherapies that concentrate on shoring up certain defense mechanisms.

It is more appropriate to conceptualize psychoanalytic psychotherapy as being on a continuum of expressive to supportive. This implies that any given treatment might employ more or less expressive and supportive interventions, depending on what is transpiring within the psychotherapeutic process. An important skill of the psychoanalytic psychotherapist, then, is the ability to employ the appropriate balance of both expressive and supportive interventions as dictated by the needs of the patient. Finally, the conceptualization of an expressive-supportive continuum also facilitates the establishment of therapeutic goals, interventional plans, and indications for individual psychoanalytic psychotherapy (Table 43–1).

TRANSFERENCE AND RESISTANCE, COUNTERTRANSFERENCE

Transference and resistance constitute the two most distinctive features of psychoanalytic psychotherapies. Transference is defined as those perceptions of and responses to a person in the here and now that more appropriately reflect past feelings about or responses to important people earlier in one's life, especially parents and siblings. Psychoanalytic psychotherapy stresses the importance of transfer-

TABLE 43–1	Comparative Interventions	
Expressive	**← Continuum →**	**Supportive**
Confrontation		Suggestion
Clarification		Reassurance
Interpretation		Advice giving
Interpretation of transference		Praise
		Environmental intervention and manipulation

ence within the treatment relationship, but it differs from psychoanalysis in that it does not, to the same degree, promote the depth and intensity of the transference.

Countertransference is variously defined as 1) the analyst's or psychotherapist's transference reactions to the patient; 2) his or her reactions to the patient's transferences; and 3) any reactions, feelings, and attitudes of the analyst or therapist toward the patient, regardless of their source. Such responses to the patient were once viewed as deviations from the ideal of a consistently bland and comfortable experiencing of the patient by the analyst or therapist. Countertransference reactions were also conceptualized as impediments to progress within the treatment, that is, as interferences in the therapist's ability to understand the patient. They are currently more broadly understood as manifestations of the requisite engagement by the therapist or analyst in the emotional process of treatment. Moreover, these reactions are a rich source of understanding the patient's experience as it touches the therapist affectively. Although countertransference feelings are at times uncomfortable for the therapist and a challenge to monitor and process, they are understood as a reflection of the glue of the relationship without which no real connection or significant change can occur.

Resistance is broadly defined as the conscious or, more often, unconscious force within the patient opposing the emergence of unconscious material. Resistance must be understood not as something the patient does to the therapist, but rather as the patient's attempt to protect herself or himself by avoiding the anticipated emotional discomfort accompanying the emergence of conflictual, dangerous, or painful experiences, feelings, thoughts, memories, needs, and desires.

Resistance occurs through the use of unconscious mental operations called defense mechanisms for which there is substantial research support (Table 43–2). The recognition, clarification, and interpretation of resistance constitute important activities of the psychoanalyst and the psychoanalytic psychotherapist, both of whom must first appreciate how a patient is warding off anxiety before understanding why he or she is so compelled.

BASIC TECHNIQUE

As noted, the analysis of transference by the repeated interpretation of resistance is the primary activity of the psychoanalyst and an

TABLE 43–2	Some Common Defense Mechanisms*
Repression	Relegation of threatening wishes, needs, or impulses into unawareness
Projection	Attribution of conflicted thoughts or feelings to another or to a group of people
Denial	Refusal to appreciate information about oneself or others
Identification	Patterning of oneself after another
Projective identification	Attribution of unacceptable personality characteristics onto another followed by identification with that other
Regression	A partial return to earlier levels of adaptation to avoid conflict
Splitting	Experiencing of others as being all good or all bad (i.e., idealization or devaluation)
Reaction formation	Transformation of an unwanted thought or feeling into its opposite
Isolation	Divorcing a feeling from its unpleasant idea
Rationalization	Using seemingly logical explanations to make untenable feelings or thoughts more acceptable
Displacement	Redirection of unpleasant feelings or thoughts onto another object
Dissociation	Splitting off of thought or feeling from its original source
Conversion	Transformation of unacceptable wishes or thoughts into body sensations
Sublimation	A mature mechanism whereby unacceptable thoughts and feelings are channeled into socially acceptable ones

*All defense mechanisms are involuntary and unconscious.

important one for the psychoanalytic psychotherapist. To promote the patient's examination of these two phenomena, both the analyst and the therapist are guided by principles that focus on the therapeutic relationship and establish a confidential, safe, and predictable environment geared toward maximizing the patient's introspection. The patient is encouraged to free-associate, that is, to notice and report as best she or he is able whatever comes into conscious awareness. In the case of psychoanalysis, the depth of the therapeutic process is enhanced by the patient's lying down, with the analyst out of the patient's visual range; by the analyst's modest level of verbal activity; and by meeting frequently, usually four or five times weekly (compared with once or twice weekly as in psychoanalytic psychotherapy) for 45 to 50 minutes for a number of years (Tables 43–3 and 43–4).

Therapeutic neutrality and abstinence are related concepts. Both foster the unfolding and deepening of the transference as well as the opportunity for its interpretation. The analyst and psychoanalytic psychotherapist assume a neutral position vis-à-vis the patient's psychological material by neither advocating for the patient's wishes and needs nor prohibiting against them. The patient is encouraged in the therapeutic relationship to develop the capacity for self-observation to the best of his or her ability. Neutrality does not mean nonresponsiveness. It is nonjudgmental nondirectiveness.

Abstinence refers to the position assumed by the analyst and psychoanalytic psychotherapist of recognizing and accepting the patient's wishes and emotional needs, particularly as they emanate from transference distortions, while abstaining from direct gratification of those needs through action. Abstinence is a principle that guards against the therapist's gratification at the patient's expense.

TABLE 43–3	Characteristics of Psychoanalysis
Goals	Personality reorganization
	Resolution of childhood conflicts
Patient's characteristics	Psychoneuroses and mild to moderate personality disorders
	Psychological mindedness
	Introspectiveness
	Can experience and learn from intense affects or conflicts without acting them out
	Reasonable object relationships
	High motivation
	Can tolerate frustration and therapeutic regression
Techniques	Use of couch
	Four or five sessions weekly
	Free association
	Neutrality
	Abstinence
	Analysis of defenses
	Analysis of transference
	Dream interpretation
	Genetic reconstruction
	Less frequent use of medication
Length of treatment	3–6 y or longer

TABLE 43–4	Characteristics of Psychoanalytic Psychotherapy
Goals	Partial personality reorganization
	Appreciation of conflicts and related defense mechanisms
	Partial reconstruction of the past
	Symptom relief
	Improved interpersonal relationships
Patient's characteristics	Includes all criteria for psychoanalysis
	Moderate to severe personality disorders (e.g., borderline)
	Some affective disorders with and without medication (e.g., major depression, dysthymia)
Techniques	Active therapeutic stance
	Face to face (sitting up)
	One to three sessions weekly
	Limited free association
	Active focus on current life issues
	Limited transference analysis
	Some supportive techniques
	Liberal use of medication
	Clarification and interpretation
Length of treatment	Months to years (may or may not be shorter than psychoanalysis)

Although it is technically proper to speak of the development of a transference neurosis only in psychoanalysis, many patients in psychoanalytic psychotherapy also develop strong transferences within their treatment experiences. By maintaining a neutral and abstinent position with respect to the patient's needs and wishes, the analyst and psychotherapist create a safe atmosphere for the experiencing and expression of even highly charged affects, the safety required for the patient's motivation for continued therapeutic work. Although there is a persistent caricature of the psychoanalyst, and to a lesser degree of the psychoanalytic psychotherapist, as working in a withholding and aloof fashion, the concepts of optimal frustration and optimal gratification imply that there is a position held by the psychiatrist that is neither sterile nor overstimulating and that promotes the establishment of a meaningful therapeutic relationship.

Two related but distinct components initially attributed to the analyst's listening process are worthy of note. First, the concept of the analyst's evenly hovering or evenly suspended attention implies that listening to the patient requires of the analyst that he or she be nonjudgmental and give equal attention to every topic and detail that the patient provides. It also embraces the notion that the effective therapist is one who can remain open to her or his own thoughts and feelings as they are evoked while listening to the patient. Such internal responses often supply important insights into the patient's concerns.

Second, empathic listening is of equal importance to both parties. Empathy permits the patient to feel understood and provides the therapist with a method to achieve vicarious introspection. Interferences to successful empathic listening are often the product of countertransference reactions, which should be suspected whenever, for example, the therapist experiences irritation, strong erotic feelings, or inattention during a treatment session.

HOW DOES PSYCHOANALYTIC PSYCHOTHERAPY WORK?

Classic psychoanalysis has held that patients are helped by the acquisition of insight into their intrapsychic conflicts. More specifically, conflict is resolved through precise and accurate transference interpretations, which permit the patient eventually to experience the analyst with fewer distortions from childhood experiences.

Psychoanalysis also helps by permitting the patient to become increasingly conscious of troublesome feelings, conflicts, and wishes that heretofore had remained out of awareness and that produced unhappiness by promoting repetitive self-defeating behaviors. Whereas insight has always been valued as a goal of psychoanalysis, insight by itself is insufficient. The process whereby insight is acquired is a lengthy and arduous one that is inextricably linked with the recall of painful affects, memories, and traumatic experiences.

For treatment to be effective then, there must be both cognitive and affective experiences for the patient. Neither a purely intellectual nor a purely cathartic experience is likely to result in relief or behavioral change. The support provided by the treatment relationship, which includes commitment, respect, reliability, honesty, and care, is a powerful factor in the curative process. It is this atmosphere that makes bearable the emotional pain that accompanies the healing of the wounds first experienced in isolation, so often inflicted by the first objects of the patient's love, need, and trust. All of these considerations are central to psychoanalytic psychotherapy as well.

The concept of working through is helpful in appreciating the lengthy and complex psychoanalytic and psychotherapeutic processes. Working through is that stage or aspect of treatment characterized by repeated identification of reenactment and reliving of earlier experiences through confrontation, clarification, and interpretation of resistance and transference that ultimately promotes the patient's self-awareness. In effect, the working through process frees the patient from the position of being at the mercy of unconscious conflicts and fears that have compromised interpersonal relationships and achievement. This is accomplished through the analysis not only of the transference but also of current interpersonal relationships outside of the analysis or psychotherapy. Ultimately, a thorough understanding of the transference and of current relationships permits the patient to appreciate their relationship to important early experiences and ultimately to ameliorate the influence of the past on the present.

Therapeutic Alliance

The *therapeutic* or *working* alliance is described in terms that relate to the real component, as distinguished from the transference component, of the therapist-patient relationship. The real component is composed of the patient's conscious, rational, and non-conflictual feelings toward the therapist that permit a collaborative relationship and that provide the motivation for working toward symptom relief.

A great deal of research in the outcome of psychoanalytic psychotherapy has focused on the importance of the therapeutic alliance. Increasing appreciation for the role of supportive factors, such as the rapport between the patient and therapist that constitutes the therapeutic relationship, has balanced the earlier, more narrowly defined position that attributed therapeutic success exclusively to insight resulting from the analyst's specific interpretive activity. The clinical consequences of appreciating the helpfulness

---

TABLE 43–5   Indications for Psychoanalysis

Psychoanalysis is the treatment of choice for repetitive, long-standing, maladaptive problems involving personality or character and chronic, repetitive behaviorial, affective, or mental disturbances or symptoms that do not respond to cheaper or quicker forms of treatment. In general, it is used for all the character disorders or personality disorders, except antisocial and schizotypal disorders, as well as numerous symptom disorders.

The chronic symptoms must reflect both

1. Intrapsychic conflict
2. Developmental arrest or inhibition

As well, the psychiatrist must expect that

3. The patient's symptoms are likely to continue unless analysis is undertaken
4. Treatments that are less intensive than analysis would likely result in excessive personal or social cost for the patient or just provide temporary relief of acute symptoms related to a current stress, without dealing with underlying issues, hence predisposing the patient to difficulties in the future.

Finally, the patient must be able to use psychoanalysis. In general, this rules out those with psychotic disorders and a number, but not all, of the borderline disorders.

From American Psychiatric Association Peer Review Manual, 3rd ed. Washington, DC: American Psychiatric Association, 1985.

of nonspecific factors have been the psychoanalytic psychotherapist's paying much greater attention to the initial phases of engaging the patient in psychotherapy and a greater respect for those positive and negative factors that the therapist brings to the working relationship. Currently, psychoanalysis and psychoanalytic psychotherapy both hold that the psychiatrist's personality and interventional technique have equal influence on the therapeutic process.

In summary, contemporary psychoanalysis and psychoanalytic psychotherapy still emphasize elucidation of the unconscious, especially within the transference, and still use interpretation as the primary clinical intervention but recognize more fully the important role of the mutual emotional engagement of therapist and patient and the curative role of this relationship as well as of other supportive factors. They adhere to a much broader perspective on human development and psychiatric disorders. Psychological problems can result not only from early intrapsychic conflict but also from developmental deficits or failures as well as from psychological trauma (Table 43–5).

HOW DOES PSYCHOANALYTIC PSYCHOTHERAPY DIFFER FROM PSYCHOANALYSIS?

Many psychiatrists find it useful to conceptualize psychoanalysis and psychoanalytic psychotherapy as residing on a therapeutic continuum. Overall, it is fair to say that psychoanalytic psychotherapy

- Places greater emphasis on the here and now in terms of the patient's current interpersonal relationships and experiences outside of the therapy, whereas in psychoanalysis, there is greater emphasis on the experiences within the analysis and the relationship between analyst and analysand
- Incorporates more than does psychoanalysis various techniques from other dynamic and behavioral psychotherapies
- Emphasizes the usefulness of focusing on current (dynamic) problems and less on genetic issues
- Establishes more modest goals of treatment

The last point is particularly important in that it facilitated the development of brief dynamic psychotherapies, which address focal problems generally in up to 20 sessions.

TASKS OF THE PSYCHOANALYTIC PSYCHOTHERAPIST

What are the challenges of the psychotherapist in performing psychoanalytic psychotherapy? First, the therapist must ensure that the patient can feel both emotionally and physically safe within the therapeutic relationship. This is accomplished by acknowledging the goals of the treatment, defining the role of the therapist, and establishing professional boundaries.

Boundaries refer to those constant and highly predictable components of the treatment situation that constitute the framework of the working relationship. For example, agreeing to meet with the patient for a specified amount of time, in a professional office, and for an established fee are some of the elements of the professional framework. Boundaries also have ethical dimensions best summarized as the absolute adherence by the therapist to the rule of never taking advantage of the patient: through sexual behavior, for personal financial or emotional gain, or by exploiting the patient's need and love for the therapist in any fashion (e.g., by using the therapy sessions to discuss the therapist's own problems). The concepts of neutrality, abstinence, and confidentiality further define the role of the therapist.

A critical task of the psychoanalytic psychotherapist is detecting when a breach in either role or boundary has occurred and restoring the patient's security through clarifying and interpreting the meaningfulness of such a breach.

Successful interpretation is based on a number of prerequisite skills: the capacity to empathize with the patient's plight, the ability to recognize the meaning of one's own fantasies about and responses to a patient (countertransference), the ability to maintain the patient's verbal flow through the use of open-ended or focused questions, and the capacity to tolerate a relatively high level of ambiguity within the therapeutic relationship. One important professional characteristic of the skilled psychotherapist is patience. Psychotherapy is often arduous, and the capacity to "stay in the chair" with the patient is critical.

Identifying repeated patterns of behavior both within the therapy and in the patient's outside life is a fundamental technique in making sense of the patient's emotional life. This of course involves the appreciation of transference and the art of knowing how and when to share this recognition with the patient. Interpretation relies on both appropriate timing and dosage. That is, the psychoanalytic psychotherapist must appreciate when the patient can best integrate the therapist's observations and must respect the patient's defenses, taking care not to overwhelm the patient by insisting that she or he confront more than is tolerable.

Psychoanalytic psychotherapy requires the successful engagement of the patient and the establishment of a therapeutic or working alliance. The alliance can be threatened by a number of phenomena including but not limited to the following:

- The therapist's countertransferences or other limitations in his or her capacity to tolerate the emotions stirred by the patient, resulting in empathic failures and mistakes
- The emergence of intense feelings and needs within the patient, for example, when an accurate well-timed intervention evokes feelings of appreciation and love accompanied by feelings of vulnerability, erotic desire, or inferiority in relation to the therapist that the patient wants to flee
- The patient is being reminded of the existence of others in the therapist's life, such as other patients or family (e.g., during interruptions due to the therapist's vacations), triggering painful and embarrassing feelings of jealousy and possessiveness

The therapist's ability to appreciate and respectfully to acknowledge to the patient the impact of these temporal events is critical to the progress of treatment.

All of the psychotherapist's skills and techniques must be embedded in a consistent and coherent theoretical viewpoint that provides the therapist with a framework to understand the etiology and meaning of a patient's symptoms and dysfunctional behaviors both in the past and in the present as well as in the beginning, middle, and termination phases of psychotherapy. This includes an organized method for understanding the therapist's unconscious and conscious responses to the patient as well. It requires that the therapist listen to the patient's communications in a manner that is markedly different from other forms of social discourse. So-called process communication speaks to the therapist on multiple levels and through displacement, through passing remarks and jokes, through shifts in topics, and through metaphors and symbols. To assist in understanding complicated process communication, psychiatrists often ask themselves, *Why is the patient telling me this now? What might the patient be trying to say about his or her uncomfortable feelings? Is something being said about the therapeutic relationship?*

Both the psychoanalytic psychotherapist and the psychoanalyst must be skillful in supporting the patient at times of emotional disequilibrium, but they may differ in the degree and manner in which support is provided to the patient. Psychoanalysis has always striven for an extensive transformation of the patient's characterological problems and a thorough analysis of the patient's transference neurosis. The psychoanalytic psychotherapist, however, must be skillful in setting more limited goals with a patient regarding the reconstruction of the patient's past. This type of treatment aims to improve the patient's quality of life largely through enhancing interpersonal relationships by promoting greater insight into perceptual distortion and intrapsychic and interpersonal conflict. Psychoanalytic psychotherapy accomplishes this objective by focusing much more on the patient's current predicaments as manifested in both life activities and the relationship with the therapist. Compared with psychoanalysis, it is less concerned with the analysis of transference and the complete discovery of the underlying genetic precursors of the patient's current psychological problems.

INDICATIONS FOR PSYCHOANALYTIC PSYCHOTHERAPY

Although current psychotherapy research attempts to ascertain what specific disorder in what type of patient is most effectively treated by what specific psychotherapeutic approach, studies have not as yet provided the answer to these questions. At this time, it is possible to speak only in generalities based on case reports and limited studies. Conditions and disorders for which psychoanalytic psychotherapy appear to be indicated are included in Table 43–6.

Psychoanalytic psychotherapy, often in combination with medication, is an appropriate intervention in a broad range of disorders, conditions, and psychiatric illnesses.

The characteristics of the patient assumed to be correlated with positive outcome in psychoanalytic psychotherapy include introspectiveness (psychological mindedness); ability to establish and maintain human relationships, even "unhealthy" ones; vocational stability; high degree of motivation; absence of formal thought

TABLE 43–6	Putative Indications for Psychoanalytic Psychotherapy

Neuroses

Personality disorders (except antisocial personality disorder)

Posttraumatic stress disorders

Adjustment disorders

Paraphilias

Mood disorders*

Anxiety disorders*

Somatoform disorders*

Sexual and gender identity disorders*

Eating disorders*

Substance abuse disorders*

Dissociative disorders*

Relational problems

Impulse-control disorders*

Psychological problems affecting medical illnesses

*Not indicated for all disorders in these categories.

disorder; and psychological resources sufficient to withstand the frustration of the treatment and its characteristic therapeutic regression and accompanying strong affects.

CONTRAINDICATIONS TO PSYCHOANALYTIC PSYCHOTHERAPY

For the most part, contraindications to any psychoanalytic psychotherapy that is heavily weighted toward the expressive end of the therapeutic continuum can be found in Table 43–7.

TABLE 43–7	Contraindications to Expressive Psychoanalytic Psychotherapy

Major ego deficits

Poor motivation

Significant cognitive deficits

Inability to obtain symptom relief through understanding

Inability to verbalize affects

Lack of psychological mindedness

Minimal impulse control

No social support network

Low frustration tolerance

Inability to form therapeutic alliance

SUPPORTIVE PSYCHOANALYTIC PSYCHOTHERAPY

Supportive psychotherapy attempts to shore up the patient's defenses and enhance his or her ability to cope with the trials of illness or psychological deficits and the challenges they impose on the patient's daily activities (Table 43–8). Not unexpectedly, it also strives to prevent decompensation and regression. As such, psychoanalytic supportive psychotherapy employs a psychodynamic understanding of the patient's difficulties but does not emphasize interpretation of the patient's internal world. Rather, supportive psychotherapy focuses on assisting the patient to address interpersonal and environmental challenges in the here and now.

Despite its noninterpretive emphasis, supportive psychotherapy can have a substantial impact in the lives of patients with significant ego deficits and those with major mental illness. These patients may include those with high levels of aggressivity, poor impulse control, overreliance on action rather than verbal expression of emotions, compromised reality testing, and limited psychological mindedness. It is also highly effective with higher functioning patients who have experienced recent psychic trauma (e.g., through natural disasters, illness, physical or sexual assault, and unexpected devastating losses).

Supportive psychotherapy techniques consist predominantly of empathically listening to the patient's feelings and experiences; giving advice and reassurance; offering suggestion and helpful coping techniques; and for some patients with severe and chronic maladaptations, gently revealing their misperceptions and how they interfere in daily functioning. Although often silent, the patient's identification with the therapist's values, ideals, and approaches to problems is exceptionally therapeutic. Environmental interventions through helping agencies and the patient's significant others are also effective supportive techniques. Although nonspecific to some degree, these interventions are nevertheless based on a comprehensive understanding of the patient's strengths and weaknesses and are frequently instrumental in curbing self-destructive and self-defeating behaviors. Transference is appreciated, but the therapist rarely interprets it in supportive psychoanalytic psychotherapy, choosing rather to foster a positive working relationship through other means.

Supportive psychotherapy can produce significant and lasting behavioral change through the reinforcement of health-promoting behaviors; increased capacity for self-reflection; anxiety reduction; and development of new defenses such as intellectualization that enable the patient to acquire a cognitive, anxiety-reducing conceptualization of her or his difficulties.

IS PSYCHOANALYTIC PSYCHOTHERAPY EFFECTIVE?

Meta-analytical studies of psychotherapy have demonstrated unequivocally that psychotherapy is effective.

Among patients treated in psychotherapy, 85% fared better on outcome measures than those receiving no treatment. Psychological growth achieved through psychotherapy is also enduring.

TABLE 43–8	Characteristics of Supportive Psychoanalytic Psychotherapy
Goals	Maintain current level of psychological functioning Restore premorbid adaptation, if possible Enhance coping mechanisms Strengthen defense mechanisms unless they are maladaptive Support reality testing Relieve symptoms Decrease mental distress

Patient's characteristics	Severe character disorders
	  Chronic ego deficits
	  Thought disorders
	  Limited psychological mindedness
	  Limited motivation
	  Poor interpersonal relationships
	  Poor impulse control
	  Low frustration tolerance
	  Regression proneness
	  Some potential for therapeutic alliance
	  Extreme passivity
	  Inability to verbalize affects
	Those in crisis situations (catastrophic loss, acute psychic trauma, medical illness)
	  Psychologically healthy
	  Effective social network
	  High premorbid adaptation
	  Flexible defenses

Techniques	Predictability and consistency of therapist Conversational style Confrontation, clarification, education Problem-solving focus Provide encouragement, advice, praise, reassurance Environmental intervention Strengthen reality testing Shore up defense mechanisms Discourage regression Infrequent genetic reconstruction Infrequent transference analysis Less therapeutic neutrality Frequent use of medication
Length of treatment	Usually once weekly or less Duration of sessions flexible Varies from brief therapy for those reactive disorders in individuals who do not need or are not motivated for further help to lifelong treatment of patients with some chronic disorders

A German study of dynamic psychotherapy and psychoanalysis found that treatment decreased medical visits by one third, lost work days by two fifths, and hospital days by two thirds. Successful outcomes were linked to longer duration of treatment.

The helpfulness of psychotherapy for those patients suffering from significant medical illness has been documented in cases of breast cancer. Patients with lymphoma, leukemia, and malignant melanoma have fared better with their illnesses when treated with group psychotherapy. Opioid-dependent patients attending community methadone maintenance programs have found expressive-supportive psychotherapy superior to counseling in its ability to maintain their gains.

At this time, the therapist is left with few data supporting the superiority of one type of psychotherapy over another for a given condition or disorder. This dilemma must be tempered by the recognition of the enormous complexity of psychoanalytic psychotherapy research.

CONCLUSION

The majority of all encounters with patients in American psychiatry involve some form of psychotherapy, and many of these interventions are based on the principles of psychoanalytic psychotherapy.

At this time, the theory and technique of psychoanalytic psychotherapy provide the most comprehensive orientation to the continuum of expressive-supportive psychotherapy. Psychoanalytic psychotherapy is a potent intervention and, as such, holds great promise when it is used for appropriate patients with appropriate psychiatric problems. Like medication, psychoanalytic psychotherapy has specific indications and contraindications. As an effective therapeutic intervention, it requires that the therapist be highly skilled in assessing the inner experience of those who come for help. It also requires extensive training and education in techniques of this treatment modality. As well, the therapist must acquire significant self-knowledge, sophistication, and dedication in working so intensively with human pain.

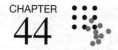

Group Psychotherapy

A broad spectrum of theoretical approaches informs therapists which aspects of the complex group behaviors they should attend to. Some focus on individuals as seen through the psychoanalytic lens of transference and resistance; others focus on interpersonal transactions in which distortions arising from childhood are played out within the group and are subject to feedback and social pressures; and others focus on properties of the group as a whole, which emphasize group dynamics and systems theories as the central organizing concepts. Learning principles are contained in almost all of these orientations and are the central emphases in cognitive-behavioral approaches. Successful integration of these approaches has not been achieved, and therapists may maintain a central theoretical orientation and pragmatically adapt elements from other orientations to address particular problems as they emerge in the treatment process.

GROUP DEVELOPMENT AND GROUP DYNAMICS

The basic science informing group psychotherapy is that of group development and group dynamics. Understanding of these concepts provides a foundation for the therapist's integration of individual, interpersonal, and intrapsychic dynamics with those of group membership.

Group Development

Groups must accomplish certain tasks as they move from a collection of individuals to a functioning and working organization. In this discussion, the focus is on developmental sequences in groups conducted along a path of psychodynamic principles (Table 44–1).

INITIAL (ENGAGEMENT, ORIENTATION) PHASE

Individuals entering a psychotherapy group are faced with two major tasks: they must determine how they will use the treatment to accomplish their goals, and simultaneously they must determine the limits of emotional safety.

REACTIVE (POWER, DIFFERENTIATION) PHASE

Many groups move into this phase by rebelliously rejecting their leader. Struggles between members emerge, and angry exchanges are not uncommon. Usual norms against expression of intense

TABLE 44–1	Stages of Group Development	
Stage	**Theme**	**Dynamics**
Orientation (forming)	Engagement	Dependency Safety Norms
Differentiation (storming)	Power	Testing Competition Autonomy
Maturation (performing)	Work	Affect tolerance Leadership Self-reflection
Termination (departing)	Separation	Loss Hope

intragroup affects are tested and modified in accordance with members' personal capacities.

MATURE (WORKING) PHASE

In this phase, groups have developed considerable cohesion. Members can tolerate differences, and they can contain anxiety and allow conflicts to emerge without having to interrupt exchanges. They have learned to provide and receive feedback from others without undue defensiveness.

TERMINATION PHASE

Ending treatment is the final stage. Often there is a regression as anxieties over departing are addressed. This provides an additional opportunity to explore the problems that emerge.

Group Dynamics

Group dynamics refer to norms and cultures that are unique to each group. They are influenced by group size; members' race, gender, and age; and the social environment. Group dynamics are a product of members' personalities, the leader's functioning, and their subsequent interactions. The dynamics emerge as members go about their tasks of determining how they will achieve their goals and maintain personal safety. Norms are rules defining what is acceptable.

THERAPEUTIC FACTORS

As in all dynamic therapies, specific and nonspecific elements contribute to therapeutic change.

Nonspecific factors are embedded in the relationship established through an accepting, nonjudgmental, supportive environment.

Groups provide a corrective emotional experience in which patients experience others responding to them differently than in their past. Patients share their stories (catharsis) and feel less isolated when others have shared similar stories (universalization); they have opportunities to help others through both cognitive understanding and emotional linking (imparting information, providing feedback, and altruism). They also see others improve, which conveys hope that they too will benefit from treatment. These elements contribute to the sense of collaboration and a willingness to adopt norms (i.e., discuss feelings about the interactions in the meeting) that further members' sense of efficacy and belonging. Taken together, these nonspecific elements contribute to group cohesion, which has been likened to the therapeutic alliance in dyadic treatment.

Additional nonspecific elements of group treatment that contribute to change are opportunities for imitative learning. Patients observe others interacting successfully and adopt those approaches themselves.

Each theoretical school emphasizes its own specific contributions to therapeutic change. In the interpersonal tradition, therapists place giving and receiving feedback about one's behaviors in the here and now as the central therapeutic factor. Other psychodynamic theorists emphasize resolution of transferences and resistances. The group is conceptualized as re-creating the family of origin, in which enactments of previous experiences with parents or siblings will emerge.

The group is organized to provide a setting in which these therapeutic factors emerge in a manner open to confrontation, clarification, and interpretation and in which members may imitate and identify with others as well as internalize their experiences that lead to change in psychic organization.

BEGINNING A GROUP

Group Organization

Starting a psychotherapy group is a complex task, and attention to organizational details will anticipate some of the potential hazards and smooth the way. Group size, duration of meetings, and time and place to meet are elements that require decisions in advance of recruiting and preparing potential members.

Recruiting, Selecting, and Preparing Patients

Few patients requesting psychotherapy consider group treatment. Gathering 6 to 10 individuals together may not be a simple task. Patients from an ongoing practice, who have a relationship with the therapist, are in an optimal position to collaborate in a decision to join a group.

In clinical settings, special attention should be paid to persons responsible for screening of new admissions. They are in a critical position to recommend group therapy when it is appropriate. Patients are more likely to agree to enter a group if the rationale is explained to them in some detail. Thus, the therapist needs to be familiar with the patient's history, coping style, symptoms, and personality configurations.

Discussion of the person's typical reactions to group situations helps engage the patient in examining his or her roles in interpersonal situations. The screening and preparatory interviews have five major tasks:

- Establish a preliminary alliance between patient and therapist
- Define the patient's therapeutic goals
- Provide information about the nature of group treatment
- Explore the patient's anticipatory anxiety
- Discuss the group agreement and gain the patient's acceptance

The Group Agreement

The agreement represents the framework in which treatment will proceed. It promotes a structure that defines boundaries between the group and the environment, among the members, and with the therapist. The elements of the agreement include the following:

- Attend all meetings, be on time, and remain throughout the session
- Actively work toward treatment goals, remain until they have been achieved, and discuss plans to stop treatment
- Observe one's inner reactions to interactions in the group and comment on them
- Use the group for therapeutic and not social purposes
- Put feelings into words and not action
- Be responsible for fees
- Protect the confidentiality of the meetings and the anonymity of members

THERAPIST'S ROLE

Clinicians begin to shape the group to provide participants a way of using their experience to learn about themselves. The therapist's focus, however, is not exclusively on in-group processes. Six foci of therapist attention are as follows:

Past------------------(here and now)------------------future
In-group--out of group
Group as a whole-(subgroup)--(interpersonal)--individual
Affect--cognition
Process---content
Understanding--------corrective emotional experience

The major, but not exclusive, focus promoting change is members learning from the here and now in the group.

Time-Limited Psychotherapy

Traditionally, time-limited psychotherapy referred to brief psychodynamic psychotherapy—that is, treatments derived directly from a psychoanalytic approach. Since the 1970s, however, a variety of time-limited treatments have gained popularity and have taken their place alongside the brief psychodynamic therapies. In this chapter, we use the construct time-limited psychotherapy to describe a range of treatment approaches that have in common several unifying features: limited duration of treatment, relatively active therapists, and focused treatment goals.

GENERAL PRINCIPLES

The Common Factors of Psychotherapy

An overview of the extant body of literature, including most psychotherapeutic modalities and a wide variety of research techniques, suggests that nonspecific "common factors" of psychotherapy significantly mediate psychotherapy treatment outcomes. These principles seem to hold for time-limited treatments as well as for long-term psychotherapies. Six therapeutic factors common to all forms of psychotherapy are as follows:

1. "An intense, emotionally charged, confiding relationship."
2. "A rationale, or myth, which includes an explanation of the cause of the patient's distress."
3. "Provision of new information concerning the nature and sources of the patient's problems and possible alternative ways of dealing with them."
4. "Strengthening the patient's expectations of help."
5. "Provision of success experiences."
6. "Facilitation of emotional arousal."

Time Limitation

By definition, time-limited treatments are prescribed for a discrete, predetermined length of time or number of sessions. Most time-limited therapies are completed within 12 to 20 sessions, with a range of 1 to 40 sessions. Meta-analysis of many studies of psychotherapy confirms that most (75%) patients achieve symptom relief within 26 sessions. Treatment frequency is generally once a week. It is important to recognize that time-limited treatment has a distinctly defined beginning, middle, and end, regardless of its absolute duration.

In time-limited treatments, the therapist must be an active participant in the treatment, helping to move the process forward in the face of an inexorably ticking clock. This calls for face to face interviews, constant attention to the focus of the treatment, and frequent redirection of the patient if the focus falters. Many treatments (e.g., interpersonal psychotherapy [IPT], cognitive-behavioral therapy [CBT]) specifically encourage the therapist to make direct suggestions to the patient when the patient is unable to solve a problem by herself or himself. In cognitive and behavioral therapies, for example, the therapist assigns homework exercises and readings.

Narrow Treatment Focus

A hallmark of time-limited therapy is careful definition of treatment goals, which are usually agreed on by the patient and therapist and often specified at the beginning of treatment. A typical and appropriate treatment goal for IPT, for example, is remission of depressive symptoms.

In conjunction with choosing a narrow focus, practitioners of time-limited treatments often make a formal or informal treatment contract, in which the patient and therapist explicitly agree to the goals and duration of treatment.

Contraindications

In the brief dynamic psychotherapy literature, time-limited treatments are generally not recommended for those individuals who might have difficulty in quickly forming a therapeutic alliance or might develop severe difficulties in the face of termination of therapy. In practice, this usually translates into a reluctance to treat borderline, suicidal, or psychotic patients with brief psychotherapy. Also excluded are acting-out, cognitively impaired, extremely dependent, or "unrestrainably" anxious patients.

Some practitioners consider severe psychopathology a contraindication to brief dynamic psychotherapy, but other time-limited treatments specifically target serious mental disorders. IPT and CBT, for example, were developed to treat major depressive disorder. These therapies and brief behavioral therapy have been used to treat a spectrum of significant pathologies, including bulimia nervosa, alcohol dependence, and paraphilias.

SPECIFIC TIME-LIMITED THERAPIES

It is beyond the scope of this chapter to describe in detail the psychotherapeutic techniques employed by each modality. Table 45–1 summarizes the interventions used in several psychotherapies.

DIFFERENTIAL THERAPEUTICS

WHO MIGHT BENEFIT FROM TIME-LIMITED THERAPY? Patients with chronic illnesses, poor premorbid functioning, extensive resources, and multiple targets of change are generally good candidates for longer treatments, and patients with

TABLE 45-1 Summary of Psychotherapeutic Techniques

Psychotherapy	Techniques	Theorists/Schools
Interpersonal psychotherapy	*Medical model** of illness Links symptoms to one of four possible *interpersonal problem areas* Individual sessions to work through an affectively meaningful problem area using role-playing, communication analysis, and direct suggestion Focuses on the *here and now* Facilitates a positive transference but does not interpret it	Klerman, Weissman/ interpersonal
Cognitive-behavioral therapy	Identifies distorted thoughts that lead to maladaptive feelings and behaviors Homework assignments to recognize, test, and challenge underlying *automatic negative thoughts* or maladaptive behaviors *Relaxation techniques* to manage anxiety Encourages *rational*, scientific collaboration between patient and therapist	Beck/cognitive and behavioral
Dialectical behavioral therapy	Individual sessions to *analyze cognitions, feelings*, and *behaviors* that lead to para-suicidal or therapy-interfering actions Group sessions and homework for *skills training* to improve relationships, regulate affect, decrease impulsivity	Linehan/cognitive and behavioral

Table continued on following page

*Italics denote key words and phrases specific to the psychotherapy described.

TABLE 45–1 Summary of Psychotherapeutic Techniques *(Continued)*

Psychotherapy	Techniques	Theorists/Schools
Supportive-expressive psychotherapy	Identifies problematical relationship themes that are resolved through *tranference interpretations* Offers *support* through the formal aspects of treatment such as regular appointments and collaboration Explores past *conflicts*, ego *defenses*, and *resistances*	Luborsky/psychodynamic
Focal psychotherapy	Identifies focal conflict Explores *triangular links* among transference relationship, current problem relationship, and past conflictual relationships Explores triangular links among anxiety, defenses, and impulses *Transference interpretations* to develop insight and resolve conflict	Malan, Balint/ psychodynamic
Time-limited psychotherapy	Selects central issue that has current relevance and past antecedents *Interpretation of transference, clarification, and defense analysis* to develop insight and permit abreaction	Mann/psychodynamic
Short-term anxiety-provoking psychotherapy	Selects an *oedipal* problem *Confronts defenses*—despite emergence of anxiety—to *uncover underlying impulse* *Transference interpretations* to develop insight and resolve conflict	Sifneos/psychodynamic
Short-term dynamic psychotherapy	Protracted initial interview to *unlock the unconscious* and establish focus *Gentle but relentless confrontation* of patient's defenses and transference resistances *Clarification and interpretation* to bring about symptom resolution	Davanloo/psychodynamic

acute illnesses, good premorbid functioning, limited resources, and focused problem areas are good candidates for shorter treatments. This scheme continues to provide a reasonable framework for assessing the indications for time-limited therapy but with four caveats:

1. Patients with acute exacerbations of some chronic illnesses (e.g., recurrent major depressive episodes) can be treated initially with full-strength time-limited psychotherapy followed by a less intensive maintenance phase of therapy.

2. Some chronic illnesses, such as dysthymic disorder, can respond to time-limited therapy even without evidence of an acute

TABLE 45–2	Time-Limited Therapies with Demonstrated Efficacy for Specific Disorders	
Disorder	**Psychotherapy**	**Efficacy**
Major depressive disorder, acute	IPT	1*
	CBT	1
Major depressive disorder, recurrent	Maintenance IPT	1
Major depressive disorder in the elderly	Cognitive therapy	2
	Behavioral therapy	2
	IPT	2
	Horowitz's stress-response psychotherapy	2
Major depression in human immunodeficiency virus–seropositive men	IPT	2
Dysthymic disorder	CBT	2
	IPT	2
Opioid addiction	Luborsky's SE psychotherapy plus drug counseling	2
	CBT plus drug counseling	2
Borderline personality disorder	DBT	2
Bulimia nervosa	CBT	1
	IPT	2
Avoidant, passive-aggressive, compulsive, or histrionic personality disorders	Davanloo's STDP	3
	Pollack and Horner's adaptational psychotherapy	3

*Tentative classification: 1, rigorously proven; 2, promising results; 3, possible efficacy.

exacerbation. In these cases, a discrete focus of treatment must be selected, even though the condition is ongoing.

3. Patients who wish to change many aspects of their lives can be encouraged to focus on a single issue in time-limited therapy and still experience improvement in self-esteem.

4. Sometimes patients with poor premorbid functioning can benefit from time-limited interventions.

ARE THERE SPECIAL POPULATIONS THAT BENEFIT FROM SPECIFIC TIME-LIMITED THERAPIES? Relying on the data that demonstrate efficacy, Table 45–2 summarizes population-specific indications for selected time-limited modalities. No doubt there are other useful but as yet untested applications of time-limited therapy. For example, many clinical anecdotal reports are available on the effectiveness of brief psychoanalytic psychotherapies, but few controlled studies have been done.

WHAT IF THERAPY FAILS? There are no data arguing against combining time-limited therapies with other treatments. Thus, in the event that a selected time-limited therapy fails, appropriate strategies include augmenting psychotherapy with medication, treating the patient with medication alone, or switching to a different psychotherapeutic modality. The order in which these options are prescribed remains at the discretion of the therapist; no studies to date have examined these critical clinical questions. Extrapolation from the psychopharmacological data, however, might reasonably suggest augmentation with medication before a psychotherapy is abandoned that has yielded at least a partial response.

Cognitive and Behavioral
Therapies

Specifically, learning theories (i.e., classical, operant, and observational models of learning) and the principles of cognitive psychology are relied on heavily in constructing cognitive-behavioral treatment models.

COGNITIVE MODEL

The basic theories of the cognitive model are rooted in a long tradition of viewing cognitions as primary determinants of emotion and behavior.

Figure 46–1 displays a simplified model for understanding the relationships between environmental events, cognitions, emotion, and behavior. This model is based on the theoretical assumption that environmental stimuli trigger cognitive processes and that ensuing cognitions give the event personal meaning and elicit subsequent physiological and affective arousal. These emotions, in turn, have a potent reciprocal effect on cognitive content and information processing, such that cascades of dysfunctional thoughts and emotions can occur. Behavioral responses to stimuli and thoughts are viewed as both a product and a cause of maladaptive cognitions. Thus, treatment interventions may be targeted at any or all components of the model.

Dysfunctional information processing is apparent at two major levels of cognition—automatic thoughts and schemas—in many psychiatric disorders. Automatic thoughts are cognitions that stream rapidly through an individual's mind, whether spontaneously or in response to some prompt or stimulus. Automatic thoughts may be triggered by affective arousal (i.e., anger, anxiety, or sadness), or conversely, affective shifts are generally accompanied by automatic negative thoughts.

Typical errors in logic (termed cognitive errors or cognitive distortions) shape the content of automatic thoughts. Examples of these processes include personalization, magnification, "mind reading," self-fulfilling prophecy, selective recall, and selective abstraction. A number of common cognitive errors are defined in Table 46–1.

Schemas are the basic assumptions or unspoken rules that act as templates for screening and decoding information from the environment. Psychological well-being may be understood in part by development of a set of schemas that yield realistic appraisals of self in relation to world (e.g., "I'm reasonably attractive, but looks aren't everything," "I can be loved under the right circumstances," or "I must work harder to compensate for an average intellect").

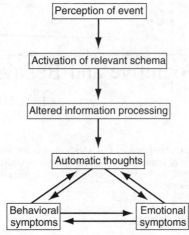

Figure 46–1 *Cognitive model of information processing.*

TABLE 46–1	Common Patterns of Irrational Thinking in Anxiety and Depression
Cognitive Error	**Definition**
Emotional reasoning	A conclusion or inference is based on an emotional state, e.g., "I *feel* this way, therefore I *am* this way."
Over generalization	Evidence is drawn from one experience or a small set of experiences to reach an unwarranted conclusion with far-reaching implications.
Catastrophic thinking	An extreme example of overgeneralization, in which the impact of a clearly negative event or experience is amplified to extreme proportions, e.g., "If I have a panic attack, I will lose *all* control and go crazy (or die)."
All-or-none (black or white, absolutistic) thinking	An unnecessary division of complex or continuous outcomes into polarized extremes, e.g., "Either I am a success at this, or I'm a total failure."
Shoulds and musts	Imperative statements about self that dictate rigid standards or reflect an unrealistic degree of presumed control over external events.

TABLE 46–1	Common Patterns of Irrational Thinking in Anxiety and Depression (Continued)
Cognitive Error	**Definition**
Negative predictions	Use of pessimism or earlier experiences of failure to prematurely or inappropriately predict failure in a new situation; also known as fortunetelling.
Mind reading	Negatively toned inferences about the thoughts, intentions, or motives of another person.
Labeling	An undesirable characteristic of a person or event is made definitive of that person or event, e.g., "Because I *failed* to be selected for ballet, I am a *failure.*"
Personalization	Interpretation of an event, situation, or behavior as salient or personally indicative of a negative aspect of self.
Selective negative focus	Undesirable or negative events, memories, or implications are focused on at the expense of recalling or identifying other, more neutral or positive information; in fact, positive information may be ignored *or* disqualified as irrelevant, atypical, or trivial.
Cognitive avoidance	Unpleasant thoughts, feelings, or events are misperceived as overwhelming or insurmountable and are actively suppressed or avoided.
Somatic (mis)focus	The predisposition to interpret internal stimuli (e.g., heart rate, palpitations, shortness of breath, dizziness, or tingling) as *definite* indications of impending catastrophic events (e.g., heart attack, suffocation, collapse).

Adapted from Beck AT, Rush AJ, Shaw BF, et al. Cognitive Therapy of Depression. New York: Guilford Press, 1979.

Although unspoken, schemas may be inferred from one's beliefs and attitudes. In the cognitive model, dysfunctional attitudes are the structural "bridge" between pathological schemas and automatic negative thoughts. A number of schemas relevant to psychiatric illness are listed in Table 46–2.

TABLE 46–2	Proposed Maladaptive Schemes
Autonomy	
Dependence	The belief that one is unable to function without the constant support of others
Subjugation–lack of individuation	The voluntary or involuntary sacrifice of one's own needs to satisfy others' needs
Vulnerability to harm or illness	The fear that disaster (i.e., natural, criminal, medical, or financial) is about to strike at any time
Fear of losing self-control	The fear that one will involuntarily lose control of one's own impulses, behavior, emotions, mind, and so on
Connectedness	
Emotional deprivation	The expectation that one's needs for nurturance, empathy, or affection will never be adequately met by others
Abandonment-loss	The fear that one will imminently lose significant others or be emotionally isolated forever
Mistrust	The expectation that others will hurt, abuse, cheat, lie, or manipulate
Social isolation-alienation	The belief that one is isolated from the rest of the world, is different from other people, or does not belong to any group or community
Worthiness	
Defectiveness-unlovability	The assumption that one is inwardly defective or that, if the flaw is exposed, one is fundamentally unlovable
Social undesirability	The belief that one is outwardly undesirable to others (e.g., ugly, sexually undesirable, low in status, dull, or boring)
Incompetence-failure	The assumption that one cannot perform competently in areas of achievement, daily responsibilities, or decision-making
Guilt-punishment	The conclusion that one is morally bad or irresponsible and deserving of criticism or punishment

TABLE 46–2	Proposed Maladaptive Schemes *(Continued)*
Worthiness *Continued*	
Shame-embarrassment	Recurrent feelings of shame or self-consciousness experienced because one believes that one's inadequacies (as reflected in the preceding maladaptation schemas of worthiness) are totally unacceptable to others
Limits and Standards	
Unrelenting standards	The relentless striving to meet extremely high expectation of oneself, at all costs (i.e., at the expense of happiness, pleasure, health, or satisfying relationships)
Entitlement	Insistence that one should be able to do, say, or have whatever one wants immediately

From Thase ME, Beck AT: An overview of cognitive therapy. In Wright J, Thase ME, Beck AT, Ludgate J (eds): Cognitive Therapy with Inpatients: Developing a Cognitive Milieu. New York: Guilford Press, 1992:9. Adapted from Young J: Schema-focused cognitive therapy for personality disorders. Unpublished manuscript, Cognitive Therapy Center of New York, 1987.

The cognitive model of psychiatric illness emphasizes the concept of stress-diathesis. From this perspective, a cognitive diathesis, such as the schema "I must be loved to have worth," might remain latent until activated by a relevant life stressor (i.e., a romantic breakup).

BEHAVIORAL MODEL

The behavioral model is based on the relatively straightforward "chain" of events and responses illustrated in Figure 46–2. In its maturity, behavioral therapy has broadened beyond an exclusive focus on observable behaviors (i.e., radical behaviorism) and now incorporates cognitive processes and other individual variables that affect one's preparedness to learn. For example, in observational learning, the stimulus-response contingency relationship is established vicariously by watching, reading about, or imagining the event in question. Reinforcement does not have to take place explicitly; it may occur vicariously, or it may simply be imagined.

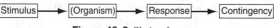

Stimulus → (Organism) → Response → Contingency

Figure 46–2 *Chain of events.*

COGNITIVE AND BEHAVIORAL TREATMENT STRATEGIES

Development of a productive therapeutic relationship and an individualized case conceptualization should always take precedence over the implementation of specific cognitive or behavioral techniques. A number of the more important CBT strategies are described briefly here.

Collaborative Empiricism

Cognitive-behavioral therapists strive for a therapeutic relationship that emphasizes 1) a high degree of collaboration and 2) a scientific attitude toward testing the validity or usefulness of particular cognitions and behavior. This therapeutic stance is referred to as collaborative empiricism.

There are several strategies for enhancing collaborative empiricism. These include 1) adjusting the therapist's level of activity to match the patient's symptom severity or the phase of treatment, 2) encouraging the use of self-help procedures, 3) attending to the "nonspecific" variables important in all therapeutic relationships (e.g., empathy, respect, equanimity, kindness, and good listening skills), 4) promoting frequent two-way feedback, 5) devising coping strategies to help deal with real losses or implementing a plan of action to address maladaptive behavior, 6) recognizing transference phenomena, 7) customizing therapeutic interventions, and 8) using humor judiciously. It is also important to recognize and account for the wide variety of individual differences in cultural backgrounds, social attitudes, and expectations that each patient brings to the therapy encounter.

Psychoeducation

Most forms of cognitive-behavioral therapy (CBT) integrate explicit psychoeducational procedures as a core element of the treatment process. Psychoeducational procedures are typically blended into treatment sessions in a manner that deemphasizes formal teaching. There is a concerted effort to teach the patient *why* it is important to challenge automatic thoughts, identify cognitive errors, and practice implementing a more rational thinking style. Behavioral interventions are also preceded by psychoeducation to convey the background for principles such as extinction, reinforcement, self-monitoring, exposure, and response prevention.

Modifying Automatic Thoughts

The first step in changing automatic thoughts is to help the patient recognize when she or he is having them! The therapist is often able to illustrate the presence of automatic negative thoughts during the initial session by gently calling attention to a change in the patient's mood. Such "mood shifts" can be vivid learning experiences that give personally relevant illustrations of the linkage between cognitions and feelings.

SOCRATIC QUESTIONING

The most frequently used and important technique for uncovering and modifying automatic negative thoughts is socratic questioning (or guided discovery). Socratic questioning teaches the use of rationality and inductive reasoning to challenge whether what is thought or felt is actually true. Typical questions include "What ran through your mind at that time?" "What is the evidence that your impression is accurate?" and "Could there be any alternative explanations?"

IMAGERY TECHNIQUES AND ROLE-PLAYING

Imagery techniques and role-playing are used when direct questioning does not fully reveal important underlying cognitions. When imagery is used, the therapist sets the scene by asking the patient to visualize the situation that caused distress. Several types of questions can be used to help frame the scene. These include inquiries about 1) the physical details of the setting, 2) occurrences immediately before the interaction, and 3) descriptions of the other people in the scene.

THOUGHT RECORDING

Thought recording is one of the most useful procedures for identifying and changing automatic thoughts. This technique is first presented in relatively simple two- or three-column versions in the early stages of therapy.

EXAMINING THE EVIDENCE

The procedure of examining the evidence is a collaborative exercise used to test the validity of automatic negative thoughts. Cognitions are set forth as hypotheses rather than established facts. The patient is encouraged to write down evidence that either supports or refutes the automatic thought using a two-column form (i.e., pros and cons).

Next, the therapist helps to guide revision of the automatic negative thought in light of the evidence (e.g., "I *often* feel inferior to others, even when there's no good evidence that they feel that way" or "I have had a number of difficulties with my teachers and employers, but not all relationships have been bad"). The process thus moves from the patient's globally negative interpretations to more specific, factually based statements.

GENERATING ALTERNATIVES

If automatic thoughts prove to be largely dysfunctional, the patient is encouraged to generate alternatives that are more accurate or factual.

COGNITIVE-BEHAVIORAL REHEARSAL

Cognitive-behavioral rehearsal is a treatment strategy that is particularly useful in patients preparing to put their experiences in CBT to work in real-life circumstances. After automatic thoughts have been elicited and modified through procedures described earlier, the therapist guides the patient in a series of rehearsal exercises to try out alternative cognitions in a variety of situations.

Modifying Schemas

The emphasis in the early phases of therapy is usually on changing automatic thoughts and resolving symptoms. However, as the patient gains knowledge of cognitive-behavioral principles and acute symptoms begin to subside, the focus of the treatment sessions shifts subtly toward work on the schema level. Because schemas serve as underlying templates for making sense of new information, they play a major role in modulating more superficial cognitions (automatic thoughts), regulating affect and self-esteem, and controlling the behavioral repertoire.

Many of the techniques used to test and modify automatic thoughts identify and revise schemas. Because schemas are so strongly held (in essence, they have helped to define reality for years), they may require intensive work in a number of therapy sessions to undergo significant change.

COGNITIVE RESPONSE PREVENTION

In cognitive response prevention, the patient agrees to complete a homework assignment in which she or he must behave in a way that is inconsistent with the pathological schema. For example, a person with perfectionistic attitudes may be engaged in an assignment in which she or he must perform in a "so-so" manner. This is intended to activate the schema, triggering automatic negative thoughts (e.g., "They'll think I'm a sloth" or "I'll never be trusted with an important assignment again"). By not responding to the perfectionistic demands dictated by the schema, the individual thus has the opportunity to cope with the automatic negative thoughts consequent to this "rule violation."

LISTING ADVANTAGES AND DISADVANTAGES

The procedure of listing advantages and disadvantages is particularly useful when a schema appears to have both adaptive and maladaptive features. Schemas that have damaging effects are often maintained because they also have a positive side. The advantages and disadvantages analysis provides the patient and therapist with essential information for planning modifications. Revised schemas are most likely to be used when they take into account both the maladaptive and the adaptive features of the old basic assumption.

BEHAVIORAL TECHNIQUES

Behavioral strategies may be folded in with cognitive methods of intervention, or they may be used without particular attention to automatic thoughts or schema. In fully integrated CBT, behavioral strategies are typically emphasized earlier in therapy and with more severely symptomatic patients.

Activity Scheduling, Graded Tasks, and Mastery-Pleasure Exercise

One key to the behavioral approach for treating depression is the interrupting of the downward spiral linking mood, inactivity, and negative cognition. Completing an activity schedule is often the first behavioral homework assignment used in CBT. The nature of the activities is examined, and deficits in activities that might elicit pleasure or feelings of competence are identified. Next, assignments are made for the patient to engage in discrete pleasurable activities (or, in the case of an anhedonic individual, activities that were rewarding before the person became depressed). If needed, a "menu" of reinforcers can be generated by having the patient fill out a Pleasant Events Schedule. Following operant principles, activities that have been "high-grade" reinforcers in the past are scheduled during times of low moods or decreased activity.

Breathing Control

An important component of CBT for anxiety disorders involves teaching the patient breathing exercises that may be used to counteract hyperventilation. Slow, deep breathing has a calming effect not unlike progressive muscle relaxation. These exercises help to distract the patient from autonomic cues. After initial instruction and practice, the deep breathing skills are then applied in progressively more anxiety-provoking situations.

Contingency Contracting and Behavior Exchange

These strategies use the principles of operant conditioning, to modify the probability of occurrence of either undesired or desired behaviors.

Contingency management programs are sometimes used across larger social systems to address the problems of a particular group, such as long-stay mental patients or unruly students. This application of operant conditioning generally targets difficulties initiating and maintaining socially desirable behaviors through the use of symbolic reinforcers, such as points, stamps, or tokens. The points or tokens are, in turn, exchanged for privileges or consumable goods on a daily or weekly basis.

Desensitization and Relaxation Training

Systematic desensitization relies on working through a progressive hierarchy of fear-inducing situations. Systematic desensitization uses the pairing of progressive deep muscle relaxation and visualization of the target behavior to decondition fearful responses. Historically, systematic desensitization is exposure to the feared situation, first in imagination and later in reality, rather than an actual counterconditioning through the relaxation response. Progressive deep muscle relaxation is also useful as a self-directed coping strategy and for treatment of sleep-onset insomnia.

Exposure and Flooding

The purpose of these strategies is to speed extinction of conditioned fear or anxiety responses. Behavioral theory dictates that fearfulness is reinforced by avoidance and escape behaviors. Because the basis of the fear or phobia is irrational, the optimal strategy is to increase exposure to the feared activity with aversive consequences. In exposure, there are at least three means of fear reduction: autonomic habituation, recognition that the fear is irrational, and explicit enhancement of morale or self-efficacy that accompanies mastering the previously dreaded activity.

In graded or progressive exposure, a hierarchy is established, ranging from least to most anxiety-provoking situations. The individual is taught one or more ways to cope with anxiety (e.g., relaxation or self-instruction), and with the help of the therapist, the items on the hierarchy are worked through, one item at a time.

Flooding, which relies on the same principles, dispatches with the hierarchical approach so that the individual is exposed to the maximal level of anxiety as quickly as possible. The rationale for this accelerated approach is that it may hasten autonomic habituation. To be effective, flooding needs to be accompanied by response prevention.

Social Skills Training

Satisfactory interpersonal relationships require a complex set of skills, including reciprocity, respect for another's opinion, appropriate modulation of self-disclosure, the tempered ability to yield on some occasions and to set limits at other times, the natural use of social reinforcers, and the capacity to express anger and resolve conflicts in a constructive manner. Many people with psychiatric disorders suffer from either a state-dependent deterioration of these social skills or lifelong deficits of such skills.

The methods employed to teach social skills include modeling (i.e., the therapist demonstrates a more effective alternative approach), role-playing and role reversal, behavior rehearsal, and specific practice assignments. Often, the interpersonal anxiety and lack of self-confidence that go hand in hand with social skills deficits lessen in response to successful mastery of targeted assignments.

Thought Stopping and Distraction

Automatic negative thoughts and repetitive, intrusive ruminations are sometimes too intense to address with purely cognitive interventions. The technique of thought stopping capitalizes on the individual's ability to use a selectively narrowed attentional focus to suppress the intrusive cognitions. For example, a ruminative individual may be asked to visualize a large red stop sign, including its octagonal shape and white lettering. The command Stop! is paired with the image. The image and command are then used to interrupt a "run" of ruminations.

Patients susceptible to panic often have a heightened awareness of otherwise normal physiological cues (e.g., heart rate, dryness in the throat, tightness in the chest, or increased peristalsis). In turn, such sensitivity triggers automatic negative thoughts about the imagined impending calamity. Distractions such as counting backward, praying, or imagining a calming scene may be applied to direct attention away from the internal stimuli. Distraction techniques thus help the individual exert some control over the symptoms, permitting greater exposure and a growing sense of self-efficacy.

FORMULATION OF TREATMENT

INDICATIONS FOR TREATMENT

The cognitive and behavioral therapies are indicated as primary treatments for adults suffering from several nonpsychotic, nonorganic Axis I disorders described in the *Diagnostic and Statistical Manual of Mental Disorders,* Fourth Edition (DSM-IV). These include dysthymia, major depressive disorder, panic disorder, and generalized anxiety disorder.

Cognitive and behavioral therapies, like most other types of treatment, have not been studied extensively in patients with Axis II disorders. Therefore, it is difficult to determine their relative rank or indication.

An adequate outpatient trial of CBT typically ranges from 10 to 20 weekly treatment sessions. Of course, deterioration or noncompliance of the patient may warrant early termination of a treatment trial, and for certain chronic conditions such as borderline personality disorder, longer courses of therapy may be indicated. In any event, outcome is defined by improvements in targeted skill areas and reductions of specific symptoms.

PREPARATION OF THE PATIENT

The cognitive and behavioral therapies explicitly incorporate strategies to increase involvement and preparedness of the patient for therapy. Patients are typically encouraged to read relevant written materials describing the theory and strategies of the therapy; for common disorders, such as major depressive disorder and panic disorder, fully developed manuals for patients are now available.

Regardless of the application mode, patients beginning CBT need to become acculturated to the following "facts of life": 1) they will be active participants in trying out new strategies; 2) they will be expected to do homework; 3) the outcome of therapy will be measured and strategies will be altered if they are not helping; 4) therapy will be focused on symptoms and social functioning and generally will be time limited in nature; and 5) the chances of success after treatment termination can be gauged by the patients' incorporation of the therapy into their day-to-day life.

PHASES OF TREATMENT

Most cognitive and behavioral therapies may be viewed as using a three-stage process. The initial phase includes the processes of clinical assessment, case formulation, establishment of a therapeutic relationship, socialization of the patient to therapy, psychoeducation, and introduction to treatment procedures. The middle stage involves the sequential application and mastery of cognitive and behavioral treatment strategies. This second stage ends when the patient has obtained the desired symptomatic outcome. The final phase of therapy is characterized by preparation for termination. The frequency of sessions is reduced, and there is a steady transfer of the responsibility for the continued use of therapeutic strategies from the therapist to the patient. This third stage of treatment also focuses on relapse prevention. Strategies used at this point include anticipation of reaction to future stressors or high-risk situations, identification of prodromal symptoms, rehearsal of self-help procedures, and establishment of guidelines for return to treatment.

INTENSITY OF TREATMENT

Outpatient CBT is normally conducted once or twice a week. In selected cases, three-times-weekly or even daily sessions may be useful, but the cost-effectiveness of such a labor-intensive approach is uncertain.

When patients are seen in a day treatment hospital or inpatient setting, sessions are typically provided on a daily or every-other-day basis. In the authors' experience, more frequent sessions help to offset symptom severity and demoralization in severely ill patients.

DURATION OF TREATMENT

In most cases, treatment is conducted in a period of 3 to 6 months. For those who begin therapy as inpatients, a similar period of aftercare is strongly recommended. Unsuccessful therapy (e.g., failure to effect significant symptomatic improvement) should generally not continue past 12 to 16 weeks for outpatients.

AUGMENTATION OF THERAPY

A major method of augmenting a cognitive and behavioral therapy is to add an appropriate form of pharmacotherapy. For example, a depressed or agoraphobic person who has not benefited much from 8 weeks or more of CBT alone should probably be considered for pharmacotherapy.

Other strategies used to enhance CBT include increasing the frequency of visits, switching emphasis (i.e., from cognitive to behavioral or vice versa), or involving the spouse or significant others in the therapy. The last strategy has been shown to be particularly useful in cases of depression associated with marital discord.

Family Therapy

Family therapy is defined in myriad ways; in practice, it ranges from individual psychoanalysis focused on the family relations of individual patients to group meetings involving large social networks of 30 to 40 persons. For the purpose of this discussion, family therapy refers to a meeting between a therapist or therapists and two or more family members with an explicit focus on *family* problems. Meetings with various family members that *may* have incidental therapeutic value (e.g., social work intake interviews) are excluded.

For the sake of completeness, the major models of family therapy are summarized in Table 47–1.

In the initial assessment, several content questions are addressed that provide an overall context for the situation. The family processes are also identified. In addition, the principles of clarity in communication, focusing attention, interpersonal validation, metacommunication, establishing generational boundaries, family problem solving, implicit contracting, normalization, mutual responsibility, and positive expectations are highlighted with, or modeled for, the family. Family therapy is perhaps most unusual in its relative disregard for psychopathological conditions. The approach of family work tends to normalize and contextualize rather than segregate and "psychopathologize" disturbed and disturbing behavior. The self-help orientation embodied by the family's defining its own solutions reinforces a sense of personal and family resourcefulness and an ability to cope. Empowering families in this way results in enhanced personal and family morale and reinforces the therapists' positive expectations.

Family theories and treatment result in an expansion of the mental health field's conceptual sights to include family and the wider social network as potentially important in the production, maintenance, and course of various psychiatric disorders. Although many questions remain unanswered and major methodological limitations prevent definitive conclusions to be drawn, it does appear that by itself, and also when added to other interventions, family therapy works. The most extensive evidence of its efficacy relates to persons with schizophrenia and their families.

It is possible, without extensive specialized family therapy training, to talk with families (in various combinations), develop rapport, enhance collaboration, extend therapists' understanding, and provide demystifying treatment-related information. If attention is given to maximizing the effects of nonspecific therapeutic factors and employing several generic intervention principles, such meetings can have important positive therapeutic effects.

Text continued on page 481

TABLE 47–1 Major Models of Family Therapy: Normality, Dysfunction, and Therapeutic Goals

Model of Family Therapy	View of Normal Family Functioning	View of Dysfunction Symptoms	Goals of Therapy
Structural			

Minuchin
Montalvo
Aponte
	1. Boundaries are clean and firm.
	2. Hierarchy with strong parental subsystem.
	3. Flexibility of system for
	  a. Autonomy and interdependence
	  b. Individual growth and system maintenance
	  c. Continuity and adaptive restructuring in response to changing internal (developmental) and external (environmental) demands
		Symptoms result from current family structural imbalance:
		  a. Malfunctioning hierarchical arrangement, boundaries
		  b. Maladaptive reaction of changing requirements (developmental, environmental)
			Reorganize family structure:
			  a. Shift members' relative position to disrupt malfunctioning pattern and strengthen parental hierarchy
			  b. Create clear, flexible boundaries
			  c. Mobilize more adaptive alternative patterns

Strategic			

Haley
Milan team
Palo Alto group
	1. Flexibility.
	2. Large behavioral repertoire for
	   a. Problem resolution
	   b. Life-cycle passage
	3. Clear rules governing hierarchy (Haley).
		Multiple origins of problems; symptoms are maintained by family's
		   a. Unsuccessful problem-solving attempts
		   b. Inability to adjust to life cycle transitions (Haley)
		   c. Malfunctioning hierarchy; triangle of or coalition across hierarchy (Haley)
		Symptom is a communicative act embedded in interaction pattern.
			Resolve presenting problem only; specific behaviorally defined objectives. Interrupt rigid feedback cycle; change symptom-maintaining sequence to new outcome.
			Define clearer hierarchy (Haley).

Behavioral-social exchange			

Liberman
Patterson
Alexander
	1. Maladaptive behavior is not reinforced.
	2. Adaptive behavior is rewarded.
	3. Exchange of benefits outweighs costs.
	4. Long-term reciprocity.
		Maladaptive, symptomatic behavior is reinforced by
		   a. Family attention and reward
		   b. Deficient reward exchanges (e.g., coercive)
		   c. Communication deficit
			Concrete, observable behavioral goals; change contingencies of social reinforcement (interpersonal consequences of behavior)
			   a. Rewards for adaptive behavior
			   b. No rewards for maladaptive behavior

Modified by Walsh F: Conceptualizations of normal family functioning. In: Walsh F (ed): Normal Family Process, New York: Guilford, 1982.

Table continued on following page

TABLE 47–1	Major Models of Family Therapy: Normality, Dysfunction, and Therapeutic Goals (Continued)		
Model of Family Therapy	View of Normal Family Functioning	View of Dysfunction Symptoms	Goals of Therapy
Psychodynamic			
Ackerman Boszormenyl-Nagy Framo Lidz Meissner Paul Stierlin	1. Parental personalities and relationships are well differentiated. 2. Relationship perceptions are based on current realities, not projections from past. Boszormenyl-Nagy: Relational equitability. a. Parental coalition b. Generation boundaries c. Sex-linked parental roles	Symptoms are due to family projections process stemming from unresolved conflicts and losses in family of origin.	1. Insight and resolution of family of origin conflict and losses. 2. Family projection processes. 3. Relationship reconstruction and reunion. 4. Individual and family growth.

Family systems therapy		

Bowen	Differentiation of self, intellectual-emotional balance.	Functioning is impaired by relationships with family of origin:
		a. Poor differentiation
		b. Anxiety (reactive)
		c. Family projection process
		d. Triangulation
			1. Differentiation.
			2. Cognitive functioning.
			3. Emotional reactivity.
			4. Modification of relationship in family system:
			   a. Detriangulation
			   b. Repair cutoffs

Experiential		
Satir Whitaker	Satir: 1. Self-worth: high. 2. Communication: clear, specific, honest. 3. Family rules: flexible, human, appropriate. 4. Linkage to society: open, hopeful. Whitaker: Multiple aspects of family structure and shared experience.	Symptoms are nonverbal messages in reaction to current communication dysfunction in system.	1. Direct, clear communication. 2. Individual and family growth through immediate shared experience.

Table continued on following page

479

TABLE 47–1 Major Models of Family Therapy: Normality, Dysfunction, and Therapeutic Goals *(Continued)*

Model of Family Therapy	View of Normal Family Functioning	View of Dysfunction Symptoms	Goals of Therapy
Psychoeducational to family management			
Fallon Leff Anderson and Hogarty McFarland	Uses information to problem solve. Clear communication. Flexible coping skills. Acknowledge, respect, and view members positively.	Dysfunctional response to offspring's illness. No, or distorted, information about the illness. Poor communication. Critical or overinvolved, or both. Unable to problem solve.	Provide information. Define problems clearly; generate and apply solutions. Reduce overinvolvement and criticism. Teach coping strategies.
Crisis intervention			
Mosher and Goldstein	Family as a system. Clarity in communication. Appropriate roles. Consensual family reality.	One member is defined as the problem. Communication deviance. Blurred generational boundaries. Rescuer, victim, scapegoat, voyeur roles; no consensual family reality.	Acknowledge the episode. Define relevant precipitants. Define unsuccessful family response. Plan alternative response. Teach metacommunication. Define appropriate roles. Evolve consensual reality.

Last, but by no means least, a family-focused view helps therapists strengthen, promote, and sustain a social institution that is central to cultures. This humanizing process is especially important in today's technology-dominated world and should be a part of every psychiatrist's work.

Couples Therapy

Relationship distress is a common and persistent source of complaint for both individuals and couples entering therapy. It has been estimated that up to 50% of all patients seeking psychotherapy primarily present with relational difficulties. Even among intact relationships, the presence of distress and dissatisfaction is disturbingly common; approximately 20% of married couples experience discord at any given point. Disruptions in interpersonal relationships are certainly among life's most stressful events and are often connected with multiple deleterious effects in functioning for both adult and child. Relationship distress is not only related to various psychological traumas but also associated with poorer physical health.

Beyond the inherent stresses of relationship difficulties, there are also serious psychological and physical traumas associated with the development of relational problems. Domestic violence represents the most devastating effect of being in a distressed relationship; approximately 4% of relationships experience severe abuse.

The scope of problems addressed by couples therapy has extended beyond traditional relational complaints, such as intimacy, sexual, and communication difficulties. Couples therapy has now been incorporated into treatments for depression, alcoholism, schizophrenia, and anxiety disorders. Table 48–1 offers a brief overview of the major models of couples therapy.

THEORETICAL MODELS

Psychoanalytic Couples Therapy

In this framework, the individual in early childhood is confronted with a series of developmental stages, tasks, and crises. The relative success of navigating through these stages largely influences the nature of future interpersonal relations.

Behavioral Approaches

BEHAVIORAL MARITAL THERAPY

BMT views a couple's distress as emanating from an imbalance in the cost/benefit ratio of the relationship; the couple is currently engaging in too many aversive behaviors relative to positive ones. Although each partner's learning history is a relevant factor, the current social environment of the couple is sufficient for understanding how each partner mutually influences and shapes the other's aversive behaviors. BMT also recognizes that certain core

TABLE 48–1 Focus and Techniques for Major Therapeutic Models

Theoretical Model	Therapeutic Goals and Techniques
Psychoanalytic Models	
Object relations	Maintain holding environment; active listening; interpretation; working through
Ego analytical	Create joint platform; explore hidden validity of responses; identify and acknowledge leading-edge feelings
Behavioral Models	
Behavioral	Change problem behaviors through homework assignments, collaborative set, behavior exchange, and communication and problem-solving skills training
Integrative Behavioral Couples Therapy	Foster acceptance and/or change of problem behaviors through emotional acceptance strategies and traditional behavioral techniques
Cognitive-behavioral	Add cognitive restructuring to behavioral goals and techniques
Premarital relationship enhancement program	Essentially behavioral techniques; focus on managing conflict and negative affect
Other Models	
Emotionally focused	Assess, acknowledge, and express underlying emotions and unmet feelings or needs; evocative or responding methods; homework
Structural-strategic	Restructure couple's boundaries; redefinition of problem behaviors; paradoxical techniques; joining

483

communication skills need to be taught to couples to change current dysfunctional behaviors.

COGNITIVE-BEHAVIORAL MARITAL THERAPY

CBMT integrates behavioral, cognitive, and affective techniques to address a couple's dissatisfaction. The behavioral techniques are essentially identical to those used in BMT. Many of the cognitive techniques used in CBMT extend from the methods used in standard cognitive-behavioral therapy. For instance, cognitive restructuring teaches couples how to recognize and modify their faulty perceptions, attributions, expectancies, assumptions, or standards.

ASSESSMENT AND COURSE OF THERAPY

To accurately evaluate a couple's relationship, it is essential to systematically evaluate the content areas of problems, the process and outcome of dyadic interaction, and individual functioning. Specific questions that inquire about presenting problems, strengths and skills of the relationship, sex and affection, social environment, individual functioning, and future prospects should be included. Table 48–2 offers an overview of the main assessment areas in marital therapy.

Treatment Planning

To some degree, the clinical picture determines the pace and direction of therapy. The emphasis on acceptance and change strategies depends on the couple's degree of distress, commitment, and motivation.

OUTCOME PREDICTORS

Although the literature so far has been riddled with contradictory and inconsistent findings, there are nonetheless several prognostic signs regarding treatment response that a therapist might consider. Younger couples, in general, appear to have better outcomes than their older counterparts. Most other demographical variables, such as education, number of previous marriages, and number of children, appear to have little relationship to outcome. Emotional disengagement may be a warning sign for poor response to couples therapy, as may polarized and highly traditional sex roles. Psychiatric illness, in the absence of marital distress, seems to also lead to poorer outcomes. The presence of negative communication and conflict engagement may not be a particularly poor prognostic sign, especially if it focuses greater attention on problem resolution. In fact, the virtual absence of any conflict engagement may itself be a negative predictor. Within therapy, couples and therapists who develop a collaborative set tend to have greater marital satisfaction at therapy termination. Also, greater emotional expression and acceptance within sessions may produce better outcomes.

TABLE 48–2	Assessment Areas in Marital Therapy

How Distressed Is This Couple?
Assess feelings, satisfaction, affection, intimacy, attraction, communication, and cooperation.
How Committed Is the Couple to Continuing the Relationship?
Assess development of relationship, events leading to therapy, motivation for therapy, expectations regarding future, reasons for continuing or discontinuing relationship, and steps taken toward separation or divorce.
What Are the Issues That Divide Them?
Assess the nature of the main complaints; include chronology of commencement and continuation, specific nature of problem, and how each partner differs and agrees on the definition and explanation of problems.
Why Are These Issues a Problem for Them?
Assess how each partner behaves before, during, and after the conflicts. Explore how conflicts evolve and how the environment maintains problem behaviors. Also, does concurrent or previous psychiatric illness play a role?
What Are the Strengths That Hold the Couple Together?
Assess strengths of the relationship and whether partners recognize and value these strengths. Assess common interests and activities as well as outside resources (such as social support, family, work). Has there been previous therapeutic work?
What Can Marital Therapy Do for the Couple?
Assess capacity and motivation to change, expectations about therapy, and possible "blocks" toward therapy (e.g., irreconcilable differences, extramarital relationship, severe psychiatric illness).

COUPLES THERAPY WITH SPECIFIC POPULATIONS

To understand whether cultural variables are responsible for relational distress, the therapist should understand each partner's cultural heritage and the context of the conflict behavior.

Multicultural understanding begins with assessment. During the interview, the therapist should be attentive to how the couple introduces or omits culturally related experiences, especially negative ones (e.g., oppression, discrimination, and adjustment to

Western culture). The therapist should pay attention to the couple's style of adaptation to the differences of their value system.

Cultural conflicts are often found in disagreements about cultural codes, cultural preferences and the permission to marry, and cultural stereotyping in stressful situations. The attempt to develop a common cultural code often occurs among couples who have recently married. This may reflect little understanding of the importance of each partner's cultural affiliation and could be remedied with acceptance work.

The second type of conflict may be a couple's struggle to establish their boundaries with extended family. Cultures have disparate understandings about what is appropriate behavior with extended family, and this may become a point of contention if each partner has different expectations about frequency of contact. Cultural stereotyping may also occur as a method to help one partner cope with stressful situations.

The therapist should be aware that different cultural groups may engage in communication styles that are normative in their culture but may be considered distressed by the therapist.

Attention to cultural context of behavior also applies to lesbian and gay couples. Understanding of the legal and social risks in declaring same-sex orientation, lack of societal customs to celebrate the stages of their relationship (e.g., engagement and marriage), and low visibility of successful role models of lesbian and gay couples can help the therapist to understand the stress that partners face already in the relationship. Specific to same-sex couples, the therapist should explore how gender role socialization has affected the relationship and whether it is an issue in the couple's distress. Therapists should be knowledgeable about the strengths and deficits of each gender role because same-sex couples may present with more defined difficulties associated with gender roles.

As with cultural minorities, therapists should be aware of how their own prejudicial views about the patient's race, views, social class, and language skills can affect the information gathered in the clinical interview. This may lead the therapist to underestimate or stereotype the impact of the culture on the relational difficulties. To minimize unintentional biases, therapists should acquaint themselves with the couple's values or be comfortable asking the patients to explain the impact of the culture on their relationship. This can promote the therapist's understanding of the context of the behavior and foster ability to identify potential reinforcers and punishing variables that maintain the distress. This can also help the therapist to provide a meaningful rationale for the patient to understand the goal of therapeutic exercises, producing results that can be generalized to the patient's natural environment.

Hypnosis

DEFINITION

Hypnosis is a psychophysiological state of attentive, receptive concentration, with a relative suspension of peripheral awareness. Hypnotic phenomena occur spontaneously, and the alteration of consciousness that hypnotized individuals experience has a variety of therapeutic applications. The hypnotic experience may be understood as involving three main factors (Table 49–1).

HYPNOSIS: WHAT IT IS AND WHAT IT IS NOT

Several principles provide guidance for the use of hypnosis in medicine and psychiatry. We attempt to clarify some of the myths and misconceptions about hypnosis by establishing what hypnosis is and what it is not in Table 49–2.

The most common modern approach to assessing hypnotizability combines a formal hypnotic induction and a series of tasks, which provide the therapist with an index of the patient's hypnotic ability. The use of such objective measurement has several advantages as shown in Table 49–3.

The Hypnotic Induction Profile allows the therapist to rate the subject on five items assessing cognitive and behavioral aspects of the single continuous but brief hypnotic experience elicited during the test. These are 1) ability to experience a sense of dissociation of the left hand from the rest of the body; 2) hand levitation, or floating of the hand back up in the air after being pulled down; 3) sense of involuntariness or unconscious compliance while elevating the hand; 4) response to the cutoff signal ending the hypnotic experience; and 5) sensory alteration in the hand or elsewhere in the body.

HYPNOSIS APPLIED

Because of its intrinsic qualities, the hypnotic state can be an effective adjunct to the treatment of various symptoms and problems both in psychiatry and in medicine generally. The first criterion to consider is the patient's level of hypnotizability. Once it has been determined that the patient has usable hypnotic capacity (defined by high scores in hypnotizability scales), a discussion about the nature of the hypnotic process follows. It is important at this point to dispel any myths and correct misconceptions the patient may have about the process. This includes the cooperative nature of the hypnotic process, rather than the "tell me what to do" that most patients expect. Finally, the therapist must decide whether the problem presented by the patient is amenable to hypnotic intervention or whether other steps should be taken instead.

TABLE 49–1	Components of the Hypnotic Process
Component	**Explanation**
Absorption	Refers to the tendency to engage in self-altering and highly focused attention with complete immersion in a central experience at the expense of contextual orientation and more peripheral perceptions, thoughts, memories, or motor activities.
Dissociation	Permits keeping out of conscious awareness many routine experiences that ordinarily would be conscious. Dissociated material may be temporarily and reversibly unavailable to consciousness, but it continues to influence conscious and unconscious experiences and behaviors.
Suggestibility	Involves heightened responsiveness to social cues. It allows subjects to suspend the usual conscious curiosity that makes us question the reason for our actions, making them more prone to accept suggestions given no matter how irrational.

Applications of hypnosis lie in four areas: general psychiatry, psychosomatic medicine, habit control, and forensic psychiatry (Table 49–4).

Hypnosis is one of the most helpful tools in the treatment of patients suffering from dissociative disorders. As a rule, these

TABLE 49–2	What Is Hypnosis?

What It Is
Hypnosis is a form of focused concentration.
Hypnotizability is a stable and measurable trait.
Hypnosis is something you do with, rather than to, a subject or patient.
All hypnosis is self-hypnosis.

What It Is Not
Hypnosis is not sleep.
There are not apparent sex differences in hypnotizability.
Hypnotizability is not a sign of weak-mindedness.
Hypnosis is not intrinsically dangerous.
Hypnosis is not therapy.
There is nothing you can do with hypnosis that you cannot do without it.

TABLE 49–3	Benefits of the Use of Hypnotizability Measures

It objectively assesses the patient's natural ability to use his or her hypnotic capacity.

It relieves performance pressure on both therapist and patient.

If provides objective data about the patient's ability to respond to treatment employing hypnosis.

It provides the therapist with scientific data to make rational treatment choices.

It provides helpful information about the subject's interpersonal style and possible psychiatric illness.

It helps predict the patient's likely response to psychotherapeutic treatment.

TABLE 49–4	Applications of Hypnosis

General Psychiatry

Anxiety disorders
  Phobias
  PTSD
Dissociative disorders
  Dissociative amnesia
  Dissociative identity disorder
Sleep disorders
  Insomnia

General Medicine

Anxiety associated with medical and surgical procedures

Pain control

Psychosomatic disorders
  Bronchial asthma
  Warts and other skin conditions
  Gastrointestinal disturbances (irritable bowel syndrome, peptic ulcer disease)
  Cardiovascular diseases

Adjuvant to chemotherapy

Emesis (chemotherapy, hyperemesis gravidarum)

Habit Control

Smoking cessation
Weight control

Forensic Psychiatry

Memory enhancement

patients experience their symptoms (i.e., fugue states, dissociated identities, and blackouts) as occurring unexpectedly and beyond their control. Hypnosis can be used formally both as a diagnostic tool and for therapeutic purposes. The hypnotic state can be seen as a controlled form of dissociation. Hypnosis is useful in the treatment of these patients, first in determining whether they have a dissociative disorder, and second in providing rapid access to these dissociated states. When used by the therapist in the context of treatment, hypnosis can demonstrate to patients the amount of control they have over this state, which they normally experience as "automatic and unpredictable." Recognizing and teaching patients with dissociative disorders how to master their capacity to dissociate are among the most important psychotherapeutic tasks in the course of their treatment.

The Condensed Hypnotic Approach

The use of hypnosis in the treatment of posttraumatic stress disorder (PTSD) and dissociative disorders can be conceptualized as having two major goals, which can be achieved by the use of six different techniques. The goals are to bring into *consciousness* previously repressed memories and to develop a sense of *congruence* between memories associated with the traumatic experience and current self-images. By bringing previously repressed memories into consciousness, the patient has the opportunity to understand, accept, and restructure them. These goals are achieved by working through six treatment stages: confrontation, condensation, confession, consolation, concentration, and control.

First the patient must *confront* the trauma. The therapist helps the patient recognize and understand the factors involved in the development of the symptoms for which help is now being sought. Hypnosis is then used to help the patient *condense* the traumatic memories. The hypnotic experience can be used to define a particularly frightening memory during the revision of the patient's history, which summarizes or condenses the main conflicts. Once memories are recovered, patients usually need to *confess* feelings and experiences for which they are profoundly ashamed. These are usually things they may never have told anyone else before; in fact, they have been running from these things all their lives. At this time, the therapist must convey a sense of "being present" for the patient while remaining as neutral as possible. This is followed by the stage of *consolation*. Here, the therapist needs to be emotionally available to the patient. This stage must be carried on with caution and in a most professional manner. Therapists should be aware that the body and emotional boundaries of these patients may have been violated in the past. Then comes the stage of *concentration*. This component of the trance experience allows patients to access or "turn on" the traumatic memories during the psychotherapeutic session and then "shut them off" once the work has been done. During the final stage, the patient comes to define herself or himself as being in *control* again.

The underlying principle to remember is that the most damaging effect of overwhelming trauma is that it renders its victims defenseless. Lacking physical and emotional control, patients activate dissociative defenses in an attempt to master their experiences. By using self-hypnosis, the therapist can model and teach the patient to regain control over her or his memories.

The task in the course of therapy is to help patients retrieve the painful memories, express them in ways that do not foster self-destructive feelings, and restructure the ways they think about themselves by reframing their memories and their self-perception. The recovery of traumatic memories helps patients to see themselves in a new light. It allows them to reassess the situation, both from the point of view at the time of the trauma (i.e., when they had no apparent control) and from their new perspective (i.e., distanced from the threat, with more information, more in control).

THERAPEUTIC PRECAUTIONS

The strength of transference during the psychotherapy of trauma victims is enormous. The use of hypnosis does not prevent development of a transference reaction; it may actually facilitate its emergence earlier than in regular therapy owing to the intensity with which the material is expressed and memories are recovered.

Reliving the traumatic experience along with patients may allow a special feeling of "being there with them" at the moment of trauma. This allows the therapist to provide guidance, support, protection, and comfort as the patient goes through the difficult path of reprocessing traumatic memories. However, this kind of *traumatic transference* between the therapist and the victim of sexual assault is different in the sense that the feelings transferred are related not so much to early object relationships but to the abuser or circumstances associated with the trauma. Instead of seeing this expressed anger at the therapist as a form of negative transference reaction, we should explore the possibility that this may be a healthy attempt for the patient to experience anger toward the perpetrator. As therapists, we should attempt not to minimize or shut off these feelings. This will only confirm the patient's former perception that there was something wrong with him or her for having these feelings, which will probably activate further use of primitive defenses, including dissociation or acting out.

A more serious complication in the use of hypnosis with trauma victims is the possible creation of *false memories.* Hypnosis, with its heightened sense of concentration, allows the patient to focus intensely on a given time or place, so it can enhance memory recall. The principle of state-dependent memory also makes it plausible that the mere entrance into this trance state can facilitate retrieval of memories associated with a similar state of mind that may have occurred during the trauma and subsequent flashbacks. However, not every memory recovered with the use of hypnosis is necessarily true. Hypnosis can facilitate improved recall of true as well as confabulated material. Suggestibility is increased in hypnosis, and information can be implanted or imagined and reported as a verdict. Because of this, therapists are warned about "believing" everything a patient is able to recall. Just as we use therapeutic judgment to analyze and interpret our patients' (nontraumatic) childhood memories, fantasies, and dreams, so we should treat hypnotically recovered material.

Applications in General Medicine

MEDICAL PROCEDURES

Because hypnosis can be used to produce a state of relaxation and to reduce anxiety, it has proved to be valuable as an adjuvant to medical procedures. Once patients have been trained in the use of self-hypnosis, they can use it both in preparation for a hospital visit and while in the clinic or hospital. It can also be used as a way of mastering the anxiety associated with potentially threatening procedures, either diagnostic (e.g., computed tomography or bone marrow aspirations) or therapeutic (e.g., chemotherapy).

PAIN CONTROL

Hypnosis can facilitate an alteration in the subjective experience of pain. Several techniques can be used to achieve this goal. Most techniques involve the production of physical relaxation coupled with visual or somatic imagery that provides a substitute focus of attention for the painful sensation.

Even though the precise mechanism for hypnotic analgesia is not known, it is suspected to have components of two complementary mechanisms: physical relaxation and attention control. Patients in pain tend to splint the painful area instinctively, which in turn increases muscle tension around the painful area, often resulting in increased pain. Therefore, creating a state of hypnotically induced relaxation may easily decrease their experience or perception of pain.

PSYCHOSOMATIC DISORDERS

Hypnosis is useful in both the diagnosis and treatment of psychosomatic illness. By using hypnosis with these patients, the therapist may assist in diagnosing the symptoms as psychosomatic. Under hypnosis, many of the symptoms may improve or be completely reversed.

In most instances, it is better if hypnosis is used as an adjuvant to any other medical treatment, including physical rehabilitation or any other modality typically used in the treatment of the "real illness." Such problems usually involve a combination of somatic and psychological symptoms. Using a rehabilitation model avoids the trap of humiliating the patient who improves with the inference that the problem was "all in the mind."

Hypnosis can be invaluable in treating a number of psychosomatic conditions. In particular, disorders affecting the gastrointestinal, such as ulcerative colitis and regional enteritis, are among those conditions in which studies demonstrated a dramatic response. Hypnosis has also been found effective in reducing the gastrointestinal side effects of chemotherapy, especially conditioned nausea and vomiting.

Applications of Hypnosis in Habit Control

SMOKING CESSATION

A number of studies demonstrate the efficacy of hypnosis as a tool to facilitate control of smoking. These studies show success rates in cigarette abstinence after treatment with hypnosis ranging from 13% to 64%. In these studies, abstinence is defined as no smoking during a follow-up time of at least 6 months.

WEIGHT CONTROL

Seldom will the use of hypnosis alone be sufficient for the treatment of weight problems. It is usually employed as an adjunct to a comprehensive dietary and exercise control program for weight reduction and management. Similar to the use of self-hypnosis in the control of smoking, the purpose in dietary control is to restructure the patient's experience with overeating. An important component of such an approach consists of teaching the patient to use self-hypnosis training to control the urge to overeat.

Applications in Forensic Psychiatry

The controversies surrounding the so-called false memory syndrome have reintensified questions regarding the validity of material recovered by the use of hypnosis. One of the most common applications of hypnosis in court and legal settings had been its use to refresh the recollection of witnesses and victims of crimes. Even though the current controversy focuses on the dangers of hypnotically induced confabulation or excessive confidence in memories, there have been some positive results.

Information retrieved with the aid of hypnosis may simply be the result of an additional recall trial; it may be new and true; or it may be a confabulation. It may indeed be a combination of all three. As a result, courts have long been unwilling to admit the testimony of a person hypnotized while testifying and have also begun to exclude testimony of witnesses who have previously been hypnotized about the event in question. Even when a subject is acting in good faith, hypnosis can amplify both truth and falsehood. A good guideline is that hypnosis increases the recovery of memories, both true and confabulated.

TREATMENT OUTCOME STUDIES IN HYPNOSIS

Most outcome studies have resulted in two main conclusions related to the therapeutic uses of hypnosis. First, there is no doubt that hypnosis is effective. Second, the degree of hypnotizability is predictive of treatment response.

Training patients in the use of self-hypnosis can facilitate the therapeutic process. This use of hypnosis can communicate the therapist's desire to enhance the patient's mastery and independence. Thus, patients can learn to use their hypnotic capacity rather than be used by it. This newly developed ability can be understood as an exercise in self-control rather than submission to the will of the therapist. It can be used to enhance control of somatic processes, reactions to anxiety-provoking stimuli, and impulsive behavior.

Behavioral Medicine

Behavioral medicine is a new subspecialty that emerged out of the realization that many medical problems have their genesis, and perhaps cure, in behavioral actions. The massive health problems triggered by smoking are some of the clearest examples.

For the three leading causes of death—heart disease, cancer, and stroke—factors that are causally related include tobacco, diet, lack of exercise, and alcohol, each the result of behavioral choices. Cigarette smoking is a proven risk factor for heart disease, malignant neoplasms, and stroke. Sedentary lifestyle has been implicated as a risk factor for many major medical diseases including coronary heart disease and diabetes. Poor dietary habits and obesity are associated with diabetes, hypertension, and coronary artery disease. Excessive consumption of alcohol is associated with gastrointestinal problems, liver disease, dementia, and fatal traffic accidents. The personal cost of these behavior-related illnesses is immense (e.g., 390,000 Americans die each year as a result of smoking), and the cost to treat these personal lifestyle choices is staggering (Table 50–1). Health attitudes and resultant behaviors have various effects on physiological characteristics of individuals—sometimes assisting their general well-being, more often posing serious adverse consequences to them.

STRESS

The most common psychosocial variable associated with illness onset has to do with the ever-elusive concept of stress, one of the most controversial and pervasive notions in health care today. Poor management of stress has been associated with an increased occurrence of heart disease, coronary artery disease, poor diabetes control, chronic pain conditions, and significant emotional distress.

Stressors have been associated with numerous pathological changes in biochemical and immunological activities. Research on the relationship of stress to the likelihood of becoming ill has clearly pointed out that exposure to stress alone is almost never a sufficient explanation for illness in ordinary human experience, just as genetics alone does not cause mental illness. Characteristics of the stressor presumed to mediate its impact include its magnitude, duration, novelty, and predictability as well as the temporal sequence of events. Relevant personal factors include biological vulnerabilities, response thresholds, age at exposure, personality style (e.g., self-efficacy, optimism, and sense of coherence), and coping styles (i.e., habitual patterns of response). In addition, the person's appraisal of the stressful situations (i.e., the degree of threat, perception of control, previous experience, and what coping resources or options are available) has been found to be critical in determining psychological

TABLE 50–1 Costs of Treatment for "Preventable" Conditions

Condition	Overall Magnitude	Intervention*	Cost per Patient†
Heart disease	7 million with CAD‡ 500,000 deaths/y 284,000 bypasses/y	Coronary bypass surgery	$ 30,000
Cancer	1 million new/y 510,000 deaths/y	Lung cancer treatment Cervical cancer treatment	$ 29,000 $ 28,000
Stroke	600,000 strokes/y	Hemiplegia treatment and rehabilitation	$ 22,000
Injuries	2.3 million hospitalizations/y 142,500 deaths/y 177,000 with spinal cord injuries in United States	Quadriplegia treatment and rehabilitation Hip fractures and rehabilitation Severe head injury treatment and rehabilitation	$570,000 (lifetime) $ 40,000 $310,000
HIV	1–1.5 million infected 118,000 AIDS‡ cases (as of 1/90)	AIDS treatment	$ 75,000

Table continued on following page

TABLE 50-1 Costs of Treatment for "Preventable" Conditions *(Continued)*

Condition	Overall Magnitude	Intervention*	Cost per Patient†
Alcoholism	18.5 million abuse alcohol 105,000 alcohol-related deaths/y	Liver transplant	$250,000
Drug abuse	Regular users: 1–3 million 375,000 drug-exposed babies	Treatment of drug-affected babies	$ 63,000 (5 y)
Low-birth-weight baby	260,000 born/y 23,000 deaths/y	Neonatal intensive care	$ 10,000
Inadequate immunization	20%–30% lack basic immunization series	Congenital rubella syndrome treatment	$345,000 (lifetime)

*Examples (other interventions may apply).

†Representative first-year costs, except as noted. Does not include nonmedical costs, such as loss of productivity to society.

‡CAD, Coronary artery disease; HIV, human immunodeficiency virus infection; AIDS, acquired immunodeficiency syndrome.

From Healthy People 2000: Washington, DC: U.S. Government Printing Office, 1991:5. U.S. Department of Health and Human Services publication (PHS) 91-S0212.

and physiological reactions to stress. Individuals who appraise situations as more threatening, important, and uncontrollable report more physical symptoms and emotional distress.

One way in which stress might lead to illness is by altering nervous, immune, or endocrine systems, creating modifications in heart rate, blood pressure, hypothalamus and pituitary activity, and other physiological processes. Physiological reactivity (particularly sympathetic nervous system reactivity) in response to stressful events has been proposed as a factor contributing to the progression of cardiovascular disease. Moreover, research in psychoneuroimmunology has demonstrated that stressors may lead to the suppression of immune functioning. Figure 50–1 diagrams some of the relationships between stress, behavior, and illness.

BEHAVIORAL MEDICINE TECHNIQUES: CLINICAL APPLICATIONS

Although behavioral medicine shares many applications and techniques with traditional medical and behavioral approaches to health care, several aspects are unique and characteristic of the

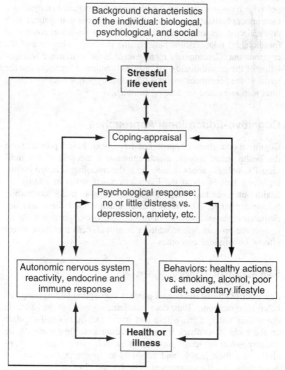

Figure 50–1 *Biopsychosocial model of stress.*

field. Five specific clinical activities have been synonymous with behavioral medicine across several areas of application and clinical populations.

Biobehavioral Assessment

Biobehavioral assessment involves the coordinated and integrated evaluation of biomedical and behavioral factors in the health status and quality of life of the patient. Careful behavioral analysis is a hallmark of this approach, with a detailed specification of the frequency, amplitude, duration, quality, and correlates of key health behaviors. Behavioral analysis emphasizes a systematic search for functional (contingent) relationships of the cues in the environment (discriminative stimuli), "signs, symptoms, or problems" (behavioral responses), and consequences of the behaviors (reinforcers).

Behavior Management

Behavior management is the use of learning principles (particularly operant and classical conditioning) to encourage and direct health behavior change. This approach emphasizes a functional analysis and contingency management to assist patients in making desired behavior change to achieve health goals. A functional analysis is a case conceptualization, similar to the case of the pain patient with an escalating narcotic intake that emphasizes empirical contingent (predictable) relationships between the person's behavior and the environment. Contingency management is the systematic manipulation of the probabilistic relationships (contingencies) between the terms of the functional analysis (i.e., discriminative stimuli, behavioral responses, and reinforcing stimuli).

Cognitive-Educational Approaches

Cognitive-educational approaches have been based primarily on the health belief model, which emphasizes the role of the individual's beliefs about health and the meaning of symptoms, including beliefs about the likely effects of behavior change on health outcomes and beliefs about the ability to make worthwhile behavior change. This model asserts that such beliefs and *anticipated* costs and benefits of health behaviors, whether accurate or not, are critical determinants of health choices that have direct effects on clinical outcomes.

Self-Control Theory

Self-control theory has been a primary conceptual underpinning of behavioral medicine. Behavioral medicine approaches are based on the notion that systems within and across individuals self-regulate on the basis of feedback from the environment. Thus, patients are encouraged to be active participants in their care, to take responsibility for their health, and to attend to appropriate feedback to assist them in self-management of health and illness.

Stress Management and Biofeedback

Stress management and biofeedback are related techniques that teach patients 1) self-regulation of arousal, 2) predictability and control of cognitive and overt responses to stressors, and 3) awareness and control of psychophysiological relationships. Biofeedback is the application of physiological monitoring for the express purpose of facilitating the patient's learning to modulate physiological responses directly. Biofeedback is often combined with perception modification techniques (e.g., relaxation training, distraction, mental visualization, and suggestion) to provide pain and symptom control.

TREATMENT FOR STRESS-RELATED ILLNESS

A person's response to stress is a complex reaction pattern with physiological, cognitive, behavioral, and social components. As a result, prevention and treatment of stress-related illness have concentrated on several important dimensions. The characteristic approach of behavioral medicine is to help individuals be more competent in managing their behaviors and emotions in reaction to taxing aspects of their environment or their medical illness. Self-management and effective command of one's health and environment depend on both possessing the necessary cognitive and behavioral skills and being able to employ those skills whenever

TABLE 50–2	Behavioral Arousal Control Methods
Progressive muscle relaxation	Systematic tensing and relaxing of major skeletal muscles
Diaphragmatic breathing	Repeated deep abdominal breathing
Autogenic training	Self-statements of rhythmical breathing, limb heaviness, and warmth
Guided imagery	Use of imagination and fantasy to visualize relaxing images
Hypnosis	Focused attention with suggestion for specific responses
Meditation	Repetitious inward attention with no specific suggestions
Biofeedback	Providing physiological information to facilitate self-regulation
Exercise	Physical activity, particularly aerobic activity
Cognitive therapy	Analysis and modification of thoughts contributing to arousal
Coping skills training	Analysis and modification of inefficacious responses to stress

necessary. Goals for treatment do not entail eliminating stress (or the medical problem) but involve helping the patient to learn the skills to function adequately despite stressful situations.

One key area of focus has been on arousal-reducing techniques, such as biofeedback, relaxation training, diaphragmatic breathing, meditation, self-hypnosis, and the use of exercise to reduce or counter stress (Table 50–2). The rationale for these stress management techniques assumes that an increased level of physiological arousal is manifested by a combination of increased muscle tension and increased sympathetic nervous system activity. In addition, specific training in reducing thoughts that increase arousal and learning more adaptive behaviors in response to a variety of stressful situations are emphasized in behavioral medicine's integrated multicomponent approach to managing stress-related illness.

Psychosocial Rehabilitation

Although the judicious use of pharmacotherapy remains essential in building a foundation for the treatment and rehabilitation of schizophrenia, psychosocial assessment and treatment must be part of an integrated biopsychosocial method for serving the needs of those with serious mental illness.

By employing the biopsychosocial approach to comprehensive care—including training in social and independent living skills, family psychoeducation, self-management of medication and symptoms, assertive clinical case management, and supported housing and employment—rehabilitation modalities can amplify the impact of medication and formal psychotherapy in fostering better outcomes and higher levels of personal functioning. There is ample evidence that optimal biopsychosocial treatment and rehabilitation, when offered in a coordinated, comprehensive, and continuous fashion, can facilitate symptomatic and social recovery from schizophrenia and other disabling mental disorders in a much greater proportion of individuals than are currently helped.

Biopsychosocial rehabilitation refers to a spectrum of services offered to an individual with a disability. These services are designed to involve the individual in selecting realistic goals that will maximize and maintain his or her optimal level of health, functioning, self-care, independence, and quality of life and minimize symptoms and impairments that are obstacles to reaching these personal goals. A set of principles that establishes a framework for the delivery of biopsychosocial rehabilitation is presented in Table 51–1.

Although these principles provide guidelines on important components of care for facilities that wish to deliver biopsychosocial treatment, they do not prescribe a specific structure or method for delivering that care. This flexibility leaves considerable room for programmatic creativity and allows service providers to determine what works best for their patients.

GOALS OF BIOPSYCHOSOCIAL REHABILITATION

The rehabilitation therapist uses the terms impairment, disability, and handicap to describe the problems faced by individuals with schizophrenia. Although the therapist is unable to change the underlying biological vulnerability or eliminate the inevitable stressors that patients are exposed to in the community, efforts can be made to build protective factors that can buffer patients from the noxious influences of vulnerability and stress. The goals of treatment and rehabilitation are to

TABLE 51-1	Principles for Biopsychosocial Rehabilitation

Individual involvement and rights

Assessment and planning

Coordination and continuity of integrated services

Provision of services

Reassessment and revision of services

Competence of providers

Evaluation and improvement of the community system for rehabilitation services

- Engage the individual in establishing personally relevant, realistic, and desired goals for life functioning
- Ameliorate positive and negative symptoms of the disorder, which are barriers to the attainment of personal goals
- Prevent or delay relapse of psychosis
- Strengthen the skills and coping capacities of the afflicated individual and natural caregivers, such as family members

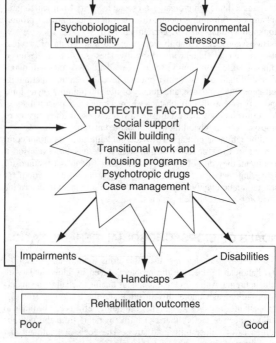

Figure 51-1 *Factors affecting serious mental disorders.*

- Remove or displace the bizarre and deviant behaviors that are intolerable for the family or community
- Provide services and compensatory community supports that enable the individual to function optimally despite continuing symptoms and disabilities

The significance of this multifactorial vulnerability-stress-protective factors model of schizophrenia (Fig. 51–1) lies in the guidelines it offers to therapists. Antipsychotic drugs buffer the psychobiological vulnerability and underlying biochemical disturbance in neurotransmitter systems; training in social and independent living skills confers coping capacities and thereby strengthens the individual's and caregivers' personal protection against stress and vulnerability; and supportive services (e.g., case management, housing, social service entitlements, supported employment) compensate for the individual's residual symptoms and deficits in functioning. Careful orchestration of pharmacotherapy, skills training, and community support services within the matrix of an effective means for flexibly delivering all interventions as changing individual needs require can significantly improve the course and outcome of the disorder as well as promote recovery in substantial numbers.

The outlook for persons diagnosed with schizophrenia is not invariably bleak but rather holds optimism that some level of recovery from the illness is possible if continuous access to treatment and rehabilitation is provided. This hopeful attitude has contributed to the growth of biopsychosocial rehabilitation techniques for schizophrenia, using new and better medications as well as improved psychosocial and behavioral treatments to accelerate remission of symptoms, recovery of social and vocational functioning, and improvement of the quality of life.

BIOPSYCHOSOCIAL ASSESSMENT OF CURRENT FUNCTIONAL STATUS

A thorough, carefully conducted assessment pinpoints the areas for rehabilitation and provides a baseline for monitoring its effects. Furthermore, assessment within the framework of biopsychosocial rehabilitation, with its emphasis on goals and functioning in addition to phase of illness and symptoms, fosters a collaborative relationship between patient and therapist that greatly enhances the treatment process.

Treatment Assessment, Planning, and Evaluation System

Client Assessment of Strengths, Interests, and Goals (CASIG) is a set of assessments and forms that help therapists plan, document, and evaluate biopsychosocial rehabilitation. CASIG is based on the model of biopsychosocial rehabilitation presented earlier, with the additional assumption that the plan for services must integrate the goals, needs, and constraints of all the relevant stakeholders—the patient, his or her significant others, individuals in the living environment, and the payor or payors.

The foundation of CASIG is the master assessment, which examines performance in 10 areas of functional living skills, subjective quality of life in 11 areas, the presence of 5 symptoms and 20 medication side effects, compliance with medication, and performance of 10 unacceptable community behaviors.

Regardless of the area being assessed or the source of the assessment information, the master assessment's items have all been designed to achieve several objectives:

- They are reliably administered by any of the paraprofessional and professional staff who typically provide services for patients.
- They can easily be incorporated into diverse staffing patterns and clinical responsibilities.
- They include multiple sources of information so that agreements and disagreements among them can be used to better plan services.
- They bridge the many facilities in which patients are served.
- With repeated administration, they monitor the progress of the individual patient's programs and, in the aggregate, monitor the effectiveness and changing characteristics of programs.

SHORT- AND LONG-TERM GOALS KEYED TO THE PHASE OF ILLNESS

The therapist and patient are guided by the continuous interaction of the patient's overall rehabilitation goals with the current stage of the disorder. During the acute, florid stage of the illness, the task for the therapist may be to assist the individual in moving from grandiose and unrealistic fantasies to articulating the more proximal and immediate realistic changes and steps that must be accomplished before the longer term goals can be reached. As the patient's symptoms stabilize and, hopefully, ameliorate, the focus shifts to helping the patient define her or his goals in terms of occupational, student, friendship, familial, and residential roles. Still another shift occurs during the late rehabilitation and recovery phase, when individuals begin to look for goals that transcend their status as patients in the capacity of patients. In this phase, the goal is to develop and nurture the wellness factors (e.g., hope, courage, self-esteem) that enable patients not only to manage but also sometimes to overcome the illness.

Long-term goals are cast in monthly to yearly time lines and should correlate with overall rehabilitation goals, serving as vehicles for achieving progress toward functional life roles. Long-term goals should be comprehensive in subserving progress in all relevant domains of life functioning (social-interpersonal, financial, recreational, medical-psychiatric, activities of daily living and independent living skills, vocational-educational, and housing-residential).

COMPREHENSIVE AND COORDINATED SERVICES FOR PATIENTS WITH SERIOUS MENTAL ILLNESS

Psychosocial rehabilitation is most efficacious when delivered in a continuous, comprehensive, and well-coordinated manner through a service delivery system. The context for integrating this treatment system is illustrated by the three dimensions of a "complex cube" of psychiatric rehabilitation. One dimension of the cube is the stage of disorder; this indicates the nature and severity of symptoms, from early signs through a full psychotic episode to remission or chronic illness. The second dimension consists of treatment and rehabilitation techniques—drug therapy, family and cognitive therapies, social skills training, and vocational rehabilitation. The third dimension consists of support programs aimed at minimizing residual handicaps; these include family support, social service entitlements, case management, and psychosocial clubs.

THE CLINICAL CASE MANAGER

Effective case management can be the vehicle for integrating bio-psychosocial treatment and rehabilitation services. Partly because of their enduring symptoms, most individuals with schizophrenia do not travel readily for medical and psychiatric appointments, nor do they eagerly embrace the social contact offered by therapeutic services. Instead, it is often necessary to deliver services through a mobile outreach form of clinical case management.

Although there is little consensus on the role of the case manager, in a biopsychosocial rehabilitation setting such a person has several specific tasks to perform. These tasks include assisting patients in building social networks, facilitating the securement of housing and employment, helping patients interact with the various service organizations to meet ongoing needs, teaching patients the skills they require for the self-management of the illness, monitoring the clinical progress of the patients, and, when necessary, undertaking timely clinical interventions.

SUMMARY

Research studies and clinical trials indicate that individuals with severe mental illness can improve their role functioning, reduce their disabilities, and achieve better-quality lives. These positive outcomes, however, are conditional. They are achieved when

- Psychopharmacotherapy is optimal and provided with full appreciation of the importance of the patient's collaboration and informed participation in drug management.
- The methods of teaching role skills are tailored to individuals' cognitive impairments and disabilities.
- There is a partnership between the teaching and the natural environment so that the one supports the other.
- The full range of needed clinical services is provided on a schedule and with an intensity that fits the ongoing course and clinical phases of each individual's illness.

Electroconvulsive Therapy

INDICATIONS FOR ELECTROCONVULSIVE THERAPY

In contrast to its origins as a treatment of schizophrenia, electroconvulsive therapy (ECT) today is generally used more frequently in patients with depression. Mania and schizophrenia account for most of the remainder of its use. The decision about when to use ECT is based on signs and symptoms of severe mental disorder that cut across diagnostic lines. These factors have been most clearly spelled out by the American Psychiatric Association's recommendations for the practice of ECT, which identified primary and secondary use of convulsive therapy. Primary indications are those for which ECT may appropriately be used as a first-line treatment. These include situations in which the patient's medical or psychiatric condition requires rapid clinical response, in which the risk of alternative treatments is excessive, or in which, based on history, response to ECT or nonresponse to medications is anticipated. If these conditions are not met, medication or other alternative treatment is recommended first, with ECT reserved for cases of nonresponse to adequate trials, unacceptable adverse effects of the alternative treatment, or deterioration of the patient's condition, increasing the urgency of the need for response. These general principles, in turn, require individualized interpretation in the presence of specific psychiatric and medical disorders.

Indications for ECT are presented in Table 52–1.

Depression

For depression the literature describes an overall response rate to ECT of 75% to 85%. Efforts to delineate subtypes of depression that are particularly responsive to ECT have yielded inconsistent results. ECT is most likely to be helpful in an acute episode of severe depression of relatively brief duration.

Psychotic depression, increasingly recognized as a distinct subtype of mood disorder that responds poorly to antidepressants alone, has emerged as a powerful indication for ECT. In this subgroup, ECT is at least as effective as a combination trial of antidepressant and antipsychotic medications. On balance, the evidence supports the early use of ECT in psychotic depression, particularly in lieu of prolonged, complicated medication trials that may be poorly tolerated in the elderly.

TABLE 52–1	Indications for Electroconvulsive Therapy

Diagnostic considerations
  Major depression
    Unipolar
      Psychotic
    Bipolar
  Mania
  Schizophrenia
    Acute
  Schizoaffective disorder
  Neurologic disorders
    Parkinson's disease
    Catatonia
    Neuroleptic malignant syndrome
Clinical considerations
  Need for rapid response on medical or psychiatric grounds
    (e.g., suicidality, inanition)
  History of treatment resistance or excessive risk or alternative treatments
  Severity of illness
  History of previous positive response to ECT
  Preference of the patient

Mania

Under certain circumstances, such as manic delirium, ECT can be lifesaving, which is a reminder that before the development of somatic treatments, mania had a mortality rate of at least 10%. Thus, in medical emergencies associated with mania, ECT should be regarded as a treatment of first choice. The same is true for medical conditions accompanying acute mania (including pregnancy) that contraindicate or render intolerable the use of psychotropic medications.

Schizophrenia

The American Psychiatric Association Task Force and the Canadian Psychiatric Association identified a role for ECT as a second-line treatment for selected patients with schizophrenia, particularly when associated with a brief duration of illness and/or affective symptoms. It has been consistently found that the patients with schizophrenia most likely to respond to ECT are those with good prognosis signs: mood disturbances, short duration of illness, predominance of positive rather than negative symptoms, and overexcitement. Diagnostic subtypes of schizophrenia associated with a positive response to ECT include acute, schizophreniform, schizoaffective, catatonic, and paranoid.

Neurological Disorders

CATATONIA

The case report literature describes the generally prompt and complete response to ECT of catatonic syndromes associated with both primary psychiatric and systemic disorders. ECT may justifiably be described as lifesaving when catatonia leads to inanition and in the often fatal malignant form of catatonia.

During the past decade, benzodiazepines have emerged as the pharmacological treatment of choice for catatonia. However, in patients unresponsive to medication, prolonged drug trials with continuing clinical deterioration should be avoided in favor of a course of ECT.

Other Considerations: Medical Illness and Age

The elderly are more vulnerable than younger individuals to the symptoms of depression—particularly psychosis, decreased nutritional intake, and suicidal ideation—and to the adverse effects of antidepressant medications; therefore, they represent a growing segment of the population base for ECT. A substantial proportion of geriatric patients with depression who are referred for ECT suffer from significant concurrent medical illness, which often precludes adequate trials of pharmacotherapy.

Even in the absence of controlled studies, the efficacy of ECT in geriatric depression is well established and is often perceived as even superior to that in younger age groups. In addition to the usual clinical criteria for recommending ECT, some have suggested that anxiety or agitation, commonly regarded as a negative prognostic sign in younger individuals, may be predictive of a good response to ECT in the older depressed patient.

Two general points should be made about the use of ECT in the elderly: 1) the physiological changes associated with ECT—cardiovascular (elevated blood pressure, arrhythmias), cognitive (confusion, memory loss), risk of traumatic injury to bones and teeth—that are benign and easily tolerated in young and middle-aged patients are prominent sources of potential ECT-associated morbidity in geriatric patients, and 2) the safety of ECT is appreciably enhanced if the foregoing effects on the older body, whether healthy or diseased, are anticipated and controlled. Thus, careful pretreatment evaluation of the patient's medical and neurological status, as well as review of concurrent use of medications and their potential impact on ECT, is crucial.

PRETREATMENT EVALUATION

Psychiatric Considerations

The pre-ECT evaluation is a good time to confirm psychiatric diagnoses, including Axis II and III disorders. Should the indications for ECT remain present, baseline assessments of mental status—including evaluation of suicidal ideation, orientation, and memory—will help to monitor changes in both therapeutic and adverse effects during the course of treatment. The history and effects of previous treatment with ECT should be obtained. At this time, decisions must also be made regarding ongoing psychotropic medications—particularly those increasing the risk of toxicity in combination with ECT (e.g., lithium) and those affecting seizure threshold (e.g., benzodiazepines, anticonvulsants)—and steps instituted to adjust, taper, or discontinue these, when appropriate.

Other Medical Considerations

The history and physical examination should focus on the cardiovascular and neurological systems, which are the areas at greatest risk. The consulting internist or other physician should advise the treatment team regarding the need for modifications in ECT technique, such as medications to moderate hemodynamic changes. The safety of possible treatment adjuncts, such as intravenous caffeine, should also be addressed when baseline cardiovascular function is compromised. Appropriate monitoring of medical conditions that may be affected by ECT, such as diabetes, should be arranged at this time.

In the uncomplicated situation, the routine laboratory work-up for ECT is the same as that indicated for any procedure involving general anesthesia: a complete blood count, serum electrolyte determination, and electrocardiogram. A chest radiograph is often obtained as well. The need for further pretreatment work-up, such as serum chemistry determinations, urinalysis, human immunodeficiency virus antibody titers, and blood concentrations of medication, is determined on an individual basis. Lumbosacral spinal films, historically routine before institution of muscle relaxation in the ECT premedication protocol, have become optional for many patients. This remains appropriate for older patients with a history of, or at risk for, osteoporosis and for any patient with a history of bone trauma. A formal anesthesiology consultation should result in an assignment of the degree of anesthesia risk and recommendations for any necessary modification in the ECT protocol. The condition of the dentition should be routinely assessed to avoid the treatment-associated risk of aspiration or fracture of loose teeth or bridgework. Especially in elderly patients, a formal dental examination may be helpful to ensure proper protection of the teeth during ECT.

Informed Consent

Among the unique features of ECT compared with other standard psychiatric treatments is the requirement for written informed consent by the patient or legal guardian or other substitute. Informed consent entails the patient's being provided the rationale for the recommendation for ECT, along with information regarding the potential benefits and risks of available alternative treatments, including no treatment. The consent form encompasses the series of treatment sessions that constitute a course of ECT, with the explicit understanding that consent may be withdrawn and treatments terminated at any point, at the patient's discretion. A separate consent form is necessary for continuation or maintenance of ECT after completion of the acute phase treatment course.

Given the transient cognitive impairments that are common in depression and during a course of ECT, it is particularly necessary to maintain a dialogue with the patient as treatment progresses to ensure that all the patient's questions and concerns are addressed, even if repetitive discourse ensues.

INITIATION OF TREATMENT

Once informed consent has been obtained, the initiation of treatment involves several decisions, including selection of the ECT device, electrode placement, dose of electricity, choice of premedications, and frequency of treatment.

In choosing electrode placement, two important factors should be considered: antidepressant efficacy and cognitive side effects. The choice of electrode placement is between unilateral placement over the nondominant (generally right) hemisphere and bifrontotemporal placement, otherwise known as bilateral placement. The advantage of unilateral placement is that there is less memory loss and confusion than with bilateral electrode placement. The disadvantage of unilateral ECT is that it appears to be less effective when the dose of electricity given is close to the seizure threshold, and the seizure threshold can vary more than 40-fold from individual to individual. For some patients, the degree or speed of response appears greater to bilateral than to unilateral ECT, requiring electrode placement to be individualized based on the relative benefits and risks for a given patient. Individuals who are unresponsive to several adequately dosed unilateral treatments may benefit from a switch to bilateral electrode placement.

A contemporary survey of ECT practices revealed that several methods for determining initial parameters for electrical dose are used in clinical practice. Some of them include adjusting dosage on the basis of age and sex to compensate for the effects of these parameters on seizure threshold. Others use a fixed set of parameters for individuals that does not take into account the range in variation of seizure threshold. The main conceptual points are that the dose of electricity *relative to seizure threshold* is an important variable (especially with unilateral electrode placement) and that optimal clinical results are most likely to be obtained when the stimulus intensity is significantly higher than the seizure threshold.

From the start of the treatment procedure, the electrocardiogram, heart rate, and blood pressure are monitored and oxygen saturation is measured via pulse oximetry. Pure oxygen by mask is typically administered after the induction of anesthesia and until the return of spontaneous respiration.

The patient is first rendered unconscious with a short-acting general anesthetic. As with any general anesthesia, the patient should be on nothing-by-mouth status for the appropriate period, prior to the treatment. Methohexital, 0.75 to 1 mg/kg, given intravenously, is the agent most commonly used. Other agents in use include thiopental, propofol, etomidate, and ketamine.

Once the patient is unconscious, a muscle relaxant is administered. Intravenous succinylcholine, 0.5 to 1 mg/kg, is almost always used for this purpose. The goal of the muscle relaxant is to dampen the tonic-clonic movements from the seizure and reduce the risk of musculoskeletal injury. The cuff technique may be applied to an ankle or forearm, preventing localized circulation of the muscle relaxant and thereby facilitating monitoring of the duration of the motor seizure.

When the patient is unconscious and relaxed, the stimulus is delivered using the desired electrode placement. Initially, the jaw will clench as a result of direct electrical stimulation. The heart rate will slow and the patient will generally have tonic contraction of the extremities. This initial period, which lasts from 2 to 5 seconds, is usually followed by a marked increase in blood pressure and heart rate. This is secondary to a centrally mediated catecholamine surge. The extremities then have tonic-clonic contractions, the intensity of which depends on the degree to which they have been modified by the muscle relaxant.

During the treatment, the seizure's duration should be monitored via one- or two-channel electroencephalography, an integral component of modern ECT devices. Combining motor movement timing with electroencephalographic monitoring yields the most reliable determination of seizure duration in the clinical setting. Although the dose of electricity relative to the seizure threshold is the important variable, an adequate seizure is generally between 20 seconds and 2 minutes in duration. Seizures lasting more than 3 minutes are considered prolonged. Should this occur, the practitioner may attempt to terminate the seizure with intravenous benzodiazepine. Diazepam given intravenously enters the brain within seconds and can terminate status epilepticus within 1 minute.

Once the seizure terminates, the patient is continuously supported and monitored until breathing occurs spontaneously, until he or she is responsive to voice commands, and until there is a return of muscle strength. The patient's vital signs are monitored every 15 minutes until they are stable.

This process is repeated for an average of 6 to 12 sessions in the treatment of depression. In the United States, ECT is usually performed three times per week, whereas in the United Kingdom and Europe a twice-weekly schedule is more common. The available data suggest that the twice-weekly schedule produces an equivalent therapeutic response with fewer treatments, but the speed of clinical improvement is slower than with the schedule of three times per week. Conversely, the more rapid therapeutic response to ECT given three times per week is accompanied by greater adverse cognitive effects than those associated with the slower rate of treatments.

Adverse Effects

The adverse effects from ECT range in severity from mild complications, such as myalgias, to serious events, such as fractured bones, to catastrophes, such as death. At present, the risk of serious complication is about 1 in 1000 patients. The risk of death is about 1 in 10,000 patients, which approximates the risk of general anesthesia for a minor surgical procedure.

Cardiac complications are the most frequent medical side effects. The arrhythmias range in severity from the common and benign sinus tachycardia to life-threatening or fatal ventricular arrhythmias. However, ECT is not associated with persistent electrocardiographic changes or myocardial damage.

Today, with careful pretreatment evaluation and consultation and the judicious use of prophylactic β-blockers and calcium channel blockers, many arrhythmias, dangerous elevations of blood pressure, and other cardiovascular complications may be avoided, even in individuals who are at high risk medically.

Confusion and memory loss are also commonly occurring side effects. These adverse effects are the major factor limiting the use of ECT. Transient confusion occurs universally as a postictal event. Memory disturbance also occurs frequently. The extent and persistence of the confusion and memory impairment are highly variable and sensitive to technical factors in ECT, such as electrode placement, electrical dosage, stimulus waveform, and frequency of treatments. In general, during the acute course of ECT, both retrograde and anterograde memory is impaired to some degree. After the treatments end, the memory difficulties gradually resolve during the ensuing weeks to months. Some patients may have permanent spottiness in memory for events that occurred in the weeks to months before, during, and after the ECT course. Rarely, patients have complained of persistent memory difficulties severe enough to interfere with social or occupational functioning, or both. However, the infrequency of this occurrence, and certain technical factors such as the lack of nondepressed pretreatment memory and other neuropsychiatric measures, have made it difficult to study these individuals systematically. Several decades of appropriately controlled animal and human studies, supplemented in more recent years by modern brain scanning techniques, have demonstrated that ECT does not cause brain damage.

Drug Interactions

Because most patients referred for ECT are already taking psychotropic medications, many ECT-drug interactions result from the inadvertent or deliberate failure to modify the preexisting medication regimen before the initiation of convulsive therapy.

The American Psychiatric Association Task Force report recommended that antidepressants be discontinued before ECT is started. The heterocyclic antidepressants are generally thought of as promoting seizures, although they have also demonstrated anticonvulsant effects. The cardiovascular effects of heterocyclic agents have been a concern when they are combined with ECT.

The standard recommendation regarding monoamine oxidase inhibitors (MAOIs) is to avoid combining them with general anesthesia. Hypertension and hypotension, as well as several other adverse effects, have been described when anesthesia is combined with MAOIs.

The few data on the newer antidepressants suggest that bupropion and the selective serotonin reuptake inhibitors may be safely combined with ECT. Despite early concerns about prolonged seizures, the initial studies and most case reports combining fluoxetine with ECT have not found a significant effect on seizure duration.

The combination of lithium and ECT has been a subject of debate. There have been several case reports indicating that the combination of the two increases the risk of delirium. Conventional clinical practice is to discontinue lithium before the institution of ECT unless a specific indication for the combination shifts the benefit/risk ratio of combination treatment for a given patient.

In contrast to lithium, the combination of neuroleptic drugs and ECT has been reported to be safe and possibly to increase the efficacy of ECT in psychotic patients.

Benzodiazepines and antiepilepsy drugs increase the seizure threshold and may decrease the efficacy of ECT. Unless there is a clinical contraindication, they should be discontinued or at least decreased before the start of ECT. If they cannot be discontinued, bilateral electrode placement may be preferred because with that technique the dose of electricity relative to the seizure threshold appears to be less important to a successful therapeutic outcome. Conversely, medications that lower the seizure threshold (such as theophylline) or prolong the seizure's duration (such as caffeine), or both, may, if given in excess, contribute to ECT toxicity, for example, status epilepticus.

CONTINUATION PHARMACOTHERAPY

The strategy of introducing or continuing antidepressant medication after a course of ECT was endorsed by British controlled studies in the 1960s that showed a significant drop in the 6-month relapse rate from 50% with placebo to 20% with continuation tricyclic antidepressant or MAOI treatment. Physicians would be best advised to use, for continuation purposes, a class of antidepressant medication or combination treatment that is different from that which failed before ECT. Few comparable data on continuation or maintenance medication exist when ECT is used for indications other than depression.

CONTINUATION-MAINTENANCE ELECTROCONVULSIVE THERAPY

Given both the logic of continuing the same treatment that achieved acute improvement to prevent relapse or recurrence and the historical reality that ECT achieved widespread use more than a decade before the introduction of effective psychotropic medications, it is not surprising that much of the literature on the use of follow-up ECT after completion of an acute course is decades old. Several studies, however, found decreased relapse rates in selected populations who received some form of maintenance ECT. Specific guidelines for decision-making regarding patient selection and course of treatment have not yet been developed.

ADEQUACY OF ELECTROCONVULSIVE THERAPY TRIAL

A course of 8 to 12 bilateral ECT treatments should be completed before any patient is declared resistant to ECT. Patients who fail to respond to several treatments with unilateral electrode placement should be switched to bilateral ECT and offered an opportunity to respond to a full trial of that modality. The treatment history of the ECT-refractory patient should be reviewed to ensure that seizures were generalized and of adequate duration. Additional ECT sessions may be required in some resistant patients for a response to occur. Adjunctive treatment—for example, intravenous caffeine to prolong induced seizures of inadequate duration—may be considered. At present, despite their frequent empirical use, no controlled study supports the use of other ECT-medication (e.g., antidepressants) combinations, which are deserving of rigorous investigation in the refractory patient.

REEVALUATION

Even in carefully selected patients, a lack of response to a course of ECT may occur in 10% to 30% of individuals. Nonetheless, this degree of refractoriness should trigger a reassessment of the patient, with confirmation of the original diagnosis. Such data may both help explain the lack of response to ECT and open avenues to further evaluation or treatment efforts.

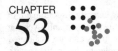

Antipsychotic Drugs

Antipsychotic drugs are effective in reducing psychotic symptoms that result from a number of disorders, including schizophrenia, schizoaffective disorder, affective disorders, and organic mental disorders.

INDICATIONS FOR ANTIPSYCHOTIC AGENTS

Antipsychotic drugs are effective for treating nearly every condition that causes psychotic symptoms.

Schizophrenia and Schizoaffective Disorder

Antipsychotic drugs are indicated for nearly all acute episodes of schizophrenia and schizoaffective disorder. This includes first episodes of psychosis as well as recurrences of chronic schizophrenia.

There may be important risks associated with an excessive delay in beginning antipsychotic drug treatment for patients with schizophrenia. Early intervention with antipsychotic drugs reduces long-term morbidity and decreases the number of rehospitalizations. In other words, even if a patient eventually recovers without drugs, it is possible that the amount of time spent in a psychotic state may be related to a worse long-term outcome.

Major Depression with Psychotic Features

Episodes of major depressive disorder are often accompanied by psychotic symptoms, including hallucinations and delusions. These symptoms often respond poorly to antidepressants when they are administered alone and usually require the use of adjunctive antipsychotic drugs. The added benefits of antipsychotic medications are most apparent for patients who are tormented by severe delusions. When the psychotic component of the episode has responded to treatment, the antipsychotic medications should be withdrawn.

Mania

Antipsychotic medications are effective in reducing manic excitement. In comparison with lithium, carbamazepine, and valproate, antipsychotic drugs have a more rapid onset of action. As a result, an antipsychotic drug may be combined with an antimanic drug during the first days of treatment of severe excited states, before the antimanic compound has its onset of action. Once lithium or another antimanic compound has become effective, the dose of antipsy-

515

chotic agent can usually be reduced and eventually discontinued. In most cases, antimanic drugs are more effective than antipsychotic agents for the broad range of manic symptoms and are associated with fewer side effects. Some studies indicate that patients with mood disorders are more vulnerable to the development of tardive dyskinesia (TD) than are patients with schizophrenia, suggesting the importance of minimizing the use of these drugs.

Tourette's Disorder

Tourette's disorder is a neurobehavioral disorder associated with motor and vocal tics. When the tics are disabling, an antipsychotic medication can be effective in reducing the severity of both motor and vocal tics. Although haloperidol and pimozide are the most commonly used agents, fluphenazine and other antipsychotic agents have also been effective. The doses used are in the common clinical range. For children 3 to 12 years old, 0.05 to 0.075 mg/kg/d is the usual dose range. Pharmacotherapy is usually unnecessary when the tics are not severe.

Borderline Personality Disorder

Some patients with severe forms of borderline personality disorder experience transient psychotic states when they are under stress. These states may be characterized by suspiciousness, ideas of reference, impulsiveness, and aggressiveness. A number of studies indicate that these individuals improve when they receive low doses of an antipsychotic agent.

Substance-Related Disorders

A number of drugs, including amphetamines, cocaine, alcohol, and phencyclidine, can cause psychotic symptoms that occur while the patient is intoxicated or during drug withdrawal. If stimulants such as amphetamines or cocaine result in psychotic symptoms that cause severe suffering or dangerous behaviors, a brief course of a high-potency antipsychotic drug is usually effective.

Antipsychotic agents are also useful for patients with hallucinations or delusions that occur with alcoholism. They should be prescribed carefully because these drugs may increase the likelihood of seizures occurring during alcohol withdrawal. As a result, benzodiazepines are more appropriate than antipsychotic drugs for uncomplicated alcohol withdrawal.

Organic Psychosis in the Elderly

Antipsychotic medications are also effective for psychotic symptoms that are secondary to organic mental syndromes. Elderly and nonelderly patients suffering from dementias often become agitated or suspicious. A number of carefully performed double-blind studies have found that antipsychotic drugs are superior to placebo for treating agitated elderly patients. Geriatric patients frequently respond to relatively low doses of high-potency medications. Low-potency medications can result in orthostatic hypotension and falling episodes. In addition, elderly patients may have an increased sensitivity to the anticholinergic effects of low-potency antipsychotic agents.

Other Organic Syndromes

Patients with Huntington's disease usually benefit from high-potency antipsychotic medications. Drug treatment can be helpful in reducing the severity of both the chorea and the psychosis that may accompany the illness. Ballismus, an illness characterized by abnormal activity of the axial and proximal musculature, is usually treated with an antipsychotic drug. Antipsychotic agents are also helpful in patients with psychotic symptoms that can result from steroids.

INITIATION OF TREATMENT

Route of Administration

In most circumstances, patients who are neither agitated nor uncooperative prefer orally administered antipsychotics to parenteral drugs. Oral drugs are usually well absorbed and reach a peak plasma concentration in 1 to 4 hours. Because these drugs have relatively long elimination half-lives (12 to 24 hours), they are effective when administered only once or twice daily. Although intramuscular medication has a more rapid onset of action, the acute calming effect of the medication—an effect that can be particularly helpful in agitated patients—is different from the antipsychotic effect, which usually takes days or even weeks to emerge. The goal during the first days is to find a dose that the patient can tolerate, to wait until a steady-state plasma concentration can be reached, and to assess the effectiveness of the treatment.

Oral administration has the disadvantage of being less dependable than parenteral administration. Drug absorption can be impaired by the administration of antacids as well as by tea or coffee. In addition, most antipsychotic drugs undergo substantial first-pass hepatic and gut metabolism, which can result in low concentrations of the parent compound reaching the circulation. Parenteral antipsychotic medications can be useful in a number of circumstances. When agitated patients refuse oral medications, an intramuscular injection may be the only form of treatment that can be administered.

Antipsychotic agents can also be administered in long-acting depot preparations. In the United States, long-acting fluphenazine and haloperidol are administered as esters dissolved in sesame oil. The oil is injected into a muscle, and the drug gradually diffuses from the oily vehicle into the surrounding tissues.

Selection of an Antipsychotic Agent

Table 53–1 gives commonly prescribed antipsychotic drugs and their side effect profiles. Although these compounds are derived from several different chemical classes, it is practical to divide them into five categories: high-potency dopamine antagonists, middle-potency dopamine antagonists, low-potency dopamine antagonists, serotonin-dopamine antagonists, and clozapine. The only currently available serotonin-dopamine antagonist is risperidone.

TABLE 53-1 Selected Antipsychotic Drugs

Drug	Routes of Administration	Usual Daily Oral Dose (mg)	Sedation	Autonomic Effects	Extrapyramidal Side Effects	Comments
Phenothiazines						
Chlorpromazine	Oral, IM*	200–1000	+++	+++	+	
Fluphenazine	Oral, IM, depot	2–20	+	+	+++	Usual dose of fluphenazine decanoate, 10–50 mg every 2–4 wk
Trifluoperazine	Oral, IM	5–30	++	+	+++	
Perphenazine	Oral, IM	8–64	++	+	+++	
Thioridazine	Oral	200–600	+++	+++	+	800 mg daily is the recommended upper limit because of the risk of pigmentary retinopathy
Butyrophenone						
Haloperidol	Oral, IM, depot	5–20	+	+	+++	Usual dose of haloperidol decanoate, 50–300 mg every 3–4 wk

Thioxanthene						
Thiothixene	Oral, IM	5–30	+	+	+++	
Dihydroindolone						
Molindone	Oral	20–100	++	+	+	
Dibenzoxazepine						
Loxapine	Oral, IM	20–100	++	+	+	
Dibenzodiazepine						
Clozapine	Oral	250–600	+++	+++	0?	Weekly blood monitoring for agranulocytosis
Benzisoxazole						
Risperidone	Oral	2–8	+	++	+	Increased risk of EPS with >10 mg/d

*IM, intramuscular.

+++, Very potent; ++, moderately potent; +, weakly potent.

For the most part, all antipsychotic drugs are equally effective in populations of patients with schizophrenia. The only possible exceptions are clozapine and risperidone, which may have advantages over other drugs. In addition, all available antipsychotic agents are equally effective for all types of schizophrenia with the exception of clozapine, which has been demonstrated to be more effective for patients who respond poorly to other drugs.

A detailed history of prior drug responses can provide information about the effectiveness and side effects of different drugs in a particular individual, as well as the patient's personal preference. A patient's report of an allergy to a particular antipsychotic drug should be carefully explored because the patient may be misinterpreting prior extrapyramidal side effects (EPS) that can be easily managed by the use of antiparkinsonian medications or more judicious dosage selection.

The selection of a drug for acute treatment may also be influenced by the long-term management strategy. If noncompliance or erratic compliance with medication has been a problem in the past for an individual, consideration should be given to the use of a long-acting depot antipsychotic drug.

As mentioned previously, clozapine and risperidone may have advantages in comparison with conventional antipsychotics. A number of controlled studies have compared clozapine to other drugs. These studies suggest that clozapine is more effective than other drugs for patients with more severe symptoms of schizophrenia who respond poorly to other drugs. However, because of clozapine's serious adverse effects, particularly agranulocytosis, its use has been limited to patients who have been clearly demonstrated to have illnesses that respond poorly to other drugs.

Risperidone is a serotonin-dopamine antagonist that may have advantages over other drugs. It is a high-potency agent that causes fewer EPS than other high-potency drugs such as haloperidol or fluphenazine. As a result, it has a favorable side effect profile with minimal sedation and anticholinergic effects. Double-blind comparisons with other drugs suggest that risperidone may result in greater improvements in positive and negative symptoms when compared with conventional drugs.

Dose of Antipsychotic Agent

Doses less than 300 mg of chlorpromazine (or 5 mg of fluphenazine or haloperidol) are likely to be too low for many psychotic patients. At the same time, doses greater than 1000 mg of chlorpromazine (or 20 mg of haloperidol or fluphenazine) are seldom necessary and may lead to substantial side effects. The only occasion for treating patients with doses outside this range is when there is evidence that a particular patient did better with a higher or a lower dose.

Patients treated with a low-potency antipsychotic drug such as chlorpromazine or thioridazine should be prescribed lower doses (e.g., 25 to 50 mg three times a day) because several days of upward titration will be required before the patient can acquire tolerance to side effects such as postural hypotension and sedation. Patients can usually reach the target of a high-potency drug within a day or two. An exception is risperidone, which usually requires 3 days or more because it can cause postural hypotension.

If the patient is able to tolerate a dose in the clinical range, that dose should be continued for at least 3 weeks. It may be important for physicians to exert patience and to avoid the temptation to escalate the dose prematurely for patients who are responding slowly.

TREATMENT RESISTANCE

A substantial proportion of patients with schizophrenia have illnesses that are to some degree resistant to antipsychotic medications. Patients with partially responsive illnesses may have stable remissions from severe episodes of schizophrenic psychosis but be left with persistent hallucinations, delusional ideas, or thought disorder. Others appear to have illnesses that are unrelieved by medications. Before a patient is considered resistant to treatment, he or she should receive an adequate dose of an antipsychotic agent—500 to 1000 mg of chlorpromazine or its equivalent—for at least 6 weeks and perhaps longer (Table 53–2). Measuring the

TABLE 53–2	**Approaches to Refractory Schizophrenia**

Acute trial

Ensure that trial is adequate.
  At least 6 wk
  Sufficient dose (500–1000 mg of chlorpromazine or its equivalent)
Ensure that compliance is adequate.

Monitor plasma concentration if feasible and adjust dose.

Consider a 2- or 3-mo trial if patient demonstrates some improvement.

If patient fails to respond

Second antipsychotic agent trial

Prescribe a conventional drug from another class or risperidone if not previously used. Perform gradual cross-tapering from first drug to second over several days—longer if first drug has low potency.

Duration and dosage should resemble those of the first trial.

Consider a trial with a depot drug if poor compliance explains poor response.

If patient fails to respond

Clozapine trial

Begin titration at 12.5 mg and raise dosage gradually until patient is receiving 300–500 mg daily in divided doses. Reduce and gradually discontinue prior antipsychotic drug as clozapine dose reaches 300 mg.

If patient fails to improve after 2 mo, consider dosage increase to 600–900 mg daily. If patient is slowly improving, maintain dose until patient is no longer improving and then consider dosage increase.

patient's plasma level of antipsychotic medication can often be useful for confirming that nonresponsiveness is not related to a lack of bioavailability.

If a patient has responded poorly to a conventional dose and if side effects are not a serious problem, raising the dose should be considered. If a high-dose trial is considered, the physician should reevaluate the clinical response after 2 to 4 weeks. If the patient has not improved, the dose should be reduced, and substitution of another drug should be considered.

In clinical practice, patients who fail to respond to an antipsychotic medication usually receive a trial of an antipsychotic agent from a different class or with a different side effect profile. In most cases, a poor response to one conventional antipsychotic drug is likely to be followed by a poor response to another antipsychotic drug. When patients respond poorly to an antipsychotic drug, physicians often choose to supplement an antipsychotic agent with a second agent. Lithium carbonate, a drug usually used for bipolar disorders, can be helpful for patients with schizoaffective disorders who continue to exhibit an excited or depressed mood despite treatment with a neuroleptic agent. Other studies indicate that adding lithium to a neuroleptic regimen is frequently helpful in patients who have no evidence of impaired affect. Other drugs that are sometimes added to a neuroleptic regimen in poorly responsive patients include carbamazepine, an anticonvulsant, and propranolol or other β-adrenergic blocker.

CLOZAPINE IN REFRACTORY SCHIZOPHRENIA

There is clear evidence that clozapine is effective for patients who have failed to respond to another antipsychotic drug. Studies carried out in both Europe and the United States indicate that clozapine is substantially more effective than conventional antipsychotic drugs for treating refractory patients.

There are three populations of patients with schizophrenia who should be considered candidates for treatment with clozapine. Patients with illnesses that are refractory to conventional drugs and risperidone should probably receive a trial with clozapine. Those who are unable to be treated with adequate antipsychotic doses as a result of a high sensitivity to EPS are also likely to benefit from clozapine. Clozapine may also be a more effective treatment for negative or deficit symptoms.

TREATMENT OF NEGATIVE SYMPTOMS

Antipsychotic drugs are only partially effective for managing negative symptoms of schizophrenia, such as affective blunting, impoverished speech, anhedonia, and apathy. The physician evaluating a patient with prominent negative symptoms is often faced with three possibilities that are difficult to distinguish: the negative symptoms may be secondary to untreated positive symptoms; they may be secondary to side effects of the patient's antipsychotic medications; or they may be enduring negative symptoms that respond poorly to antipsychotic agents. Since negative symptoms such as emotional withdrawal or impoverished speech may be secondary to positive symptoms, the physician should consider whether the psychotic illness has been adequately treated.

The physician should also consider whether negative symptoms, particularly akinesia, are related to EPS. Improving the management of EPS by reducing the drug dose, adding an antiparkinsonian drug, or changing to a drug with less EPS liability, such as clozapine or risperidone, may be helpful.

If the previously mentioned causes of secondary negative symptoms have been ruled out, the patient is likely to be demonstrating a type of enduring negative symptoms that are difficult to manage. Although both clozapine and risperidone have been shown to be more effective than conventional agents in treating negative symptoms, it is unclear if these effects are related to a reduction in EPS or to an effect on primary negative symptoms.

ANTIPSYCHOTIC MEDICATIONS FOR GERIATRIC PATIENTS

Antipsychotic drugs are frequently prescribed for geriatric patients with a number of conditions. Patients with schizophrenia almost always require treatment with antipsychotic drugs for both acute symptoms and long-term maintenance. Others with bipolar disorder and major depressions with psychotic symptoms may benefit from these drugs if the psychotic symptoms are disabling. In addition, patients with psychotic symptoms that are secondary to organic mental illness usually benefit from antipsychotic medications.

Geriatric patients should be treated with substantially lower doses than are used in nongeriatric patients. A useful guideline is to prescribe about half the usual dose administered to nonelderly adults. The need for lower doses is explained by the slowed metabolism and increased volume of distribution in the elderly.

Elderly patients are also more likely to experience EPS, particularly parkinsonism. These patients are particularly sensitive to the side effects of anticholinergic antiparkinsonian medications, including impaired memory, constipation, difficulty urinating, and blurred vision. As a result, side effects are usually best managed by lowering the dose of antipsychotic medication. The elderly are also more likely to experience TD and less likely to demonstrate a remission of TD if their antipsychotic medication is discontinued.

MONITORING PLASMA LEVELS OF ANTIPSYCHOTIC DRUGS

Monitoring the plasma level of a drug may be useful when a patient has received an antipsychotic drug for an adequate time—perhaps 4 to 6 weeks—and has not demonstrated an adequate response. A low level (e.g., less than 5 ng/mL of haloperidol, 1 ng/mL of trifluoperazine, or 1 ng/mL of fluphenazine) suggests that raising the dose may be helpful. A higher level (e.g., greater than 15 ng/mL of haloperidol) may indicate that side effects are interfering with therapeutic response and that lowering the dose may be helpful. Monitoring plasma levels may also be helpful when physicians are reducing the dose of a drug during maintenance therapy. A blood level that is too low under these conditions may indicate that a patient is being placed at too great a risk for psychotic relapse.

A plasma level may also be useful when patients are receiving certain drugs such as heterocyclic antidepressants, fluoxetine, β-blockers, and cimetidine, which may increase plasma levels by competing for enzyme binding sites, or barbiturates and carbamazepine, which may decrease plasma levels by enhancing metabolism of the antipsychotic agent.

ADVERSE EFFECTS

Acute Extrapyramidal Side Effects (Dystonia, Parkinsonism, Akathisia)

All antipsychotic medications, with the exception of clozapine, are associated with serious and often disabling neurological side effects. The most common is a group of EPS that include dystonia, parkinsonism, and akathisia. This group of acute EPS appears relatively soon after the initiation of antipsychotic drug treatment and remits soon after the drugs are discontinued. In contrast, tardive syndromes occur after months of treatment and often persist after medications are discontinued.

Dystonias are the most dramatic form of acute EPS. They are intermittent or sustained muscular spasms and abnormal postures affecting mainly the musculature of the head and neck but sometimes the trunk and lower extremities. Dystonias can lead to gait disturbances that may be confused with hysteria. These reactions usually appear within the first few days of therapy. The most common dystonias are torticollis, contractures of the tongue, trismus, and oculogyric crisis. Laryngeal dystonias are the most dangerous.

Dystonias almost always respond rapidly to antiparkinsonian medications and can usually be prevented either by pretreatment with antiparkinsonian medications or by limiting the neuroleptic dosage prescribed. Dystonic reactions occur in about 40% of patients treated with high-potency drugs without prophylactic antiparkinsonian medications.

Patients with drug-induced parkinsonism may demonstrate stiffness, tremor, and shuffling gait that is indistinguishable from idiopathic parkinsonism. Examination will usually reveal a positive glabella tap. This motor disturbance affects about 30% of patients who receive chronic treatment with traditional antipsychotic medications.

In its mildest form, drug-induced parkinsonism is manifested as apathy, unspontaneous speech, difficulty in initiating usual activities—so-called akinesia, and a decrease in spontaneous gestures. These symptoms may be difficult to distinguish from the negative or deficit symptoms of schizophrenia.

The most common side effect of conventional antipsychotic agents is akathisia, a form of EPS consisting of a subjective feeling of restlessness. Patients who experience severe akathisia often pace continuously or move their feet restlessly while they are sitting. Some complain that they are unable to feel comfortable regardless of what they do. One study found that as many as 75% of patients treated with a conventional dose of haloperidol experience some degree of akathisia. Others found that 25% of patients experience akathisia. This condition can be difficult to assess and is frequently misdiagnosed as anxiety or agitation.

EPS is treatable in most patients. The anticholinergic antiparkinsonian drugs such as benztropine or trihexyphenidyl are by far the most commonly used drugs for EPS. Many physicians prescribe these drugs routinely for patients receiving neuroleptic agents—particularly potent neuroleptics. Unfortunately, these drugs also have side effects, including dry mouth, constipation, urinary retention, and blurry vision. More recent studies indicate that anticholinergic antiparkinsonian drugs can also result in some loss of memory. This side effect is dose dependent and remits when the drug is stopped.

Other drugs for treating EPS include amantadine, a drug that is effective against parkinsonism, and propranolol, which is effective in managing akathisia. Both of these drugs can be administered with anticholinergic antiparkinsonian drugs.

Tardive Dyskinesia and Other Tardive Syndromes

Patients who are chronically exposed to an antipsychotic medication—usually for months or years—may experience a form of TD, which frequently consists of mouth and tongue movements, such as lip smacking, sucking, and puckering as well as facial grimacing. Other motions may include irregular movements of the limbs, particularly choreoathetoid-like movements of the fingers and toes and slow writhing movements of the trunk. Younger patients with TD tend to exhibit slower athetoid movements of the trunk, extremities, and neck. Prevalence surveys indicate that approximately 20% of patients who receive chronic treatment with conventional antipsychotic medications exhibit symptoms of TD.

Elderly patients, particularly elderly women, are more vulnerable to TD. Individuals who are more sensitive to acute EPS appear to be more vulnerable to the development of TD. Patients with organic mental illness and affective disorders may be more vulnerable to TD than are those with schizophrenia.

All conventional antipsychotic drugs are associated with a risk of TD. Clozapine, however, is associated with a substantially lower risk than are other antipsychotic medications. The risk of TD with risperidone administration is unknown.

Early observations of the course of TD suggested that the disorder was inevitably progressive and irreversible. However, when antipsychotic drugs are discontinued, a substantial proportion of patients with TD have a remission. This is more likely for those with a recent onset. Unfortunately, withdrawal of antipsychotic agents is seldom an option for patients with serious psychotic illness.

The American Psychiatric Association task force on TD issued a report in which a number of recommendations were made for preventing and managing TD. These include 1) establishing objective evidence that antipsychotic medications are effective for an individual; 2) using the lowest effective dose of antipsychotic drug; 3) prescribing cautiously for children, elderly patients, and patients with mood disorders; 4) examining patients on a regular basis for evidence of TD; 5) considering alternatives to antipsychotic drugs, obtaining informed consent, and also considering a reduction in dosage when TD is diagnosed; and 6) considering a number of options if the TD worsens, such as discontinuing the antipsychotic medication, switching to a different drug, or considering a trial of clozapine.

Perhaps the most important part of the strategy is regular monitoring. Patients who have an increased risk for TD, including elderly patients, patients who are sensitive to EPS, and individuals with affective illness, should be examined for evidence of abnormal movements as often as every 2 or 3 months. Individuals at a lower risk should be examined every 3 to 6 months. The Abnormal Involuntary Movement Scale includes both an examination procedure for TD and a method for documenting abnormal movements.

Neuroleptic Malignant Syndrome

The neuroleptic malignant syndrome (NMS) is an uncommon side effect of antipsychotic drugs that includes 1) severe muscle rigidity; 2) autonomic instability including hyperthermia, tachycardia, increased blood pressure, tachypnea, and diaphoresis; and 3) changing levels of consciousness. The syndrome most often presents as muscle rigidity and progresses to elevated temperature, fluctuating consciousness, and unstable vital signs. Plasma levels of creatine kinase are usually elevated in patients with NMS. Elevations in liver transaminase levels, leukocytosis, myoglobinemia, and myoglobinuria are less frequent. Mortality in well-developed cases has been reported as ranging from 20% to 30% and may be higher when depot forms are used.

NMS is usually associated with use of high-potency antipsychotic agents and often occurs when the dose is being increased. Physicians should be concerned about patients who demonstrate severe muscle rigidity and a rising body temperature because early diagnosis and treatment can be lifesaving.

If NMS is suspected, antipsychotic agents should be discontinued and supportive and symptomatic treatment started. Treatment may include using antiparkinsonian medications for EPS, correcting fluid and electrolyte imbalances, treating fevers, and managing cardiovascular symptoms such as hyper- or hypotension. If the patient's temperature is elevated to higher than 101°F, treatment with dopamine agonists such as bromocriptine should be considered, along with intensive medical monitoring if the temperature exceeds 103°F. If these treatments are inadequate, administration of dantrolene or benzodiazepines should be considered.

Patients who have recovered from NMS can usually be treated with a different antipsychotic drug or even the same drug that caused the disorder. Patients who experience NMS recurrently with both high-potency and low-potency antipsychotic agents may be candidates for a trial with clozapine. However, there are case reports of patients experiencing NMS while receiving clozapine.

Neuroendocrine Effects

All antipsychotic drugs, with the exception of clozapine, elevate serum prolactin levels. Although some patients acquire tolerance to this elevation after several weeks, most have chronic elevations. Elevated prolactin levels in women can lead to menstrual abnormalities, including anovulatory cycles and infertility, menses with abnormal luteal phases, or frank amenorrhea and hypoestrogenemia. Women have also reported decreased libido and anorgasmia. Galactorrhea is due to the direct effect of prolactin on the breast tissue; it may be uncomfortable but is seldom of any medical significance.

In men, elevated prolactin levels can lower testosterone levels and result in impotence. Men frequently report ejaculatory and erectile disturbances, which are probably related to the autonomic effects of the antipsychotic medication. These problems tend to be most prominent with low-potency drugs and are usually dose related.

Cardiovascular Effects

Low-potency antipsychotic medications such as chlorpromazine or thioridazine can cause orthostatic hypotension through α_1-adrenergic blockade. As a result, patients who are prescribed these drugs should have the dose gradually increased over several days because most patients develop a tolerance to this side effect. Elderly patients are particularly vulnerable to this side effect and, as a result, many clinicians prefer to treat elderly patients with high-potency compounds.

Chlorpromazine may cause prolongation of the QT and PR intervals, ST depression, and T-wave blunting, and thioridazine may cause QT and T-wave changes. Both should be used cautiously in patients who exhibit increased QT intervals.

It is unclear if antipsychotic drugs are associated with an increased prevalence of sudden deaths due to cardiac events. At this stage, it is probably safe to conclude that whatever role antipsychotic medications play in increasing the risk, it is probably small.

Gastrointestinal Effects

The anticholinergic effects of antipsychotic drugs can result in dry mouth and constipation (as well as urinary retention and blurry vision). These effects are relatively common with low-potency drugs and are dose related. Patients with severe dry mouth may be helped by frequent rinsing of the mouth or by use of sugarless gum or drops. Constipation can usually be managed with stool softeners or laxatives. Constipation from clozapine can be a serious problem if it progresses to paralytic ileus. For this reason, physicians should monitor the bowel status of clozapine patients as the dose is being titrated upward.

Hepatic Effects

Antipsychotic medications may cause transient elevations in liver function tests. These are seldom a serious concern. Cases of jaundice have been reported with phenothiazines but are uncommon. Nevertheless, patients receiving antipsychotic drugs who have nausea, rash, fever, and abdominal pain should have their liver function evaluated.

Hematological Effects

Treatment with traditional antipsychotic drugs may result in transitory leukopenia. This commonly occurs early in treatment and resolves spontaneously. Agranulocytosis resulting from antipsychotic drugs other than clozapine is rare.

Agranulocytosis is a serious risk for patients treated with clozapine. Approximately 1% of patients treated with clozapine for a year experience agranulocytosis. Agranulocytosis from clozapine is reversible if the drug is withdrawn. As a result, patients given clozapine in the United States must be registered in a program that ensures that they receive weekly monitoring of their white blood cell count. The drug is prescribed on a weekly basis unless the white blood cell count is less than 3500/mm^3 or if there is a substantial drop in the white cell count. If the white blood cell count is between 3000 and 3500/mm^3 and the granulocyte count is greater than 1500/mm^3, patients should be monitored twice weekly. If the white blood cell count falls to less than 3000/mm^3 or the granulocyte count falls to less than 1500/mm^3, clozapine treatment should be disrupted and patients should be monitored daily. If the white blood cell count drops to less than 2000/mm^3 or the granulocyte count drops to less than 1000/mm^3, clozapine should be discontinued and bone marrow aspiration should be considered. When this occurs, the patient requires immediate medical attention because agranulocytosis can be fatal.

The risk of agranulocytosis is greatest early in treatment, usually 6 weeks to 6 months after treatment is initiated. Nevertheless, new cases have appeared after 1 or 2 years of treatment. As a result, current guidelines require weekly monitoring for as long as clozapine is prescribed and for 1 month after it is discontinued.

Other Side Effects

Antipsychotic drugs, particularly low-potency ones such as chlorpromazine, may cause photosensitivity reactions consisting of severe sunburn or rash. As a result, patients should be instructed to use sunscreen.

Patients receiving long-term treatment with chlorpromazine may develop granular deposits in the anterior lens and posterior cornea. These deposits, visualized on slit-lamp examination, seldom affect the patient's vision. Thioridazine can result in retinal pigmentation when it is prescribed in doses greater than 1000 mg daily. Affected patients can have serious visual impairment or blindness. As a result, thioridazine should not be prescribed at doses greater than 800 mg daily.

Antipsychotic drugs can also lower the seizure threshold. This is more common with low-potency agents. Clozapine has the greatest liability for causing seizures, particularly at higher doses. It is estimated that 5% of patients treated with clozapine for a year will experience a seizure.

ANTIPSYCHOTIC MEDICATIONS AND PREGNANCY

All antipsychotic drugs can cross the placenta. When feasible, physicians should attempt to discontinue antipsychotic drugs during the first trimester of pregnancy, and during the entire pregnancy if possible. For some patients, the risk of severe psychosis will not permit discontinuing medications. Whenever possible, physicians should discontinue antipsychotic agents during the weeks that immediately precede delivery because of impaired drug clearance in newborns.

These drugs are secreted in breast milk; therefore, mothers who are receiving antipsychotic medications should be instructed not to breast-feed.

DRUG INTERACTIONS AND ANTIPSYCHOTIC AGENTS

Clinically important pharmacokinetic interactions can occur when other drugs affect hepatic enzymes that are necessary for the biotransformation and eventual elimination of an antipsychotic medication. For most antipsychotic drugs, this will involve the cytochrome P-450 enzymes. One of the more common interactions occurs when antipsychotic agents are combined with selective serotonin reuptake inhibitors. Most of these inhibitors—particularly fluoxetine and paroxetine—are potent inhibitors of hepatic enzymes. As a result, plasma levels of the antipsychotic drug are likely to be increased. The result may be an increase in EPS for conventional antipsychotic drugs or a greater risk of sedation or seizures with clozapine. Other drugs that may similarly increase plasma concentrations of antipsychotic medications include heterocyclic antidepressants, β-blockers, and cimetidine.

Other drugs—particularly phenytoin, carbamazepine, and barbiturates—can reduce plasma concentrations of antipsychotic drugs by increasing the metabolism of the antipsychotic agent. This is particularly important for carbamazepine, which is commonly combined with antipsychotic medications and can reduce the plasma concentration of haloperidol by 50%. Cigarette smoking can also reduce the plasma levels of antipsychotic drugs.

There are other common interactions that will concern physicians. Antacids can decrease the absorption of the antipsychotic agent from the gut. Antipsychotic drugs antagonize the effects of dopamine agonists or levodopa when these drugs are used to treat parkinsonism. Chlorpromazine, haloperidol, and thiothixene can block the antihypertensive effects of guanethidine. Antipsychotic medications may also enhance the effects of central nervous system depressants such as analgesics, anxiolytics, and hypnotics. If patients require preanesthetic medication or general anesthetics, the doses of these drugs may need to be reduced.

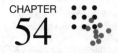
Mood Stabilizers

ACUTE MANIA

General Management Considerations

Before treatment is initiated (Table 54–1), it is important to determine whether a patient is suffering from primary mania, indicative of bipolar disorder, or secondary mania, resulting from an organic dysfunction. Primary mania seldom occurs for the first time after age 40 years, but many organic factors—stroke, neoplasms, epilepsy, infections (e.g., acquired immunodeficiency syndrome), metabolic and endocrine disturbances, substance abuse—can precipitate secondary mania.

Pharmacotherapy

LITHIUM

For many patients with hypomania, lithium by itself can induce a total remission. For patients with full-blown mania, however, an adjunctive antipsychotic or antianxiety agent may be required to treat intolerable psychosis or excitement.

Lithium is rapidly and completely absorbed after oral administration. It is not protein bound and does not undergo metabolism. Peak plasma levels are achieved within 1.5 to 2 hours for standard preparations or 4 to 4.5 hours for slow-release forms. Lithium's plasma half-life is 17 to 36 hours. Ninety-five percent of the drug is excreted by the kidneys, with excretion proportionate to plasma concentrations. Because lithium is filtered through the proximal tubules, factors that decrease glomerular filtration rates will decrease lithium clearance. Because sodium is also filtered through the proximal tubules, a decrease in plasma sodium can increase lithium reabsorption and lead to an increase in plasma lithium levels. Conversely, an increase in plasma lithium levels can cause an increase in sodium excretion, depleting plasma sodium.

Tests that should be done before lithium is started include a complete blood count, electrocardiography, electrolyte determinations, and renal and thyroid panels. Lithium dosage is usually based on a plasma concentration sampled 12 hours after the last dose. As with any drug, approximately five half-lives must elapse for steady state to be achieved. For an average adult, this takes about 5 days (longer in the elderly or in patients with impaired renal function). To treat acute mania, plasma concentrations should typically be greater than 0.8 mEq/L. To avoid toxic effects, the level should not usually exceed 1.5 mEq/L. It is important to know what other medications a patient may be taking, because many drugs can interact with

TABLE 54–1	Treatments for Acute Mania	
Treatment	**Advantages**	**Disadvantages**
Lithium	Efficacy: 70%–80%	Side effects, low therapeutic index
Antipsychotics	Rapid onset of action	Not as effective as lithium in stabilizing mood
Anxiolytics	Good as adjunctive sedatives, wide margin of safety	Probably not specifically antimanic
Valproate	Comparable to lithium	Side effects
Carbamazepine	Possibly comparable to lithium	Side effects
Other drugs (e.g., verapamil)	Not adequately studied	
Electroconvulsive therapy	Efficacy: ~80%, safe for patients unable to take medication	More difficult to administer

lithium and lead to increased or decreased lithium levels or an increase in adverse effects (Table 54–2).

To reach therapeutic levels rapidly in healthy younger patients with normal renal and cardiac function, the psychiatrist may prescribe 300 mg of lithium carbonate four times daily from the outset, sampling the first plasma level after 5 days (or sooner should toxic signs become apparent). Thereafter, the dose should be adjusted to achieve a 12-hour plasma concentration between 0.8 and 1.3 mEq/L at steady state.

In a patient with mild hypomanic symptoms, by contrast, it may be wiser to begin with a lower lithium dose, such as 300 mg twice a day, taking longer to achieve therapeutic levels but, at the same time, minimizing side effects that could trouble the patient and hamper cooperation.

The most common acute adverse effects from lithium are nausea, vomiting, diarrhea, postural tremor, polydipsia, and polyuria. If troublesome, these can usually be mitigated by a slower dosage increase. Other medications may be helpful for side effects that persist despite dosage adjustment (e.g., propranolol, 20 to 160 mg/d, for tremor; diuretics, such as thiazide or loop, for polydipsia or polyuria). Gastrointestinal problems may be alleviated by taking lithium with food or switching to a different preparation. More severe symptoms and signs, including confusion and ataxia, may herald toxic plasma levels and should prompt an immediate blood assay and, if necessary, temporary discontinuation or dosage reduction.

Many skin reactions have been described in association with

TABLE 54–2	Drug Interactions with Lithium

Increase Levels of Lithium

Angiotensin-converting enzyme
Alprazolam (Xanax)
Amiloride (Midamor)
Antipsychotic agents?
Ethacrynic acid (Edecrin)
Fluoxetine (Prozac)
Ibuprofen (Motrin)
Indapamide (Lozol)
Indomethacin (Indocin)
Mefenamic acid (Ponstel)
Naproxen (Naprosyn)
Phenylbutazone (Butazolidin and others)
Some antibiotics
Spironolactone (Aldactazide, Aldactone, and others)
Sulindac (Clinoril)
Thiazide diuretics
Triamterene (Dyazide, Dyrenium)
Zomepirac (Zomax)

Decrease Levels of Lithium

Caffeine
Carbonic anhydrase inhibitors
Laxatives
Osmotic diuretics
Theobromine diuretic (Athemol)
Theophylline (Tedral and others)

Increase Adverse Reactions

Antithyroid effects: carbamazepine (Tegretol), iodine
Cardiovascular toxicity: hydroxyzine (Atarax, Vistaril, and others)
Confusion: electroconvulsive therapy
Extrapyramidal symptoms: neuroleptics
Hypertension: methyldopa (Aldomet and others)
Neurotoxicity: diltiazem (Cardizem), verapamil (Calan and others), clozapine (Clozaril)
Seizures: fluvoxamine (Luvox)
Somnambulism: antipsychotic agents
Toxic symptoms with normal blood levels: methyldopa (Aldomet and others)

lithium therapy, including atopic dermatitis, acne, psoriasis, and hair loss. These can usually be treated by standard dermatological means but occasionally are severe enough to force the discontinuation of therapy. Electrocardiographic effects of lithium are also usually benign and tolerable. Rarely, however, an effect such as slowing of the sinus node can lead to severe bradycardia and syncope.

ANTIPSYCHOTIC AGENTS

The chemistry and pharmacology of antipsychotic drugs are presented in detail in Chapter 53, and the adverse effects and precautions for these agents are the same in the treatment of acute mania as they are for acute schizophrenia (see Chapter 25). In double-blind controlled trials, investigators have found chlorpromazine, haloperidol, pimozide, thioridazine, and thiothixene to be effective in the treatment of acute mania but, in general, not as effective as lithium. However, although lithium has been found better in stabilizing mood and ideation, antipsychotics have been found to be superior in controlling hyperactivity and to have a more rapid onset of action.

ANXIOLYTIC AGENTS

The pharmacology, adverse effects, and precautions associated with anxiolytic drugs are covered in Chapter 56. Among anxiolytic agents currently available, the benzodiazepines are selected unquestionably as adjuncts in the treatment of acute mania because of their safety and efficacy. Although some have claimed specific antimanic efficacy for clonazepam or other benzodiazepines, most psychiatrists are more impressed with their benefits as adjunctive sedatives than with more specific antimanic activity.

VALPROATE

After rigorous clinical investigation, the anticonvulsant valproate (in the form of divalproex sodium) has been approved in the United States for treatment of the acute mania of bipolar disorder. At least 16 uncontrolled and 6 controlled studies have shown valproate to be effective in treating acute mania.

Valproate is available in the United States as valproic acid (Depakene) or divalproex sodium (Depakote), a compound containing equal parts valproic acid and sodium valproate. Divalproex is better tolerated than valproic acid, has been studied more extensively, and is more commonly used. All valproate preparations are rapidly absorbed after oral administration, reaching peak plasma levels within 2 to 4 hours after ingestion. Food may delay absorption but does not affect bioavailability. Valproate is rapidly distributed and highly bound (90%) to plasma proteins. Its half-life ranges from 9 to 16 hours, depending on whether it is taken alone or with other medications, and it takes 1 to 4 days to attain steady state.

Valproate is metabolized by the hepatic cytochrome P-450IID6 system. Unlike carbamazepine, it does not induce its own metabolism or hepatic metabolism in general, but it does appear to inhibit the degradation of other drugs metabolized in the liver. Valproate inhibits drug oxidation and may increase serum levels of concomitantly administered drugs that are oxidatively metabolized, such as phenobarbital, phenytoin, and tricyclic antidepressants. Coadministration of carbamazepine, or other microsomal enzyme-inducing drugs, will decrease plasma levels of valproate, and drugs that inhibit the P-450 system (such as selective serotonin reuptake inhibitors) can increase them. The coadministration of other highly protein bound drugs, such as aspirin, can increase free valproate blood levels and precipitate toxic effects.

Although experts rank lithium as the treatment of choice for a patient with classic mania—probably owing to more clinical experience, greater supporting literature, and lower cost—divalproex is an acceptable first-line alternative. It may be used singly in patients who cannot tolerate lithium. For patients who do not respond to lithium, there are no secure data on whether divalproex should be added as an adjunct or substituted, but most knowledgeable psychiatrists would choose the former in a patient who appears to respond at least partially to lithium and the latter in patients for whom lithium seems to afford no benefit.

Before initiating divalproex, the psychiatrist should obtain a comprehensive medical history and perform a physical examination, paying particular attention to suggestions of liver disease or bleeding abnormalities. Baseline liver and hematological functions are measured before treatment, every 1 to 4 weeks for the first 6 months, and then every 3 to 6 months. Evidence of hemorrhage, bruising, or a disorder of hemostasis-coagulation would indicate a reduction of dosage or withdrawal of therapy. The drug should be discontinued immediately in the presence of suspected or apparent significant hepatic dysfunction.

The typical starting dose for healthy adults is 750mg/d in divided doses. The dose can then be adjusted to achieve a 12-hour serum valproate concentration between 50 and 125 µg/mL. The time of dosing is determined by possible side effects, and if tolerated, once-a-day dosing can be employed. As with lithium, the antimanic response to valproate typically occurs after 1 to 2 weeks.

Adverse effects tend to appear early in the course of therapy, are usually mild and transient, and tend to resolve in time. Gastrointestinal upset is probably the most common complaint in patients taking valproate and tends to be less of a problem with the enteric-coated divalproex sodium preparation. Other common complaints include tremor, sedation, increased appetite and weight, and alopecia. Less common are ataxia, rashes, and hematological dysfunction, such as thrombocytopenia and platelet dysfunction. Platelet count usually recovers with a dosage decrease, but the occurrence of thrombocytopenia or leukopenia may necessitate the discontinuation of valproate. Serum hepatic transaminase elevations are common, dose related, and usually self-limiting and benign. Fatal hepatotoxicity is extremely rare, usually is restricted to young children, and generally develops within the first 6 months of valproate therapy. Other serious problems include pancreatitis and teratogenesis. If the side effects of valproate become intolerable, the psychiatrist may need to discontinue it and try one of the other treatments described in this section as an alternative. If valproate is tolerated but not totally effective, the psychiatrist might use one of the other treatments as an adjunct.

CARBAMAZEPINE

In light of the less well substantiated evidence for the efficacy of carbamazepine, the authors' preference would be to place this anticonvulsant third as an antimanic choice, behind lithium and valproate. The decision to move on to carbamazepine and whether to use it alone or in addition to lithium or valproate (or even both) will hinge on the same considerations listed for considering valproate instead of or in addition to lithium. If a patient has been treated with one or more of these agents in a previous manic episode, that experience should be used to guide treatment of a current episode.

Concomitant administration of drugs that inhibit the cytochrome P-450 system (see Table 54–3) will increase plasma levels of carbamazepine. Concomitant administration of phenobarbital, phenytoin, or primidone could cause a decrease in carbamazepine levels through induction of the cytochrome P-450 enzymes.

Before carbamazepine is started, baseline blood and platelet counts, urinalysis, and liver and kidney function tests are in order. Although earlier guidelines called for routine monitoring of some or all of these indices, and some psychiatrists still obtain blood counts once or twice during the first few months of treatment and when plasma concentrations are sampled, a more general consensus at present is to instruct patients and family members

TABLE 54–3	Drug Interactions with Carbamazepine

Increase Levels of Carbamazepine

Cimetidine (Tagamet)
Diltiazem
Erythromycin
Fluoxetine (Prozac)
Fluvoxamine (Luvox)
Isoniazid (INH and others)
Propoxyphene (Darvon and others)
Valproate
Verapamil

Decrease Levels of Carbamazepine

Phenobarbital
Primidone
Phenytoin (Dilantin and others)

Carbamazepine Decreases Levels of

Antipsychotics
Benzodiazepines (except clonazepam)
Corticosteroids
Hormonal contraceptives
Thyroid hormone
Tricyclic antidepressants

Others

Lithium + carbamazepine may increase neurotoxic effects

to contact the psychiatrist immediately if petechiae, pallor, weakness, fever, or infection occurs. At that time, the psychiatrist should order relevant tests.

Used as a monotherapy, the typical starting dose for carbamazepine is 200 to 400 mg/d in three or four divided doses, increased to 800 to 1000 mg/d by the end of the first week. If clinical improvement is insufficient by the end of the second week, and if the patient has not had intolerable side effects to the drug, increases to as high as 1600 mg daily may be considered. Although there are no good studies of the correlation between blood level and clinical response, knowledgeable psychiatrists often target a range of 4 to 15 ng/mL. If carbamazepine is combined with lithium or neuroleptics, psychiatrists often prefer to use lower doses and blood levels. If valproate and carbamazepine are administered simultaneously, blood levels of each should be monitored carefully because of complex interactions between the two agents.

When the dose of carbamazepine is built up rapidly, side effects are more likely. The most common effects in the first couple of weeks are drowsiness, dizziness, ataxia, diplopia, nausea, blurred vision, and fatigue. These tend to diminish in time or to respond to a temporary reduction in dose. Less common reactions include gastrointestinal upset, hyponatremia, and a variety of skin reactions, some of which are severe enough to require discontinuation of carbamazepine. About 10% of patients experience transient leukopenia, but unless infection develops, carbamazepine may be continued. More serious hematopoietic reactions, including aplastic anemia and agranulocytosis, are rare.

PHARMACOTHERAPY IN ACUTE DEPRESSION

There is a widespread clinical impression that administering an antidepressant to a bipolar patient can trigger a switch into mania. Some experts also believe that antidepressants speed up mood cycles, although this point is more controversial. Because of both concerns, some psychiatrists prefer to be cautious about prescribing an antidepressant at the first sign of depression in a bipolar patient

TABLE 54–4	Predictors of Poor Response to Lithium Prophylaxis
Rapid or continuous cycling	
Mixed states or dysphoric mania	
Alcohol or drug abuse	
Noncompliance with treatment	
Cycle pattern of depression-mania-euthymia	
Personality disturbance	
History of poor interepisode functioning	
Poor social support system	
Three or more prior episodes	

who is being maintained with lithium, an anticonvulsant, or a combination. If symptoms are mild and short-lived, therefore, the psychiatrist might consider watchful waiting while maintaining close contact to detect any more severe deterioration.

When a patient is known to have bipolar disorder, administration of an antidepressant to reverse an acute depression is almost always used together with one of the mood-stabilizing agents, usually lithium, valproate, or carbamazepine (or a combination). Most bipolar patients will be taking these drugs in maintenance therapy. Moreover, mood stabilizers may enhance the effectiveness of the antidepressant and might protect against the possibility of a switch into mania.

The predictors of poor response to lithium treatment are presented in Table 54–4. The adverse effects, pharmacology, and interactions of antidepressants are covered in Chapter 55.

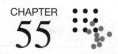
Antidepressants

Although the bulk of this chapter describes the use of antidepressants in the treatment of major depression, they are also used to treat a number of other conditions. Some uses have gained general acceptance, whereas others rely on moderate or preliminary evidence. A summary of various indications is presented in Table 55–1.

SELECTION OF AN ANTIDEPRESSANT

The decision whether to treat depressive symptoms with pharmacotherapy requires an assessment of both the need for intervention and the likelihood that treatment will be successful. Assessing the need for intervention involves longitudinal and cross-sectional factors. Assessing the likelihood that treatment will be successful is somewhat more difficult but may rely on clinical, demographical, and biological factors.

The physician should consider the course and duration of previous episodes of depression, as well as the severity of symptoms and the degree of functional impairment. Suicidal ideation is of particular concern and needs rapid and intensive treatment.

Selection of a Particular Agent

Although, as noted earlier, the various antidepressants seem to have equal efficacy in the treatment of depression, a given patient may respond preferentially to one or to a class of agents. Again, cross-sectional and longitudinal factors should be taken into account.

Longitudinal factors include a history of response to a particular agent, a family history of good response, a history of prior side effects (particularly if they resulted in drug discontinuation), and a history of symptoms that could suggest mania (or more minor variants of manic episodes).

Cross-sectional factors include data from the physical examination and laboratory work-up that might suggest susceptibilities to certain antidepressant agents or contraindications based on physical illness.

PREPARATION OF THE PATIENT

Side Effects of Antidepressants

Comprehensive lists of side effects in the *Physicians' Desk Reference* and in textbooks can be overwhelming. If such lists are unaccompanied by a discussion of the rarity of most adverse

TABLE 55–1	Indications for Antidepressant Use

Major Depression

Acute depression
Prevention of relapse
Other depressive syndromes
  Bipolar depression
  Atypical depression
  Dysthymic disorder

Other Uses

Tricyclic Antidepressants

Strong evidence
  Panic disorder (most)
  Obsessive-compulsive disorder (clomipramine)
  Bulimia nervosa (imipramine, desipramine)
  Enuresis (imipramine)
Moderate evidence
  Separation anxiety
  Attention-deficit/hyperactivity disorder
  Phobias
  Generalized anxiety disorder
  Anorexia nervosa
  Body dysmorphic disorder
  Migraine (amitriptyline)
  Other headaches
  Diabetic neuropathy, other pain syndromes (anitriptyline,
    doxepin)
  Sleep apnea (protriptyline)
  Cocaine abuse (desipramine)
  Tinnitus
Evidence for but rarely used for these disorders
  Peptic ulcer disease
  Arrhythmias

Monoamine Oxidase Inhibitors

Strong evidence
  Panic disorder
  Bulimia nervosa
Moderate evidence
  Other anxiety disorders
  Anorexia nervosa
  Body dysmorphic disorder

Atypical Agents

Trazodone
  Insomnia
  Dementia with agitation
  Minor sedative-hypnotic withdrawal
Bupropion
  Attention-deficit/hyperactivity disorder

Table continued on following page

TABLE 55–1	Indications for Antidepressant Use *(Continued)*

Serotonin Reuptake Inhibitors
Strong evidence
Obsessive-compulsive disorder (high-dose fluoxetine, sertraline)
Bulimia nervosa (fluoxetine)
Moderate evidence
Panic disorder
Obesity (high-dose fluoxetine)
Substance abuse
Impulsivity, anger associated with personality disorders
Pain syndromes
Preliminary evidence
Obsessive jealousy
Body dysmorphic disorder
Hypochondriasis
Behavioral abnormalities associated with autism and mental retardation
Anger attacks associated with depression
Depersonalization disorder
Social phobia
Attention-deficit/hyperactivity disorder (as an adjunct)
Chronic enuresis
Paraphiliac sexual disorders
Nonparaphiliac sexual disorders

reactions, it is unlikely that any rational person would use antidepressants at all. Thus, it is more important to discuss the likely side effects of a medication rather than all possible side effects.

Conversely, it would be an error to prepare a patient inadequately for the likely side effects of a given antidepressant. Side effects, even relatively benign ones, are a major cause of treatment noncompliance. Proper preparation and reassurance about side effects can help reduce this rate. It should help to reassure the patient that many of the side effects diminish with time or with an adjustment of dose. It may also help to frame side effects in a positive light, as they represent concrete evidence that the medication is exerting its effect on the body. A number of common, uncommon, and hypothetical side effects are given in Table 55–2 and are discussed here.

The dietary restrictions required when using monoamine oxidase inhibitors represent the major limitation to widespread use of these effective antidepressants. Nonselective inhibition of monoamine oxidase prevents the normal hepatic metabolism of tyramine-containing foods or sympathomimetic agents. The increased level of tyramine in the circulation stimulates the release of norepinephrine from sympathetic terminals. This sudden increase in norepinephrine is the basis for the "tyramine-cheese" reaction, so named because cheese is the most common source of the tyramine that causes this reaction. In fact, other pressor amines, such as levodopa, can also cause the reaction, but tyramine, a natural product of food

TABLE 55–2   Side Effects (Common, Uncommon, and Hypothetical) of the Antidepressants

Predictable Side Effects

Muscarinic Effects

Gastrointestinal effects
 Decreased salivation
  Drying of the mucous membranes
  Gum disease, dental caries
 Decreased peristalsis
  Constipation
  Paralytic ileus
Inhibition of bladder contraction
 Urinary hesitancy
 Urinary retention
Visual effects
 Accommodation paresis
  Blurry vision
  Mydriasis
 Pupillary dilatation
  Precipitation of acute narrow-angle glaucoma
Cardiac effects
 Decreased vagal tone
  Tachycardia
Central nervous system effects
 Impaired memory and cognition
 Delirium
 Exacerbation of tardive dyskinesia

Histamine Effects

H_1
 Sedation
 Orthostatic hypotension
 Weight gain
 Impairment of psychomotor coordination, risk of falling
 Cognitive impairment
H_2
 Decreased gastric acid

Norepinephrine Effects

Increased norepinephrine
 Anxiety
 Tremors
 Diaphoresis
 Tachycardia
 Constriction of the bladder neck and urethra
Receptor blockade
 Postural hypotension
 Ejaculatory delay or impotence
 Reflex tachycardia
 Memory dysfunction

Table continued on following page

TABLE 55–2	Side Effects (Common, Uncommon, and Hypothetical) of the Antidepressants *(Continued)*

Serotonin Effects

Reuptake blockade
 Gastrointestinal effects
  Anorexia
  Nausea
  Vomiting
  Diarrhea
 Central nervous system effects
  Anxiety
  Akathisia
  Insomnia (more common) or sedation
 Sexual functioning effects
  Anorgasmia
  Ejaculatory delay
  Spontaneous orgasms

Receptor antagonism

Hypotension

Ejaculatory disturbance

Weight gain or carbohydrate craving

Dopamine Effects

Reuptake blockade
 Antiparkinsonian effects
 Psychomotor agitation
 Psychosis
Receptor antagonism
 Extrapyramidal symptoms
 Tardive dyskinesia
 Endocrine effects
 Sexual dysfunction

Monoamine Oxidase Inhibition Effects

"Tyramine-cheese" reaction
 Hypertensive crisis

Increased standing systolic blood pressure

Hypotension

Sedation

Psychomotor stimulation

Membrane-Stabilizing Effects

Effects on cardiac conduction
 Dysrhythmia
 Asystole

TABLE 55–2	Side Effects (Common, Uncommon, and Hypothetical) of the Antidepressants *(Continued)*

Idiosyncratic Side Effects

Allergic Reactions

Dermatological effects	Hematological effects
Rashes	Agranulocytosis
Urticaria	Bleeding
Photosensitivity	Inflammation
Stevens-Johnson syndrome	Systemic vasculitis
Pigmentation changes	

Hepatic Effects

Abnormal liver enzymes

Seizures

Precipitation of Mania and Rapid Cycling

Sexual Dysfunction

Decreased or increased (less common) libido
Ejaculatory delay or anorgasmia
Impotence
Priapism

Other Effects

Tremors
Diaphoresis
Syndrome of inappropriate antidiuretic hormone secretion
Alopecia
Headaches (including precipitation of migraine)
Stupor

fermentation and bacterial decarboxylation, is the most common in foods. The result of a tyramine-cheese reaction can be a hypertensive crisis. Thus, patients should be well educated as to the foods that must be avoided while using monoamine oxidase inhibitors.

In the past, there has been a tendency toward conservative dietary restrictions, often based on single case reports or indirect analogies. More research and experience have suggested that not all the foods commonly restricted are equally likely to precipitate a reaction. Better compliance is likely if a more reasonable diet is prescribed.

Drug-Drug Interactions (Table 55–3)

As with the diet, any medication that increases tyramine can precipitate a hypertensive crisis when monoamine oxidase inhibitors (MAOIs) are used. Such medications include numerous over-the-counter preparations for coughs, colds, and allergies. The same rule applies to sympathomimetic drugs (such as epinephrine and amphetamines) and dopaminergic drugs (such as antiparkinsonian medications).

TABLE 55–3	Drug-Drug Interactions of Antidepressants

Tricyclic Antidepressants (TCAs)

Additive effects
  Other anticholinergic agents
  Other soporific agents
  Other cardiac-active or vasodilating agents
Pharmacokinetic effects
  Inhibition of TCA absorption
    Cholestyramine
  Inhibition of TCA metabolism
    Fluoxetine
    Antipsychotic agents
    Methylphenidate
    Cimetidine
  Induction of TCA metabolism
    Phenobarbital
    Carbamazepine
    Nicotine
Pharmacodynamic concerns
  Guanethidine (relies on neuron reuptake)
  Clonidine

Monoamine Oxidase Inhibitors

Agents that can increase tyramine (many over-the-counter cough, cold, and allergy preparations)
Sympathomimetic agents
Dopaminergic agents
Serotonin-potentiating agents (serotonin syndrome)
  Serotonin reuptake inhibitors
Central serotoninergic dysregulators
  Meperidine
  Propoxyphene
  Diphenoxylate hydrochloride and atropine sulfate (Lomotil)

TABLE 55–3	Drug-Drug Interactions of Antidepressants *(Continued)*

Atypical Agents

Trazodone
  May increase other drug levels (digoxin, phenytoin, warfarin)

Bupropion
  Dopaminergic agents

Serotonin Reuptake Inhibitors

Pharmaockinetic effects
  Inhibition of cytochrome P-450 enzymes
    May slow the metabolism of other drugs metabolized by that system, including TCAs, carbamazepine, antipsychotics, opiates, certain benzodiazepines, bupropion, verapamil, diltiazem, cimetidine

Serotonin syndrome
  Occurs in combination with other serotonin agonists: monoamine oxidase inhibitors, pentazocine, L-tryptophan, lithium, carbamazepine

The combination of monoamine oxidase inhibitors and narcotics, particularly meperidine, may cause a fatal interaction. The reaction can vary from symptoms of agitation and hyperpyrexia to cardiovascular collapse, coma, and death. A similar reaction has also been reported when propoxyphene and diphenoxylate hydrochloride and atropine (Lomotil) are used with MAOIs.

THE SEROTONIN SYNDROME

This syndrome occurs when a serotonin reuptake inhibitor is combined with another drug that can potentiate serotonin, such as MAOIs, pentazocine, and L-tryptophan. It has also been reported with the adjunctive use of less obvious serotoninergic drugs, such as lithium and carbamazepine. This creates a toxic effect with symptoms of abdominal pain, diarrhea, diaphoresis, hyperpyrexia, tachycardia, hypertension, myoclonus, irritability, agitation, epileptic seizures, and delirium. In its severest form, it can result in coma, cardiovascular shock, and death. For this reason, a clearance period is required before switching between a serotonin reuptake inhibitor and an MAOI. Switching from fluoxetine to an MAOI is particularly difficult, given fluoxetine's long clearance time—about 6 weeks. Clearance is considerably more rapid for sertraline or paroxetine, and a 2-week washout period is advised when changing from one of these agents to an MAOI. Occasionally, case reports have suggested that some patients tolerate a quicker switch; however, a full waiting period remains the most prudent course.

INITIATION OF TREATMENT

Choosing a Drug

On the average, all antidepressants are equally effective. Although an individual patient may preferentially respond to a certain antidepressant, it is difficult to predict this in advance. Without a personal or family history of such a response, side effects are the most influential factor in choosing an agent. Side effects may be particularly relevant in the following groups of patients.

CARDIOVASCULAR PATIENTS

The major cardiovascular side effect of tricyclic antidepressants is orthostatic hypotension. This can be clinically significant in both the hypertensive patient and the elderly patient. Some tricyclic medications may have a lower risk of orthostatic hypotension, notably nortriptyline and doxepin. The evidence for nortriptyline's causing little or no hypotension is convincing; for doxepin it is weaker.

Tricyclic antidepressants do not show a negative inotropic effect and do not seem to worsen congestive heart failure. Patients with congestive heart failure may, however, be at a higher risk for orthostatic hypotension. Again, nortriptyline is the safest tricyclic antidepressant in this case.

Certain findings may further limit the role of tricyclic medications in heart disease. As with all type IA antiarrhythmic agents, tricyclic antidepressants are believed to have a beneficial effect on certain cardiac arrhythmias, particularly ventricular premature depolarization. However, a large multicenter study of ventricular arrhythmias after myocardial infarction found that type IA antiarrhythmics can increase the risk of mortality among patients with ventricular arrhythmias. Data also suggest that antiarrhythmic drugs cause increased mortality in atrial fibrillation as well. Thus, we recommend caution when using tricyclic antidepressants in all patients with ischemic heart disease, particularly patients with ventricular arrhythmias that follow a myocardial infarction.

SEROTONIN REUPTAKE INHIBITORS. The serotonin reuptake inhibitors differ from the tricyclic antidepressants in that they do not prolong the PR or QRS interval. Thus, they probably lack any of the proarrhythmic and antiarrhythmic activities associated with tricyclic antidepressants. They do not cause orthostatic hypotension. Therefore, to date the serotonin reuptake inhibitors have shown no significant cardiac effects, particularly those attributable to tricyclic antidepressants. Further investigation is needed in patients with serious cardiac disease.

ELDERLY PATIENTS

Two pharmacokinetic changes are of greatest importance in aging patients: decreased efficiency of the hepatic microoxidase system and a decreased muscle-fat ratio. Decreased efficiency of hepatic microoxidases results in the slower metabolism of antidepressants. Normal increases in body fat and a loss of muscle mass result in an alteration of the volume of distribution for a substance. Thus, lipophilic drugs, including all antidepressants, are more widely distributed in the elderly body.

Both the resulting slower metabolism and the increased volume of distribution increase the half-lives of the various antidepressants. The elderly, therefore, are likely to have a greater incidence of side effects.

The half-lives and steady-state concentrations of the serotonin reuptake inhibitors are only minimally affected by age. Paroxetine may be an exception to this, and it may have an increased half-life in the elderly.

Starting Doses

TRICYCLIC ANTIDEPRESSANTS

Tricyclic antidepressants are usually begun at a relatively low dose. For the majority of tricyclic antidepressants, including imipramine, amitriptyline, desipramine, maprotiline, and doxepin, the initial starting dose is in the range of 50 to 70 mg/d. Notable exceptions include nortriptyline and protriptyline, which are more potent agents. In the case of nortriptyline, the usual starting dose is 25 to 50 mg/d, and for protriptyline, 10 to 15 mg/d. The lower doses are preferred in patients who are elderly. In the frail elderly, further dose reductions may be needed (about one half or less of the usual starting dose).

Once a medication is initiated, it is gradually increased to a therapeutic level. A number of strategies have been suggested for this increase. Most tricyclic antidepressants can be increased to 150 mg/d by the second week and then to a range of 300 mg/d by the third or fourth week. This can be achieved through small daily increments of 25 mg or by weekly increases of 75 mg. Younger patients tolerate larger and more rapid increases, whereas the elderly benefit from smaller (25 mg/d) and less frequent (every other day) increases with a lower target dose (150 mg/d).

MONOAMINE OXIDASE INHIBITORS

Phenelzine is usually begun at a dose of 30 mg/d. It is increased by 15 mg after 3 days, then weekly to a target range of 45 to 90 mg/d. Tranylcypromine is started at 20 mg/d. It is increased by 10 mg after 3 days, with additional daily increases of 10 mg after 1 week, to a target range of 30 to 60 mg/d.

ATYPICAL ANTIDEPRESSANTS

Trazodone is generally dosed in a manner similar to tricyclic antidepressants, with starting doses of 50 to 75 mg and target ranges of 150 to 300 mg, with doses not exceeding 400 mg in outpatients and 600 mg in inpatients. Unlike many of the tricyclic antidepressants, trazodone's short half-life requires divided doses, usually twice daily.

Bupropion, like trazodone, requires divided doses. It should be started at 100 mg twice a day and increased to 100 mg three times a day after a few days. The recommended dose of the medication is 300 mg/d; however, patients not responding at that dose can be increased to 450 mg/d. Patients should be instructed to avoid taking more than 150 mg in a single dose. In the elderly, a usual starting dose is 75 mg/d. This is then increased to 75 mg twice a day.

SEROTONIN REUPTAKE INHIBITORS

Although dosing strategies are less well understood with these agents, the wisest choice is to start a patient at the lowest effective dose and increase as indicated by clinical response. Reasonable doses are 20 mg for fluoxetine (10 mg for patients who find 20 mg difficult to tolerate), 50 mg for sertraline, and 20 mg for paroxetine. For children, adolescents, and the elderly, 50% reductions in these doses are reasonable starting doses.

THERAPEUTIC DRUG MONITORING

Although blood levels are available for many antidepressants, those for imipramine, desipramine, and nortriptyline have been best established. Imipramine and desipramine appear to have a curvilinear dose-response curve with an optimal range of 150 to 300 ng/mL. Nortriptyline appears to have a therapeutic window in the range of 50 to 150 ng/mL. These blood levels are nominal, as some patients do respond above or below these ranges, and blood level monitoring should not be a substitute for clinical observation.

Drug levels have not been well established for the MAOIs and the serotonin reuptake inhibitors.

RESPONSE PERIOD

The time to response varies with the patient. Few patients show a significant response before 2 weeks. The usual range for response is 3 to 4 weeks; however, it can take 6 weeks or longer. For patients who complete a satisfactory treatment regimen, the response rate for antidepressants is about 60% to 70%, although some of these responses will be partial. Response rates may be as high as 80% with tricyclic antidepressants if blood levels are monitored.

There is little benefit in making treatment changes before 3 weeks (except to mitigate side effects). Changes in treatment strategy should be considered after the physician is satisfied that the patient has been treated with an adequate dosage of the antidepressant for an adequate time. In the case of tricyclic antidepressants, this can be confirmed with blood levels. In the case of serotonin reuptake inhibitors and MAOIs, there are fewer data available to confirm an adequate dose. For the patient showing inadequate response, these medications are increased to the limit of side effect tolerance.

In patients showing an inadequate response after a reasonable time, the physician must decide whether to continue with the same medication and augment with an additional agent or to switch medications altogether. This decision depends on an assessment of whether the patient has shown any response to the current strategy. Partial responders may be more likely to benefit from treatment augmentations, whereas patients who show no response or worsen during treatment warrant a new agent.

Antidepressant Augmentation

Typical augmentation strategies (Table 55–4) include the addition of lithium carbonate, thyroid hormone, or a stimulant.

TABLE 55–4 Antidepressant Augmentation Strategies*

Agent	Dosing Strategy	Length of Trial	Reported Response Rate	Comments
Lithium carbonate	Start at 300 mg b.i.d. increase to therapeutic blood level (0.8–1.2 mEq/L)	3–6 wk	As high as 65%	Best documented strategy; has been combined with most agents
Triiodothyronine	Start at 25 µg/d, may increase to 50 µg/d	At least 3 wk	At 25%	Equal to lithium in one placebo-controlled trial
Stimulants (methylphenidate dextroamphetamine)	†	†	†	Few systematic data
Combined antidepressant therapy	May need lower doses than usual (due to enzyme inhibition)†	†	†	Mainly open trials; controlled studies in progress
Psychotherapy	N/A	Varies by therapy	Varies by therapy	Good data for both cognitive-behavioral therapy and inter-personal therapy

*N/A, not applicable.

†Inadequate data.

549

LITHIUM AUGMENTATION

The blood level of lithium necessary for adjunctive use has not been well established. It is probably best to start at a low dose (300 mg or less twice a day) and to increase to a therapeutic blood level (0.8 to 1.2 mEq/L) if there is no response. The trial may take 3 to 6 weeks for augmenting effect.

THYROID AUGMENTATION

For thyroid hormone supplementation, the starting dose is 25 µg/d of triiodothyronine, which can be increased to 50 µg/d in a week if there is no response. The trial should continue for at least 3 weeks.

STIMULANT AUGMENTATION

Among the stimulants, methylphenidate and dextroamphetamine have been used for antidepressant augmentation, but there are few systematic data regarding the proper dose or length of treatment for this potential use.

COMBINED ANTIDEPRESSANT THERAPY

Open trials have supported the use of combined therapy of a tricyclic antidepressant and a serotonin reuptake inhibitor in patients for whom either class alone has failed. Controlled trials of this strategy are in progress. When antidepressants are combined, it is important to remember that the serotonin reuptake inhibitors can potentiate tricyclic antidepressant levels, and this should be monitored carefully. MAOIs have also been used in combination with tricyclic antidepressants, although this should be monitored closely given the risk of potential toxic interactions. Given the risk of a serotonin syndrome, MAOIs should not be combined with serotonin reuptake inhibitors (see section on serotonin reuptake inhibitors under drug-drug interactions).

Changing to a New Agent

For the patient who shows no response or whose condition deteriorates during therapy, the physician should initiate a new trial of an alternative single agent. It is unlikely that another agent from the same class as the failed agent will be more successful, and therefore it is best to choose from a different class. One should differentiate between nonresponse with an adequate trial and failure to respond owing to intolerance of the drug—the first case probably warrants a change to another class of agent, whereas the second case merely warrants a change to a similar agent with a different side effect profile.

When the switch involves an MAOI, sufficient time must be given for medication clearance. Although seldom used, MAOIs may be strikingly effective in patients not responsive to other classes of antidepressants. Generally, 10 to 14 days for either medication is required for clearance of tricyclic antidepressants and MAOIs. Fluoxetine requires a much longer period—6 weeks—whereas sertraline and paroxetine require about 2 weeks in the switch to an MAOI.

CONTINUATION PERIOD

This period usually lasts 5 to 8 months after the end of the acute treatment period. The goal at this phase is the prevention of relapse. There is a high risk of relapse if treatment is discontinued after the acute treatment phase.

Once a patient has responded to a medication, the medication should be continued for a minimum of 4 to 6 months, beginning from the point of initial response. The World Health Organization recommended 6 months as a minimal period for continuation of treatment after the acute phase, and the American Psychiatric Association recommended a minimum of 16 to 20 weeks of treatment after the full remission of symptoms. This period should be lengthened for the patient with a history of longer depressive episodes.

DISCONTINUANCE OF TREATMENT

After the continuation period, somatic therapy is usually discontinued in the patient with a single episode of major depression. Before discontinuing, however, it is important to remember that depression is a lifelong disease with a chronic course. One should always weigh the benefits of discontinuance against the risks of recurrent depression.

Tapering and Withdrawal

For the tricyclic antidepressants, the usual strategy is to taper the medications at a rate of 25 to 50 mg every 2 to 3 days. Too rapid a discontinuation may produce symptoms of cholinergic "rebound" or supersensitivity. Such a rebound includes severe gastrointestinal symptoms (nausea, vomiting, and cramping), other signs of autonomic hyperactivity (diaphoresis, anxiety, agitation, headaches), and insomnia (often with vivid nightmares).

MAOIs may also have a withdrawal syndrome, including symptoms of psychosis, on abrupt withdrawal; however, this syndrome is much more rare than that seen with tricyclic antidepressants.

Fluoxetine has a long half-life, and abrupt discontinuation should be permissible. Sertraline and paroxetine, with shorter half-lives of about a day, may require a 7- to 10-day taper. A true withdrawal associated with serotonin reuptake inhibitors remains unconfirmed.

On discontinuance, the goal is to enable early intervention should symptoms recur. A first episode of depression has a high risk of recurrence (~50%), and the risk of relapse is even higher in patients who show only partial response to medication. The patient should be educated to recognize symptoms of depression. The patient's own history suggests which symptoms were prodromal to the patient's full depressive episode.

PROPHYLACTIC, OR MAINTENANCE, PERIOD

The goal of the prophylactic period is to prevent the recurrence of depression.

There are a number of reasons to consider long-term prophylactic therapy for depression rather than medication withdrawal. Depression is a lifelong disease, with recurrence being the norm rather than the exception. As the number of acute episodes increases, the risk of future episodes increases as well, and the interval between episodes shortens. Each subsequent episode carries a higher morbidity and disability.

The best predictors of the likelihood of recurrence appear to be older age at onset and number of episodes. It has been proposed that long-term continuation is the treatment of choice for the following groups of patients: 1) those who were 50 years old or more at the time of the first depressive episode, 2) those who were 40 years old or more at first episode and have had at least one subsequent recurrence, and 3) anyone who has had more than three episodes.

Anxiolytic Drugs

GENERAL APPROACH TO USING ANXIOLYTICS

For anxiety disorders, selection of a medication as part of the treatment is based on 1) the efficacy of the medication for the particular disorder, as demonstrated by appropriate clinical trials; 2) the time to onset of therapeutic effect, because a faster acting medication may be preferred in patients with high distress and disability; 3) the effectiveness of the anxiolytic in any comorbid conditions; 4) the side effect profile of the medication, including its potential for dependence and abuse; and 5) the potential for interaction between the anxiolytic and any other therapy required.

BENZODIAZEPINES

Indications

Benzodiazepines are thought to potentiate the activity of γ-aminobutyric acid, an inhibitory neurotransmitter system widely distributed in the central nervous system, with a role in muscle relaxant, anticonvulsant, anxiolytic, antiaggressive, and sedative actions. The efficacy of benzodiazepines in relieving anxiety symptoms has been amply demonstrated by countless clinical trials. Their advantages for the treatment of anxiety include strong anxiolytic effect, rapid onset of action (within 1 to 2 days), excellent safety profile, fairly rapid development of tolerance for sedative side effects, lack of tolerance for anxiolytic effect, and low risk of interaction with other medications.

Benzodiazepines are indicated for the management of clinically significant anxiety and agitation in a broad range of situations. They are used as general sedatives, administered as needed, sometimes parenterally and in high doses, in psychiatric and medical emergencies, before surgical and stressful medical procedures, and in severe life crises. They are also used as ongoing adjunctive treatment for pain, especially associated with muscle spasm; a variety of chronic medical conditions, such as hypertension and duodenal ulcer; convulsive disorders; involuntary disorders of movement; certain psychotic conditions; certain mood disorders; and withdrawal from alcohol and other substances of abuse.

Benzodiazepines, usually prescribed in a consistent regimen, are indicated as first-line pharmacotherapy for anxiety disorders listed in the *Diagnostic and Statistical Manual of Mental Disorders,* Fourth Edition (DSM-IV), especially generalized anxiety disorder and panic disorder with or without agoraphobia. Social phobia can be treated with benzodiazepines, and they may be used for obsessive-compulsive disorder, especially when anxiety is a prominent symptom. They may help reduce hyperarousal in posttraumatic stress disorder, but they do not seem to address the core symptoms. Persistent requests for increased dosage may be associated with comorbid substance abuse. Therefore, attention to current and past abuse of addicting drugs is important for developing a strategy of treatment with the individual patient.

Selection of a Specific Benzodiazepine

There is little evidence for differential effectiveness among the benzodiazepines, particularly in generalized anxiety, although the effects of many of these compounds have not yet been systematically explored in most of the anxiety disorders as we classify them today.

Initiation of Treatment

The large therapeutic index of the benzodiazepines simplifies their administration. Nevertheless, the response among patients is variable and requires individual adjustment for best results. Three useful principles for initiating treatment with a benzodiazepine are 1) begin with a low dose; 2) raise dosage slowly, allowing sufficient time to assess the effect of each increment; and 3) use the lowest *effective* dose (Table 56–1).

Treatment may be initiated with a single dose in the evening, when sedation presents no serious problem. If, for example, diazepam is to be used and the patient's level of generalized anxiety is only moderate, a 2.5-mg dose may be appropriate. If the anxiety level is high, the starting dose may be 5 mg. This dose may be administered twice daily on the second day, three times daily on the third day, and four times daily on the fourth day. Any significant sedation, however, is a signal to pause in the dose escalation plan until this subsides. The first target dose level is usually 10 to 20 mg daily, but some patients with severe generalized anxiety ultimately may require 40 mg or more daily.

The most satisfactory strategy in the treatment of panic is to aim for complete prevention of attacks through a regular regimen of medication. The dosage of alprazolam for panic disorder should begin at 0.25 mg two to three times a day, with titration up by 0.5 mg daily every 3 days. Some patients experience blockade of panic attacks at a dose as low as 2 mg/d; most require 4 to 6 mg/d in divided doses for full effect, and a few require 10 mg daily or more.

The introduction of a benzodiazepine, like its withdrawal, is better managed more slowly than has generally been recognized. After a dosage increment, initially strong anxiolytic and sedative effects may wane for a period as long as 2 weeks. During this phase, treatment induction, this is not a signal to abandon the medication on the presumption that tolerance has developed.

Short-Term Adverse Effects

Common short-term side effects include sedation, fatigue, ataxia, slurred speech, amnesia, and impaired cognitive and motor performance. Patients should be cautioned to assess their alertness

TABLE 56–1	Principles of Benzodiazepine Therapy

Assess the patient's condition, including principal diagnosis; comorbid psychiatric and general medical problems; use of alcohol, caffeine, and drugs; severity of distress; level of disability; chronicity of disorder; and life situation.

Educate the patient about the nature of the disorder and the therapeutic options, with their advantages and drawbacks.

Negotiate the details of the treatment plan.

Aim to completely *prevent* symptoms by using a regular regimen.

Initiate treatment with a low dose.

Caution the patient to monitor alertness before operating dangerous equipment.

Escalate dosage *slowly*, allowing up to 2 weeks to assess the anxiolytic and sedative effects of each increment.

Continue dose escalation if tolerance to the anxiolytic effect develops.

Consider other therapeutic options if doses greather than alprazolam 6 mg daily (or equivalent) produce no effect, *especially* if the patient requests increasing dosages.

Maintain the lowest *effective* dose for several months, depending on the chronicity of the disorder.

Periodically reduce or discontinue medication to assess the need for continued maintenance.

Counsel the patient to plan ahead to avoid abruptly stopping medication.

Discontinue benzodiazepines by tapering *slowly*, allowing up to 4 weeks for stabilization after each decrement.

Begin the taper with decrements of 25% of the ongoing dosage, but use smaller decrements later, especially after the dose has been reduced by half.

Substitute a benzodiazepine with a longer half-life if there is persistent symptom breakthrough between doses.

carefully before driving or operating dangerous equipment, especially just after a dosage increment. They should also be warned that the effects of alcohol and benzodiazepines are additive. Tolerance to sedation usually occurs within 1 or 2 weeks of upward dosage adjustment. Otherwise, sedation can be controlled by decreasing the dose. The lethality of benzodiazepines is low, and overall they are among the safest classes of medication.

Patients with a history of alcohol and drug abuse are at increased risk for abuse and dependence with benzodiazepines, so these compounds should be used with care in this population. Patients with no history of substance abuse appear to be at low risk for abusing benzodiazepines.

Continuation and Maintenance Treatment

Although the long-term use of benzodiazepines has been controversial, the importance of planning some type of ongoing or intermittent treatment for long periods for patients with anxiety (except for some adjustment disorders) is now more generally accepted. Ballenger (1991), for example, recommended maintenance treatment of panic disorder for 3 to 12 months after stabilization to allow the patient to return to a normal lifestyle.

Long-Term Adverse Effects

The most important potential adverse effects of benzodiazepines administered for long periods are dependence and abuse. Although tolerance to the sedative effects of benzodiazepines develops rapidly, there is some evidence that subtle deficits in attention and psychomotor, cognitive, and memory functions may persist indefinitely during a consistent regimen of benzodiazepine treatment.

Discontinuation of Treatment and Dependence

Although anxiety disorders are characteristically chronic, the course varies among patients. The decision to discontinue treating a particular patient who has responded well remains ultimately an individual one. Most experts believe that there is no substitute for periodically discontinuing medication to assess whether it is still required.

In this context, the major disadvantage of benzodiazepines becomes apparent: anxious patients consistently treated 4 months or longer are at risk for rebound and withdrawal symptoms (as well as relapse) on discontinuation of the medication.

Rebound is defined as a prompt, brief recurrence, after sudden discontinuation of anxiolytic medication, of the same anxiety symptoms that originally brought the patient to treatment, at a severity higher than at baseline level. In a study of alprazolam in panic disorder, 27% of patients met these criteria.

The withdrawal syndrome is defined as the development of more persistent anxiety symptoms after reduction or discontinuation of anxiolytic medication, often with symptoms that were not present originally. These typically include confusion, clouded sensorium, heightened sensory perception, paresthesias, muscle cramps, muscle twitches, blurred vision, diarrhea, decreased appetite, and weight loss in some combination in 35% of patients whose medication was tapered in a period of 4 weeks. The frequency of the withdrawal syndrome varies from 5% to 95% in different studies, depending on several factors: the half-life of the anxiolytic, the daily dosage and duration of treatment, and the rate of taper.

To minimize the risk of rebound and withdrawal symptoms, discontinuation of a benzodiazepine after extended use, especially a compound with a short half-life such as alprazolam or lorazepam, should be *gradual,* one eighth to one fourth of the total dose every few weeks, with careful monitoring for side effects.

Abuse Potential

The abuse potential of benzodiazepines has been, if anything, of even greater concern than their tendency to produce dependence, particularly among patients with comorbid substance abuse or personality disorder. Careful evaluation of anxious patients for these conditions, therefore, is necessary, even though they are not absolute contraindications for benzodiazepines.

BUSPIRONE

Indications

Concern about the problems of sedation, dependence, and abuse potential with benzodiazepines led to a search for medications that relieve anxiety without these adverse effects. One such medication, buspirone (BuSpar), appears to meet these criteria.

Although the evidence for the effectiveness of buspirone is not as extensive as for the benzodiazepines, there are now a substantial number of placebo-controlled studies to support its use in generalized anxiety disorder, especially with associated depressive symptoms.

Initiation of Treatment

To minimize side effects, buspirone should be initiated at 5 mg three times a day, titrated up weekly by 15-mg dosage increments to a maximum of 60 mg daily in divided doses. Because the response is delayed for several weeks, buspirone may be preferred for patients with chronic anxiety who are not responding to acute stresses. Because patients often come for treatment when anxiety is at a peak level, the delayed onset can result in dissatisfaction with and discontinuation of therapy.

Patients who switch from a benzodiazepine to buspirone are likely to experience rebound and withdrawal symptoms, because buspirone is not cross-tolerant with the benzodiazepines. In addition, the therapeutic effects of buspirone require several weeks to develop. Preparation of the patient for these events and a slow taper of the benzodiazepine before or during treatment with buspirone may make for an easier transition.

Adverse Effects

Buspirone, as indicated before, is free of the major adverse effects of benzodiazepines: sedation, psychomotor impairment, dependence, withdrawal syndrome, and abuse potential. Buspirone does not interact with alcohol. Adverse effects include nausea, dizziness, headaches, and fatigue.

β-BLOCKERS

Indications

Several studies have documented the effectiveness of β-blockers (propranolol and atenolol) in reducing the peripheral manifestations of anxiety (particularly palpitations, tachycardia, tremor, and sweats) in performance anxiety, a specific, limited form of social phobia. Performing artists have used β-blockers extensively.

Initiation of Treatment

For performance anxiety, propranolol, 10 to 40 mg, may be taken in a single dose about 1 hour before a performance. A test dose given before an important performance, with monitoring of pulse and blood pressure, may be useful. For a consistent regimen, propranolol can be initiated at 10 mg two or three times a day and can be titrated upward to as much as 240 mg/d in divided doses. The effectiveness of a specific dose can be assessed within a few days. Atenolol, a long-acting β-blocker, is effective at 50 to 100 mg given in the morning.

Adverse Effects

Adverse effects of β-blockers include fatigue, mild gastrointestinal distress, and insomnia. The more lipophilic β-blockers, such as propranolol, that enter the central nervous system may cause depression. β-Blockers are contraindicated in patients with cardiogenic shock, sinus bradycardia and greater than first-degree block, bronchial asthma, bronchospasm, and congestive heart failure.

Advantages of long-acting β-blockers such as atenolol are once-a-day dosing, less plasma level variability, more cardioselectivity, and less likelihood of bronchial constriction. A benefit of all β-blockers is their lack of dependence and abuse potential.

Discontinuation

After β-blockers have been taken on a regular basis, rebound hypertension can occur on abrupt discontinuation. In this situation, a gradual taper is recommended. The taper does not have to be as slow as that for benzodiazepines and can be monitored effectively by recording vital signs of blood pressure and pulse.

Sedative-Hypnotics

One of the most frequent indications for the use of sedative-hypnotic agents is primary insomnia. Primary insomnia refers to those sleep disturbances in which no other known sleep disorder (e.g., narcolepsy, obstructive sleep apnea), medical condition (e.g., depression, hyperthyroidism), medication (e.g., stimulants), or substance use (e.g., cocaine, caffeine) accounts for the symptoms. Sedative-hypnotic medications will typically be considered for, or requested by, patients with primary insomnia or with circadian rhythm sleep disorders.

Treatment should always be preceded by an appropriate diagnostic evaluation. This fosters inquiry into and attention to environmental and emotional stressors (e.g., noise, prebedtime arguments). Improving sleep hygiene may be sufficient to address the insomnia of some patients.

Although effective sleeping pills may provide real short-term benefits for some, there is little evidence to recommend their general long-term use. Some, but not all, studies suggest that some degree of tolerance typically develops after weeks or a few months of nightly use. Abrupt discontinuation, which either deliberately or inadvertently happens all too often (e.g., a patient is admitted to a hospital and does not disclose a history of use), can result in transient rebound insomnia or a withdrawal (abstinence) syndrome when prior use has been prolonged or at high doses. It should be remembered that about 30% of insomniacs use alcohol as a hypnotic.

SELF-PRESCRIBED REMEDIES

Over-the-Counter Drugs

OTC drugs are the most widely used sleeping pills. They typically contain the histamine H_1 receptor antagonist diphenhydramine (e.g., Sominex, Compoz) or some other antihistamine (e.g., doxylamine) with sedating properties. In the past, chlorpheniramine maleate and methapyrilene were frequently used. Diphenhydramine and doxylamine are also available in prescription-strength compounds (e.g., Benadryl, Unisom). The sedation or drowsiness resulting from H_1 receptor antagonists may produce enough relaxation to promote sleep, but this effect may often be more subjective and indirect than from a direct effect on sleep architecture.

Compliance with the OTCs, in general, is higher than with prescribed hypnotics. However, because antihistamines are not short acting, many people complain of next-day drowsiness or "thick-headedness" or an OTC drug "hangover." During sleep, diphenhydramine may increase motor activity. Anticholinergic effects,

559

including dry mouth, urinary retention or difficulty urinating (hesitancy), or confusion may also occur. These complications are of particular concern for the elderly. Tolerance usually develops to the sedating properties of antihistamines within days to weeks.

Alcohol

Alcohol (ethanol) is probably the most frequently used self-prescribed sleep inducer. What most people do not realize, however, is that whereas alcohol (e.g., brandy) may promote sleep onset, it typically fragments subsequent sleep architecture. Most alcohol-aided sleep is not as restorative, or at least not as restful, as unaided sleep. Many persons who consume alcohol at bedtime sleep deeply and soundly for a few hours and then awaken and are unable to fall back to sleep.

PRESCRIPTION MEDICATIONS

Benzodiazepines

Benzodiazepines are the more consistently effective than self-prescribed treatments for people who cannot sleep because of transient stress. Benzodiazepines induce drowsiness, relax muscles, and decrease mental agitation. As doses and consequently brain concentrations are increased, drowsiness and relaxation shift into decreased wakefulness and then sleep. It appears that marketed benzodiazepine hypnotics are more alike than different except for duration of action and time of onset of action. They clearly work well for transient and especially situational insomnias that would otherwise clear up with time.

Six benzodiazepines are marketed as hypnotics in the United States (Table 57–1). There is little convincing evidence that

TABLE 57–1	Benzodiazepine Receptor Agonists Marketed in the United States as Hypnotics		
Generic Name	Trade Name	Dosage Strength(s) (mg)	Relative Duration of Action
Trizolam	Halcion	0.125, 0.25	Shorter
Zolapidem	Ambien	5, 10	Shorter
Temazepam	Restoril and generics	7.5, 15, 30	Intermediate
Estazolam	ProSom	1, 2	Intermediate
Flurazepam	Dalmane and generics	15, 30	Longer
Quazepam	Doral	7.5, 15	Longer

TABLE 57–2	Some Unwanted Effects* Common to Most Sedative-Hypnotic Agents

Motor impairment and falls
Anterograde impairment of memory and new learning (recall)
Discontinuation syndromes (e.g., rebound insomnia, withdrawal reactions)
Tolerance and physical dependence
Respiratory depression
Interactions (additive or synergistic) with alcohol (ethanol)
Architecture of sleep is altered
Daytime drowsiness and other carryover effects

*Ordered to fit the mnemonic MAD TRIAD rather than frequency of occurrence or clinical significance.

distinguishes among the marketed benzodiazepine hypnotics in terms of efficacy or safety when they are administered appropriately (i.e., amounts, dosing intervals, and duration of use).

Rebound insomnia is common after several nights of use of shorter half-life benzodiazepine hypnotics. Some patients find that their sleep after discontinuation seems worse than their original problem. Rebound insomnia may in fact be transiently more marked or exaggerated than the original insomnia problem. It rarely lasts, however, for more than a few nights, and it can generally be avoided by dose tapering rather than abrupt discontinuation or by using lower dosages during treatment.

Some patients receiving shorter half-life benzodiazepines complain of increased wakefulness during the terminal hours of sleep (i.e., the last 2 to 3 hours). This is similar to what may happen when alcohol is used as a hypnotic. Another concern experienced by some patients taking shorter half-life benzodiazepine hypnotics is increased daytime anxiety, particularly during the morning.

The elderly, particularly elderly women, are major consumers of benzodiazepine hypnotics. They receive more than a third of all prescriptions even though they represent 10% to 15% of the population.

Table 57–2 lists some of the unwanted direct or indirect pharmacological effects that may occur to a greater or lesser degree with specific benzodiazepine hypnotics as well as with other nonbenzodiazepine sedative-hypnotics. The mnemonic MAD TRIAD (see Table 57–2) may help one remember these effects.

Chloral Hydrate

Chloral hydrate (Aquachloral, Noctec, Welldorm) was among the earliest sleeping pills. It is reasonably effective, however, in dosages between 0.5 and 1.5 g (Table 57–3). The elimination half-life of 6 to 8 hours for its active metabolite, trichloroethanol, is consistent with a minimal likelihood of next-day performance impairment.

Chloral hydrate's drawbacks include a narrow therapeutic index

TABLE 57–3	Nonbenzodiazepine Sedative-Hypnotics Commonly Available in the United States		
Generic Name	**Trade Name***	**Dosage Range (mg)**	**Class†**
Pentobarbital	Nembutal	100–200	II
Secobarbital	Seconal	50–100	II
Butabarbital	Butisol	50–100	III
Phenobarbital	Luminal	100–300	IV
Ethchlorvynol	Placidyl	500–1000	IV
Chloral hydrate	Noctec	500–1500	IV
Meprobamate	Miltown Equanil	400–1600	IV
Hydroxyzine hydrochloride	Atarax	50–400	
Hydroxyzine pamoate	Vistaril	50–400	

*Only trade names originally associated with the product are listed.

†Class refers to the current U.S. Drug Enforcement Agency controlled substances schedule designation.

(toxic dose–therapeutic dose), gastric irritation leading to nausea and vomiting, and gastric necrosis with high dosages. As with other sedative-hypnotics, dependence and tolerance may develop. It may also displace other drugs from their protein binding sites, and during prolonged dosage it may be a hepatic microsomal enzyme–inducing agent.

Zolpidem

Zolpidem (Ambien) is marketed as a nonbenzodiazepine alternative to benzodiazepine hypnotics. Based on limited use to date, zolpidem in comparison to marketed benzodiazepines may have a slightly reduced likelihood of producing tolerance or withdrawal syndromes. Its abuse potential may also be somewhat lower than with benzodiazepines, but it clearly has some cross-tolerance with alcohol at higher-than-standard hypnotic dosages.

Other Hypnotics

A variety of other oral hypnotic agents are also available. Most widely used outside the United States are the barbiturates. Three are most commonly prescribed: butabarbital, phenobarbital, and secobarbital. Most barbiturates are scheduled as class II drugs (see Table 57–3), cause induction of hepatic oxidative metabolism, and are dangerous in overdosages.

Other agents used as hypnotics include hydroxyzine, meprobamate, and ethchlorvynol. None of the latter agents nor the barbiturates have comparable efficacy and safety to the benzodiazepines. Their use is not encouraged by the author, even though health care cost pressures and other forces have led to a resurgence in their use in some settings.

Some physicians employ small doses (i.e., 25 to 50 mg) of sedating antidepressants (e.g., amitriptyline, trazodone, trimipramine) as hypnotics. These may be appropriate alternatives for certain patients (e.g., those with depression), but the risks from the adrenergic and cholinergic properties of some of these agents must be considered.

DRUG INTERACTIONS

The majority of drug interactions are predictable and reflect the additive effects of two (or more) drugs with sedative properties. The effect of taking a benzodiazepine while drinking alcohol is an example.

In addition to these easily understood and anticipatable interactions, some interactions occur as the result of the second drug acting as an inhibitor of the other drug's metabolism.

SUGGESTED GUIDELINES FOR PRESCRIBING MEDICATIONS

It is clinically useful to provide patients with information on good sleep hygiene practices (e.g., see Table 57–4). It also helps to advise patients to take any sedative-hypnotics on an empty stomach and with ample fluids (e.g., a full glass of water) to promote rapid dissolution and absorption and onset of effect. One should always caution patients about potential impairments of memory, coordination, or driving skills, and about unsteadiness if they are awakened

TABLE 57–4	Helpful Hints for Better Sleep Hygiene

Do not go to bed to try to sleep when you are not tired.

Avoid napping during the day, even when you are tired. Also avoid early-evening naps.

If possible, take an appropriate medication to relieve any physical pain you may be having. Pain interferes with sleep.

Eat selectively. Being hungry when you go to bed may disrupt your sleep. Avoid a heavy meal too close to bedtime. Avoid caffeine and other methylxanthines (e.g., chocolate, colas, coffee, tea) after 4:00 PM. A warm, noncaffeinated beverage and a small carbohydrate snack before bedtime may be soothing and enhance drowsiness.

Exercise at least two or three times per week. Avoid strenuous exercise too close (i.e., 4–5 hr) to bedtime. A short early-evening walk or a bicycle ride may be relaxing.

Table continued on following page

| TABLE 57–4 | Helpful Hints for Better Sleep Hygiene *(Continued)* |

Try to keep stress and conflict out of the bedroom. Enhance relaxation whenever possible (e.g., a warm bath, a massage, comforting sexual experiences, meditation, reading a good [but not too exciting] book). Try deep-breathing methods (e.g., abdominal breathing in which slow inhalation is linked to the downward movement of the diaphragm and slow exhalation is linked to the upward movement of the diaphragm). Do this for 10 breaths, working to slow your breathing rate progressively. Repeat as necessary while trying to relax the rest of your body. Focus on a relaxing image and try to capture the whole scene, including scents and temperature. Read about or consult someone, if necessary, to learn about other aspects of stress management and relaxation strategies.

Develop comfortable nighttime rituals or routines. Try to go to bed at a regular time. If you do not fall asleep after a half hour or so, read a book or watch a pleasant television program for a while. With this in mind, it is likely that watching the late (e.g., 11:00 PM) news is not a good habit. When possible, it may be better to leave the bedroom if you do not readily fall asleep and return only when tired. Keep your arising time as regular as possible as well. Keep the room temperature comfortable for you. A hot room may increase awakenings (>24°C [75°F]), and a cold room may promote an increase in unpleasant dreams (<12°C [56°F]). Some fresh air may be helpful. Humidify your bedroom if it is too dry. Try to use a firm mattress. Sometimes an adjustable bed should be considered because having the knees bent may decrease lower back muscle strain and pain. Avoid noise, unless it is a form of white noise that is soothing to you.

after having taken a sleep aid. A safe practice is for patients not to keep more than one night's dose by their bedside to avoid the temptation to take more. It is also important to remind them that if they use medication for more than a few nights, some pattern of tapering should be followed when they stop.

Universally accepted guidelines for dosing and duration of use for hypnotics are not established. Both dose and duration must be individualized, with the goal of finding the lowest dose and the shortest duration.

Short-term treatment (i.e., from 1 or 2 nights to 1 to 2 weeks) is reasonable for most patients. However, some patients with chronic insomnia may benefit from longer term use provided that there is careful monitoring by the prescribing physician. Because no criteria are presently available to identify this subpopulation, it seems reasonable to consider several short-term trials, with gradual tapering at the end of each period and a drug-free interval between each period, to establish the patient's need for, and the appropriateness and value of, continued therapy. The drug-free time interval between the initial periods should range from 1 to 3 weeks, depending on the half-life of the agent and of its active metabolites and the rapidity of the taper schedule. Reevaluation of such a patient's continued need for hypnotic medication at 3- to 6-month intervals is also reasonable. Because the elderly are particularly susceptible to falls or confusion from hypnotic use, use of the lowest available dosage strength is advisable.

Psychostimulants

Psychostimulants are powerful treatment agents and have been used for the treatment of adults with depression, attention-deficit/hyperactivity disorder (ADHD), neurasthenia, and acquired immunodeficiency syndrome dementia. Although the psychostimulants have become the medications of choice for the treatment of children with ADHD, their central mechanisms of action, whereby motor activity is reduced, sustained attention is increased, and impulsivity is reduced, are unknown.

Numerous studies have shown that relative to placebo, psychostimulants improve the performance of children with ADHD on a variety of laboratory measures of cognitive function. Psychostimulants reduce excessive motor behavior in children with ADHD.

More recent studies of treated children with ADHD have shown that psychostimulants enhance arithmetical productivity, efficiency, and accuracy. These studies employed optimal experimental procedures, including standardized medication dosages and relevant dependent measures.

A number of double-blind, placebo-controlled crossover studies have reported variable reductions in aggressivity in children with ADHD from stimulant treatment. This is a critical area, because aggressivity in children predicts future morbidity.

Maternal responses to methylphenidate (MPH)-treated children with ADHD show increases in warmth, decreased maternal criticism, and greater frequency of verbal interactions. Rates of friction with siblings were also lower when the ADHD children were responsive to MPH.

Children with ADHD often have impaired peer relationships. Their impulsive interpersonal style leads them to be intrusive, abrasive, and loud and to relate to others with high intensity. Direct observations of boys with ADHD in the classroom, playground, and lunchroom have produced a picture of social interaction failure, aggressivity, and peer rejection.

In a linear dose-response manner, higher dose MPH (0.6 mg/kg) produced improved peer ratings. MPH at that dosage reduced noncompliance, the number of episodes of verbal and physical aggression in both classroom and playground, to the level of that of the control subjects. MPH also reduces ADHD boys' verbal aggression in unstructured lunchroom environments. Still, not all interpersonal problems shown by children with ADHD respond to medication interventions.

SUBSTANCE ABUSE OF STIMULANTS

Psychostimulants have been abused by adults, but the risk for addiction by children with ADHD is low. Klein (1991) found that the psychostimulants differ in their ability to induce euphoria, with "dextroamphetamine the most euphorigenic, methylphenidate, less so, and magnesium pemoline, hardly at all." Adolescents and young adults with ADHD do not list the psychostimulants among medications used recreationally, whether or not they had received treatment with psychostimulants. Adolescents previously diagnosed as having ADHD during their school-age years are at greater risk for substance abuse than control subjects, but those who do abuse medications tend not to pick stimulants.

PREVALENCE OF PSYCHOSTIMULANT USE IN THE UNITED STATES

Psychostimulant medication has grown to be a ubiquitous treatment modality for ADHD in the United States. This is due, in part, to the prevalence of the disorder. ADHD has been estimated to afflict up to 5% of children in primary school in the United States. The cardinal features of ADHD, which are present as early as age 3 years, include excessive gross motor activity, disorganization of behavior, distractibility, low frustration tolerance, and inability to sustain attention or remain on task. These core clinical signs lead to impairment in functioning with peers, with parents, and on academic tasks.

MPH has become the most frequently prescribed medication used in the treatment of ADHD, accounting for more than 90% of stimulant use in the United States. The increasing popularity of MPH probably has to do with its efficacy in ameliorating the target symptoms of ADHD, reducing gross motor overactivity, decreasing off-task behavior, increasing compliance with adult requests, and decreasing aggressivity, as reported in multiple controlled studies. Not only is MPH effective; it is safe, showing a low incidence of side effects in the short trials and long-term follow-up studies. Its rapid action, its relatively low-priced generic form, the frequency with which the ADHD diagnosis is made, and the wide range of tolerated doses are other reasons for the popularity of this treatment agent in this country.

WHAT IS BEING TREATED

The *Physicians' Desk Reference* (PDR) has two main indications for the use of MPH: narcolepsy and ADHD. Other stimulants differ somewhat, with the indications for methamphetamine (Desoxyn) including ADHD and obesity and for pemoline including only ADHD.

NARCOLEPSY: ANOTHER CHILD AND ADOLESCENT INDICATION FOR STIMULANT TREATMENT

Narcolepsy is a chronic neurological disorder that presents with excessive daytime sleepiness and various problems of rapid eye movement physiology, such as cataplexy (unexpected decreases in muscle tone), sleep paralysis, and hypnagogic hallucinations (intense dream-like imagery before falling sleep). Treatment can include a regular schedule of naps; counseling of family, school, and patient; and use of medications, including stimulants and rapid eye movement–suppressant drugs, such as protriptyline. Dahl recommended beginning with standard, short-acting stimulants, such as MPH, 5 mg twice a day, and increasing the dose up to 30 mg twice a day if need be.

SELECTION OF A STIMULANT MEDICATION AS A TREATMENT MODALITY

Deciding to Use Medication

The decision to use medication for any child psychiatric condition depends on a balance of risks and benefits. Risks must be examined not only in terms of the drug used, but also in terms of if the drug is *not* used and the child continues to be impaired in social and academic functioning. Before stimulants can be used to treat a behavioral problem, the child must meet the *Diagnostic and Statistical Manual of Mental Disorders,* Fourth Edition (DSM-IV) criteria for ADHD.

There are few children with ADHD for whom monotherapy is sufficient—parent training and pedagogical and behavioral classroom interventions are often indicated; therefore, multimodal therapy is usually the best treatment. When medication treatment is presented in this fashion, including a frank discussion of potential risks and benefits, most parents are willing to give it a try, especially if reassured that the decision to continue medication will be made on empirical grounds.

Preparation of the Patient

Physicians can explain the reasons for taking pills and how the pills can prove helpful in school and at home. Children often have negative attitudes about treatment, thinking of treatment as a punishment. Pill taking thus can be the visible sign of the child's continued punishment and can be socially stigmatizing if the daily trip to the nurse generates peer ridicule. Discussing the public nature of in-school pill administration may be the only topic that the child wishes to talk about. It is prudent to include the patient in all discussions about dosing and changing of doses. At best, it may improve compliance, particularly when the parent is not there to check on pill taking.

Consideration of Side Effects

Stimulant side effects are dose dependent and range from mild to moderate in most children. Most stimulant side effects are related to their adrenergic activity. These side effects include insomnia, anorexia, irritability, weight loss, abdominal pain, and headaches. When side effect reports have been gathered on ADHD children taking placebo, anxiety, staring, disinterest, and sadness were reported; only parents' reports of decreased appetite, stomachaches, and insomnia differentiated ADHD children given placebo from those given medication. In that study, less than 4% of children had to stop taking stimulants because of these side effects.

The management of stimulant-related adverse effects generally involves a temporary reduction of dose or a change in time of dosing. MPH has an excellent safety record, probably because the duration of action is so brief. The management of specific side effects is covered in the following sections and summarized in Table 58–1.

COMMON SIDE EFFECTS

Common psychostimulant side effects include insomnia, decreased appetite, weight loss, headache, heart rate elevation at rest, and minor increases in systolic blood pressure. Many of these side effects can be managed with temporary dose reduction. Severe insomnia can be managed by changing time of dosing, with most of the medication given early in the day. Complaints of stomach upset, nausea, or pain sometimes respond to giving the medication in the middle of the meal; otherwise, the problem can be treated symptomatically with antacid tablets or by switching to sustained-release MPH, which is absorbed more slowly.

ACUTE WITHDRAWAL: REBOUND. One adverse effect, commonly known as behavioral rebound, appears when children experience psychostimulant withdrawal at the end of the school day. Children present with afternoon irritability, overtalkitiveness, noncompliance, excitability, motor hyperactivity, and insomnia some 5 to 15 hours after the last dose. If rebound occurs, many physicians add a small afternoon dose of MPH or tricyclic antidepressant.

COGNITIVE CONSTRICTION. Another effect reported, but not consistently documented by controlled studies, is psychostimulant-related "cognitive constriction." This effect is a dose-related but subtle adverse reaction that becomes more obvious at high doses of psychostimulants. The stimulant is thought to interfere with cognitive tasks that call for changes of set or divergent thinking.

RARE SIDE EFFECTS

Stimulant-related toxic psychosis, including MPH-induced mania and MPH-induced delusional disorders, is a rare phenomenon in children, with fewer than 30 cases reported. Psychosis is a contraindication for psychostimulant use. The physician should avoid dispensing psychostimulants to agitated children with psychotic symptoms and consider neuroleptics instead. The addition of a neuroleptic to the treatment regimen of a severely disturbed child with ADHD raises the possibility that the child's hyperactivity and poor attention span were secondary to an underlying psychotic condition.

SEIZURE DISORDERS. A commonly held notion is that stimulants lower the seizure threshold. Both ADHD and seizure disorders are quite prevalent and may occur in the same individuals, so the question of the risk of stimulant treatment may frequently arise. A study suggests that stimulant treatment of children with ADHD maintained on effective anticonvulsant doses produced no increase in seizure frequency, no changes in the electroencephalogram waveforms, or no difficulty in regulating anticonvulsant blood levels. Current practice is to give children with ADHD and epilepsy a combination of anticonvulsant and MPH. Plasma levels of the anticonvulsant should be monitored to avoid toxicity resulting from

TABLE 58–1 Stimulant Side Effects and Management

Side Effect	Management
For all side effects	Unless severe, allow 7–10 d for tolerance to develop.
	Evaluate dose-response relationships.
	Evaluate time-action effects and then adjust dosing intervals or switch to sustained-release preparation.
	Evaluate for concurrent conditions, including comorbidities and environmental stressors.
	Consider switching stimulant drug.
Anorexia or dyspepsia	Administer before, during, and after meals.
	With pemoline, consider drug-induced hepatitis.
Weight loss	Give drug after breakfast and after lunch.
	Implement calorie enhancement strategies.
	Give brief drug holidays.
Slowed growth	Apply weight loss remedies.
	Give weekend and vacation (longer) drug holidays.
	Consider another stimulant or nonstimulant drug.
Dizziness	Monitor blood pressure and pulse.
	Encourage adequate hydration.
	If associated with only T_{max}, change to sustained-release preparation.

Insomnia or nightmares	Administer earlier in day.
	Omit or reduce last dose.
	If giving sustained preparation, switch to tablet drug.
	Consider adjunctive antihistamine or clonidine.
Dysphoric mood or emotional constriction	Reduce dose or switch to long-acting preparation.
	Switch stimulants.
	Consider comorbidity requiring alternative or adjunctive treatment.
Rebound	Switch to sustained-release preparation.
	Combine long- and short-acting preparations.
Tics	Firmly establish correlation between tics and pharmacotherapy by examining dose-response relationship, including no-medication condition.
	If tics are mild and abate after 7–10 d with medications, reconsider risks and benefits of continued stimulant treatment and renew informed consent.
	Switch stimulants.
	Consider nonstimulant treatment (e.g., clonidine or tricyclic antidepressant).
	If tic disorder and ADHD are severe, consider combining stimulant with a high-potency neuroleptic.
Psychosis	Discontinue stimulant treatment.
	Assess for comorbid thought disorder.
	Consider alternative treatments.

MPH's competitive inhibition of metabolic pathways, boosting the plasma levels of both drugs.

Long-Term Stimulant Effects: Growth Velocity Reductions

The growth effects of MPH appear to be minimal. Sixty-five children followed up to age 18 years showed an initial growth loss during MPH treatment but caught up during adolescence and reached heights predicted from their parents' heights. These results confirmed the observations by Roche and associates (1979) that psychostimulants have mild and transitory effects on weight and only rarely interfere with height acquisition. Height and weight should be measured at 6-month intervals during stimulant treatment and recorded on age-adjusted growth forms to determine the presence of a drug-related reduction in height or weight velocity. If such a decrement is discovered during maintenance therapy with psychostimulants, a reduction in dosage or change to another class of medication can be carried out.

Continuing Stimulant Treatment in Patients with Tic Disorders

The PDR suggests that the presence of tics is a contraindication to stimulant usage. With the comorbidity of ADHD in children with Tourette's disorder estimated to fall between 20% and 54%, there is a concern that a stimulant's dopamine agonist action will unmask, trigger, accelerate, or provoke irreversible Tourette's symptoms.

Drug Interactions

Mixing psychostimulants with other psychotropic medications is generally not advisable. Most serious is the addition of a psychostimulant to a monoamine oxidase inhibitor antidepressant regimen, a potentially lethal combination that can elevate blood pressure to dangerous levels.

INITIATION OF TREATMENT

Medication treatment begins with a choice of medication. Although the three psychostimulants, MPH, dextroamphetamine (DEX), and pemoline, have roughly equal efficacy, MPH is often used first. If pemoline is to be used, liver function studies should be done and repeated at 6-month intervals.

The titration phase serves two purposes: acclimatization of the child to the drug and determination of his or her best dose. School-age children should be started with low doses to minimize adverse effects. Psychostimulant medication should be taken at or just after mealtime to lessen the anorectic effects; studies have shown that food may enhance drug absorption. MPH treatment can be initiated with a single 5-mg dose at 8:00 AM for 3 days; then a 5-mg dose at 8:00 AM and at noon for the next 3 days; then 10 mg at 8:00 AM and 5 mg for 3 days; and finally 10 mg at 8:00 AM and

10 mg at noon are given and maintained for at least 2 weeks. Preschoolers may start as low as 2.5 mg at 8:00 AM but build to the same total daily 20-mg dose of MPH. The dosing instructions should be written down for the parent, with dates and times specified in detail. A photocopy of the instructions should be kept in the patient's chart.

Table 58–2 is an inventory of stimulant drugs and doses. DEX is usually started at 2.5 to 5 mg a day and gradually increased in 2.5- to 5-mg increments; MPH is usually started at 5 mg twice a day and then titrated in increments of 5 mg/dose every 4 to 7 days. Peak behavioral effects are noted 1 to 3 hours after ingestion and dissipate in 3 to 6 hours for both MPH and DEX. Pemoline is usually started at 37.5 mg each morning and titrated in 18.75-mg increments to maximal clinical effectiveness. Most children respond at a total daily dose of 56.5 or about 2 mg/kg/d in a single dosing. Although the PDR states that steady state is reached within 3 days, traditional practice was to use pemoline for 2 to 4 weeks before clinical benefit becomes apparent.

EARLY PROGRESS ASSESSMENT

Progress assessment is handled by a schedule of *regularly scheduled visits to the physician's office.* These visits allow the physician to observe the child's activity level and attentiveness, to collect information on beneficial effects and adverse reactions, and to review the teacher's reports on the patient's academic and social progress. Clinical progress is reviewed so that the physician can track ADHD signs and symptoms, academic progress, and success with peers. Any counseling, therapy, or educational guidance can be given at that time.

Maintenance plans should include schedules for the regular collection of information that constitutes the child's therapeutic drug monitoring. Each child's response to psychostimulants is different. Likewise, each family's needs are different. Plans for medication vacations and weekend and after-school dosing must be individualized.

Medication *compliance* should be monitored at each visit. The parent is instructed to bring the medication bottle along so that pill counts can be done monthly and compared with the prescription dates. Height and weight should be taken every 6 months, and the child's pediatrician can be requested yearly to perform a complete physical examination and blood work (complete blood count, liver function studies).

Plasma Level Monitoring

Plasma level measures of MPH concentrations have provided research data but are not practical for use in the day-to-day clinical care of children with ADHD to guide titration or dose adjustments during maintenance treatment. MPH plasma levels do not correlate with clinical response and provide no more predictive power than teacher and parent global rating forms, because therapeutic drug monitoring efforts are hampered by MPH's short half-life and its tendency to degrade unless strict collection and storage methods are used.

TABLE 58–2	Stimulant Drug and Doses		
Parameter	**Dextroamphetamine**	**Methylphenidate**	**Pemoline**
Dose formulations	5-, 10-, 15-mg tablets 5-, 10-, 15-mg spansules	5-, 10-, 20-mg tablets 20-mg sustained-release tablet	37.5-mg tablet
Dose range	5–60 mg/d in split doses	5–80 mg/d in split doses	18.75–112.5 mg/d
Dose schedule	b.i.d. or t.i.d.	b.i.d. or t.i.d.	every morning or b.i.d.

Treatment duration should be planned on an individual basis. One method is to plan in single school year units, starting with the present and projecting treatment to last through the present school year plus at least one additional month into the following academic year. Once the child has responded to an initial level of medication, maintenance doses can be set slightly lower. Treatment can be continued, if need be, and the next decision point can be set for the following fall.

This provides a framework for the second concept, a trial off medication. This can be used to determine if treatment should be continued for another year. Medication can be discontinued during some stable period in the school year. This should not be at the beginning of the school year or during crucial placement examinations. Placebo tablets are no longer available from the companies producing MPH, so the psychostimulants are simply discontinued. Most children do not need to taper their dose of medication at discontinuation, unless they show signs of marked afternoon rebound.

Index

Note: Page numbers in *italics* indicate illustrations; those followed by t indicate tables.